D1357992

Scientific Basis of Athletic Conditioning

Scientific Basis of Athletic Conditioning

A. Garth Fisher, Ph.D.

Director, Human Performance Research Center
Brigham Young University
Provo, Utah

Clayne R. Jensen, P.E.D.

Professor and Dean
College of Physical Education
Brigham Young University
Provo, Utah

THIRD EDITION

Lea & Febiger Philadelphia London

1990

Lea & Febiger
200 Chester Field Parkway
Malvern, Pennsylvania 19355-9725
U.S.A.
(215) 251-2230
1-800-444-1785

Lea & Febiger (UK) Ltd.
145a Croydon Road
Beckenham, Kent BR3 3RB
U.K.

First Edition, 1972
Reprinted, 1975
Reprinted, 1977
Second Edition, 1979
Third Edition, 1989

Library of Congress Cataloging in Publication Data

Fisher, A. Garth.
Scientific basis of athletic conditioning / A. Garth Fisher, Clayne R. Jensen.—3rd ed.
p. cm.
Jensen's name appears first on the earlier edition.
Bibliography: p.
Includes index.
ISBN 0-8121-1238-5
1. Sports—Physiological aspects. 2. Physical fitness.
I. Jensen, Clayne R. II. Title.
RC1235.F55 1989
612′.044—dc20 89-12285
CIP

Reprints of chapters may be purchased from Lea & Febiger in quantities of 100 or more.

Copyright © 1990 by Lea & Febiger. Copyright under the International Copyright Union. All Rights Reserved. This book is protected by copyright. No part of it may be reproduced in any manner or by any means without written permission from the publisher.

PRINTED IN THE UNITED STATES OF AMERICA

Print number: 5 4 3 2 1

Preface

Humans are naturally competitive and ambitious for excellence in athletic performance. Throughout recorded history, man has strived to run faster, jump higher, throw farther and exhibit greater strength, endurance and skill.

In 776 B.C., Coroebus, a lowly cook of little native ability, became the Olympic champion in the stade (from which came the word stadium), a 200-yard straight run. The account of his feat tells that he trained vigorously by running up and down hills. Among other early Olympians was Polydamas of Thessaly, who is said to have gained so much strength from lifting stones that he could kill a lion with his bare hands. Arrachian supposedly developed enough skill by wrestling beasts to win the Olympic pancratium (wrestling) crown 5 times before he was finally defeated and lay dead in the stadium. According to legend, Milo of Croton, a renowned athlete of the 6th century B.C. lifted a calf above his head every day until it was full grown. He became so strong that he was 6 times Olympic champion.

Due to practical experience, combined with recent scientific experimentation, many of the old methods of preparation for athletic competition, though fascinating and rich in tradition, have been discarded and replaced by new methods based on greater insight and understanding. For centuries, the evolution toward better methods was slow, but in recent years dramatic changes have occurred to bring about some astounding results in performance. Fortunately, our knowledge continues to grow relative to the functioning of the body systems during training and performance, and how to develop and apply such characteristics as strength, endurance, power, agility, speed, and specific skills. Further, we have learned much about the effects of diet, drugs, altitude, warm-up and other influencing factors, and we continue to gain new knowledge about almost every aspect of conditioning and performance.

Recognizing the increased emphasis being placed on athletic participation, we prepared the first edition of this text book in 1972, and the improved second edition appeared in 1979. Those early editions brought together under one cover the most important up-to-date information and presented it in a manner that was highly useful to both coaches and athletes. But during the last decade, an abundance of improved information has become known, and we have become more perceptive about the particular content that should be included. As a result, the third edition of *Scientific Basis of Athletic Conditioning* is considerably different and much improved over the second edition. The principal ideas and concepts are presented more clearly and the total content is highly readable.

In Part I, the basic physiologic information that relates to performance is presented in a logical sequence, yet at the same time, each chapter is written in such a way that it can be taken out of sequence and used effectively.

Part II, which explains the application of physiologic principles to performance, has been refined and updated to give maximum help to the reader in applying the principles of Part I to real situations. The principles are presented in a manner that will help the student apply them in a wide variety of situations. Again special care has been taken to present the content both clearly and concisely.

Part III covers additional factors that affect performance. For instance, certain substances are taken by athletes to enhance performance. Some are helpful, while others are not. And some substances are even detrimental and dangerous. Foods and diet also affect performance as do altitutde and other factors. The differences in trainability and performance between males and females are also discussed.

The new edition is well illustrated with 174 figures that have been carefully selected or prepared to add clarity and meaning to the written content. Also, certain tests of athletic characteristics are included. This new updated edition can provide a truly meaningful experience for students who are dedicated to the application of the best scientific information to athletic conditioning and performance.

We recognize the contributions of all those who have written books we have read, taught classes we have taken, and done research in exercise science, and thank them for their influence on this book. We wish to point out that a major goal in writing this text was to present a clearly written and understandable summary of the basic concepts of the science of exercise; it was not to present an up-to-date critical review of the latest literature. Because of this, we have attempted to avoid extensive documentation of the concepts with research data that may have affected the readability of the text. Those who desire further information on a specific topic can review some of the articles listed in Selected Readings at the end of each chapter or request a computer search of that topic from a library.

We wish to thank certain individuals who helped in the gathering of information and the preparation of the manuscript, particularly Evan Thomas, Pat Vehrs, Teresa Peugnet, and Donna Winterton. Also, appreciation is expressed for ongoing support by our wives, Jerry and Elouise. Special acknowledgement is extended to Dr. Robert K. Conlee, for his most valuable input and critiques in connection with the content.

Provo, Utah A. Garth Fisher, Ph.D.
Clayne R. Jensen, P.E.D.

Contents

Part I

Basic Physiologic Principles

Central to all performance is the contraction of muscle, for muscles are attached to the bony levers and no movement of these levers occurs unless muscles pull on them. Because of the importance of muscle contraction, it is discussed first. However, skeletal muscles will not contract unless stimulated by motor neurons, and stimulation will do no good unless energy is available. To carry this idea a step further, energy cannot be produced unless oxygen and nutrients are supplied to the muscle and this is done by the cardiovascular system—and it cannot carry oxygen unless the lungs supply it in the alveoli. This thought process is the basis for our approach to the discussion of each of the physiologic principles contained in Part I. The only deviation from this approach is in the discussion of nutrition. For some, nutrition would be discussed immediately following the discussion of the energy systems. Since nutrition is not a "basic physiologic principle" in the same way as muscles, nerves, metabolism, cardiovascular and pulmonary systems, we chose to include it in Part III, "Factors Affecting Performance." For those who like, nutrition could be discussed immediately following metabolism. In fact, any of the topics could be discussed in any order, depending on the background and thought processes of each individual who uses this text, for each topic is complete within itself. However, some ideas are necessarily presented sequentially, and the reader may run across some ideas that have not been discussed before if he/she chooses to rearrange the order.

Why do we present Basic Physiologic Principles in Part I? We could surely learn to coach or participate in certain activities simply by learning and applying "techniques" used by great coaches or athletes. However, this approach is fraught with danger. In fact, this has been the main approach used by many athletes and coaches in the past. A better approach, in our minds, is to learn *principles*, and to use these principles as the basis for the decisions we make about conditioning. Thus, Part I gives us the "scientific basis of athletic conditioning."

1

Skeletal Muscle

All voluntary movements, whether as complex as a golf swing or as simple as scratching your nose, require the contraction of muscles. These muscles act on the bony levers of the body, and the movement we desire occurs. Of course, skeletal muscle requires a signal from the motor areas of the brain, and availability of energy in the form of ATP or no contraction will occur. The other types of muscles—smooth and cardiac—relate to the body functions that support muscular contraction, but cannot be controlled in the same way that skeletal muscle is controlled.

Exercise physiology in its simplest sense is the study of the various factors that trigger or support muscular contractions. Because of the central role of muscles to any type of activity, it seems reasonable to study them first.

TYPES OF MUSCLES

In terms of structure, there are two basic types of muscle in the human body, *smooth* and *striated*. Striated muscle can further be classified into skeletal and cardiac muscle. Thus, three kinds of muscle exist: *smooth, cardiac,* and *skeletal*. All three kinds possess the basic characteristics of muscle tissue: *extendibility*— the ability to stretch; *elasticity*—the ability to return to normal length when the stretching force is removed; *excitability*—the ability to be excited by or respond to stimuli; and *contractility*—the ability to apply tension.

Smooth muscle is located in the walls of blood vessels and most internal organs (viscera) and is involuntarily controlled. It aids in the regulation of autonomic functions such as blood pressure control and digestion and is characterized by smooth appearing (nonstriated) muscle cells, smaller than most skeletal muscle cells which are slender and tapered toward both ends (Fig. 1–1A, B, and C).

Striated muscle includes both skeletal and cardiac muscles. That is, a repeating pattern of light and dark stripes are seen when viewed through a microscope. Physiologically, skeletal and cardiac muscle differ in several inportant ways. (1) Skeletal muscle cells must receive an impulse from a motor neuron to contract, whereas many cardiac muscle cells are autorhythmic and will contract by themselves whether or not nerves are connected. (2) Skeletal muscle cells are functionally separated from each other, where the firing of one cell will have no effect on a neighboring cell. Cardiac cells, on the other hand, form a *functional syncytium*. That is, when one cells fires (contracts) the impulse spreads through all of the other cells in each portion of the heart. This is accomplished through specialized connections between cells called *intercalated discs*. (3) A skeletal muscle fiber is also *all-or-none*. If it contracts, the muscle contracts with all the force it can exert or not at all. Increased force, therefore, depends on an increase in the number of fibers fired. Since all the cardiac fibers in the ventricles of the heart fire each time any one of the fibers fires, an increase of contractile force requires a different mechanism. In cardiac muscles, an increase in the amount of calcium available in the fiber increases the contractile force of that fiber. Therefore, cardiac fibers are not all-or-none. (4) Skeletal muscle fibers can be *tetanized* by increasing the frequency of stimulation. Cardiac muscle recovers slowly after a con-

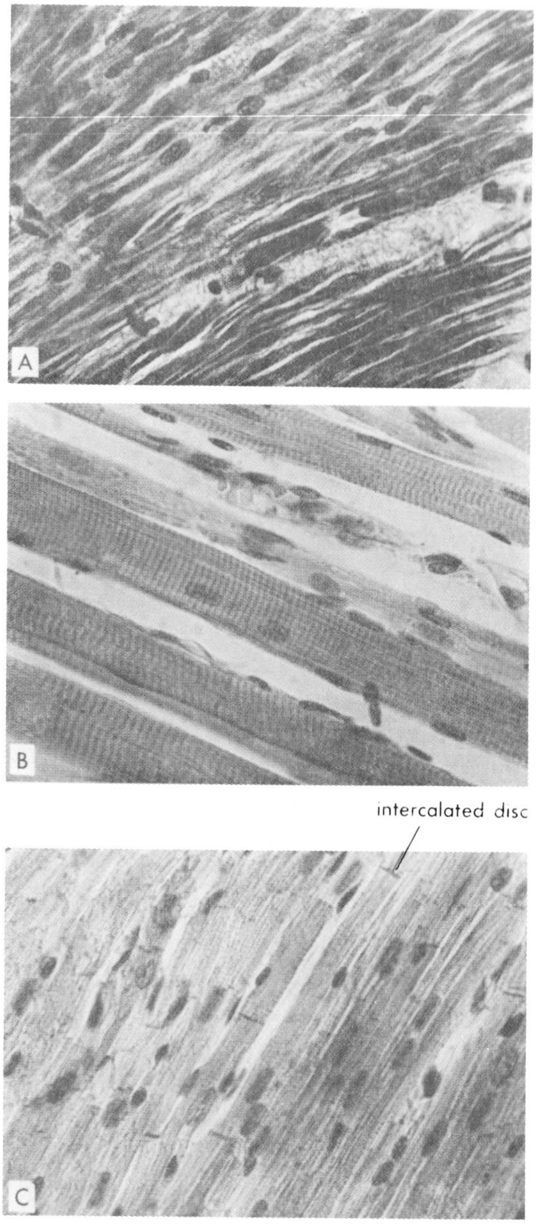

Fig. 1–1. *A–C.* Electron micrographs of smooth, skeletal, and cardiac muscles. Shown in longitudinal section. (From Crouch, J.E. *Functional Human Anatomy*, 4th Ed. Courtesy of Lea & Febiger, 1985.)

traction so *tetany* will not occur. No blood can be pumped from the heart unless the muscle relaxes for a short time between contractions so that the ventricles of the heart can fill.

Because of the role of skeletal muscle in movement, most of the emphasis of this section will concentrate on this type of muscle.

GROSS STRUCTURE OF SKELETAL MUSCLE

The basic unit of skeletal muscle is the muscle cell or fiber, a long cylindrical structure containing numerous nuclei. The thickness of the muscle cell may vary from 10 to 100 microns (μ), and the length can vary from only a few centimeters (cm) to more than 30 cm in a muscle such as the human sartorius. Each muscle cell is enclosed by a cell membrane known as the *sarcolemma* (*sarc*—meaning flesh, and *lemma*—meaning husk) that is a functional part of the cell. The cell membrane separates the internal structure of the cell from the surrounding body fluid and determines, to a large extent, what enters and leaves the cell. It also creates a small electrical charge that is necessary for skeletal muscle contraction. Since muscle cells must apply their force across the movement of bony levers, and since many of the individual muscle fibers are shorter than the entire muscle, each muscle-cell is encased in a complex network of *connective tissue.* The connective tissue around the cell, just outside the sarcolemma, is called the *endomysium.* Groups of these muscle fibers are surrounded by a sheath of tissue called *perimysium.* These groups are known as *fasciculi* (singular = fascicle) and are visible to the naked eye. The muscle as a whole is surrounded by a layer of connective tissue called *epimysium* (Fig. 1–2A and B).

This connective tissue network binds together the single contractile units and groups of units, and integrates their actions while allowing a certain degree of freedom and autonomy among the cells. It is also this connective tissue that fuses to form the tendons that attach the muscles to the bone.

Capillaries and nerves are also found in the connective tissue between muscle cells. Capillaries carry oxygen and nutrients to the cells and carbon dioxide and waste products away from them. Nerves are important because contraction cannot occur without a signal from a motor neuron (Fig. 1–2C).

SKELETAL MUSCLE—SHAPES

Structurally, humans are highly versatile, in that they can walk, run, hop, climb, jump,

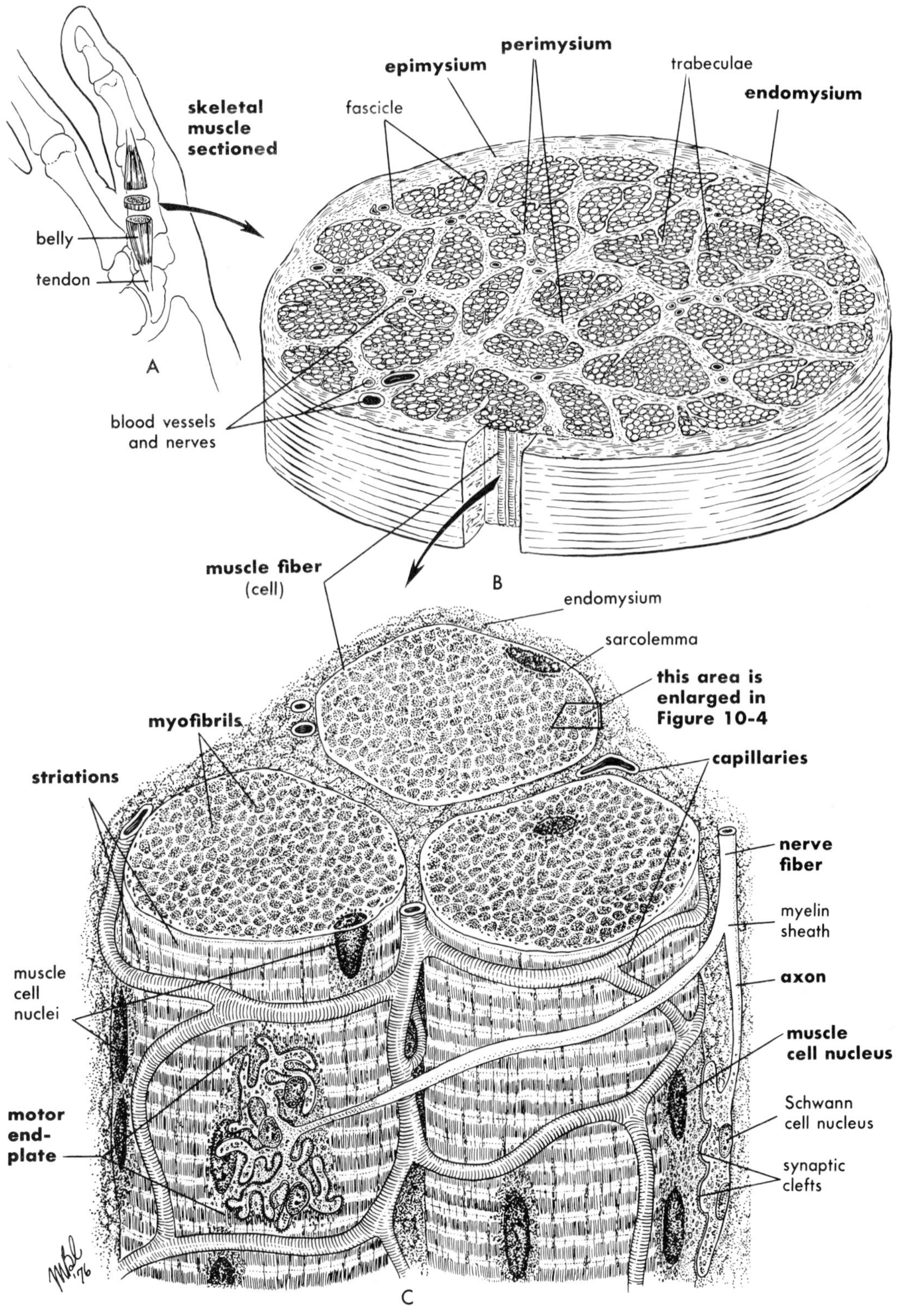

Fig. 1–2. *A. and B.* Schematic diagram showing different levels of connective tissue in a skeletal muscle. *C.* Detail of three skeletal muscle fibers and related structures. (From Crouch, J.E. *Functional Human Anatomy*, 4th Ed. Courtesy of Lea & Febiger, 1985.)

swing, swim, throw objects, and manipulate implements.

Because muscles are called upon to perform such a large variety of movements, they also vary greatly in their shapes. Some are long and slender; others are short, stubby, round, flat, or fan-shaped. Most muscles are *uniceps*, meaning that they taper into only one tendon at each end (one-headed). For example, the brachioradialis is a unicep muscle. A muscle is a *biceps* (two-headed) muscle when it is divided at one end to form two tendons. The muscle in the front of the arm between the shoulder and elbow (biceps brachii) is an example of a biceps muscle (Fig. 1–3A). A *triceps* (three-headed) muscle is one that divides to form three tendons at one end, such as the triceps brachii muscle in the back of the upper arm (Fig. 1–3B).

Muscles also vary greatly in the arrangement of the individual fibers within them in order for the body to be able to create the intricate movements required for the myriad of activities it performs. The arrangement of the muscles can be divided into three major categories;(1) *longitudinal* or *parallel,* (2) *convergent,* and (3) *pinnate.* Longitudinal or parallel muscle fibers lie parallel to the line of action of the entire muscle, and will act in a purely translational motion. In other words, the forces induced by the fibers parallel the overall force at the tendon. These muscles are relatively large, weak, strap-like muscles that contract over a great distance, and are usually good for endurance exercises (e.g. sartorius). Convergent muscles can be roughly classified as a type of parallel muscle and are powerful because they converge to maximize the force of contraction to one point. Examples of convergent muscles are the deltoid and pectoralis. Pinnate (feather-like) muscle fibers lie at an angle to the line of action of the entire muscle and the angle of "pinnation" may differ among muscles in different locations. The major difference between parallel and pinnate muscles is that parallel muscle fibers pull directly through the tendon, while pinnate-fibered muscles will rotate about their origin, changing the angle of pinnation as they shorten. Thus, the difference in the two is not so much the angle at which they connect to the surfaces of origin and insertion, but whether they rotate upon activation. An example is the parallel fibers of the sartorius which originate and insert at angles to their attachments, but induce forces parallel to the overall force at the tendon. In contrast, the seemingly parallel fibers of the pinnate medial gastrocnemius change their angle of insertion as they shorten (Fig. 1–4).

THE MUSCLE CELL

A single muscle cell is surrounded by the sarcolemma, or cell membrane and filled with the cell fluid or *sarcoplasm*, which provides the watery medium for the chemical processes of the cell. It also contains many small organelles, or subcellular components such as *mitochondria* (the cellular organelles responsible for producing oxidative energy for muscular contraction) as well as *ribosomes* (for the production of protein), *fat droplets, glycogen* (muscle sugar used by the mitochondria to produce energy), *myoglobin* (a reddish oxygen-carrying compound much like hemoglobin in the blood), *ATP* and *CP* (high-energy phosphate molecules waiting to be used), and hundreds of thin protein strands called *myofibrils,* which support its function as the contractile component of the system.

The muscle cell also has a net-like system of small longitudinal tubules and vesicles surrounding the myofibrils (the sarcoplasmic reticulum) which gives the interior components of the cell a communicative tie (Fig. 1–5). The *transverse tubules (T-tubules)* are small tubules in the cell extending from openings in the sarcolemma that are probably responsible for spreading the nervous impulse from the muscle cell membrane (sarcolemma) into the deeper portions of the cell, allowing all the contractile elements to be triggered at the same time. On each side of the T-tubules are small structures called *terminal cisternae,* (or lateral sacs) which store larger quantities of calcium (Ca^{++}), an important component to the contractile process. The point at which the T-tubules and terminal cisternae meet is referred to as the *triad* (Fig. 1–5). Interestingly, the T-tubules are in different locations in different muscles. For instance, in mammalian skeletal muscle, they are small and located at the A-I junction (see next section) whereas in

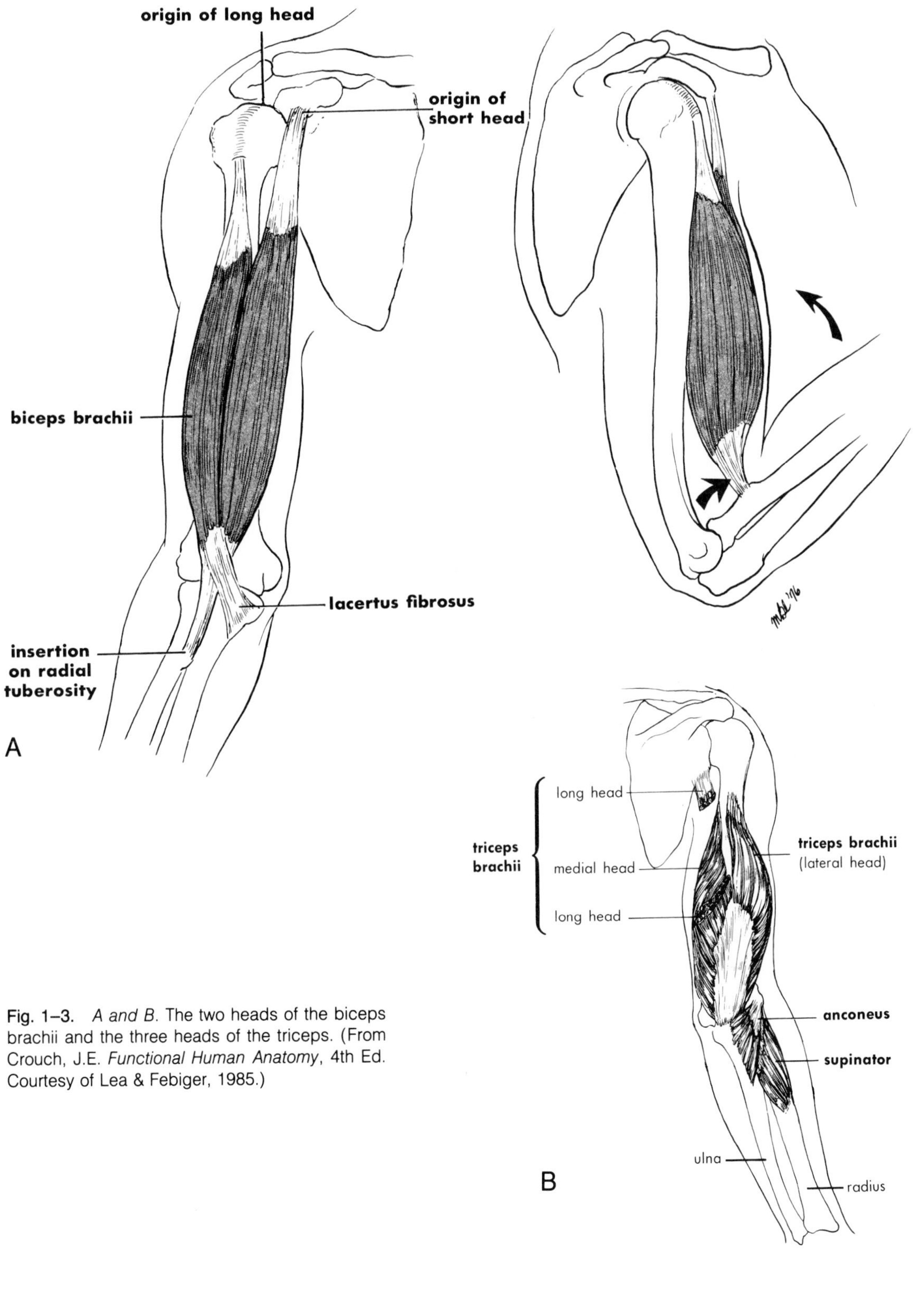

Fig. 1–3. *A and B*. The two heads of the biceps brachii and the three heads of the triceps. (From Crouch, J.E. *Functional Human Anatomy*, 4th Ed. Courtesy of Lea & Febiger, 1985.)

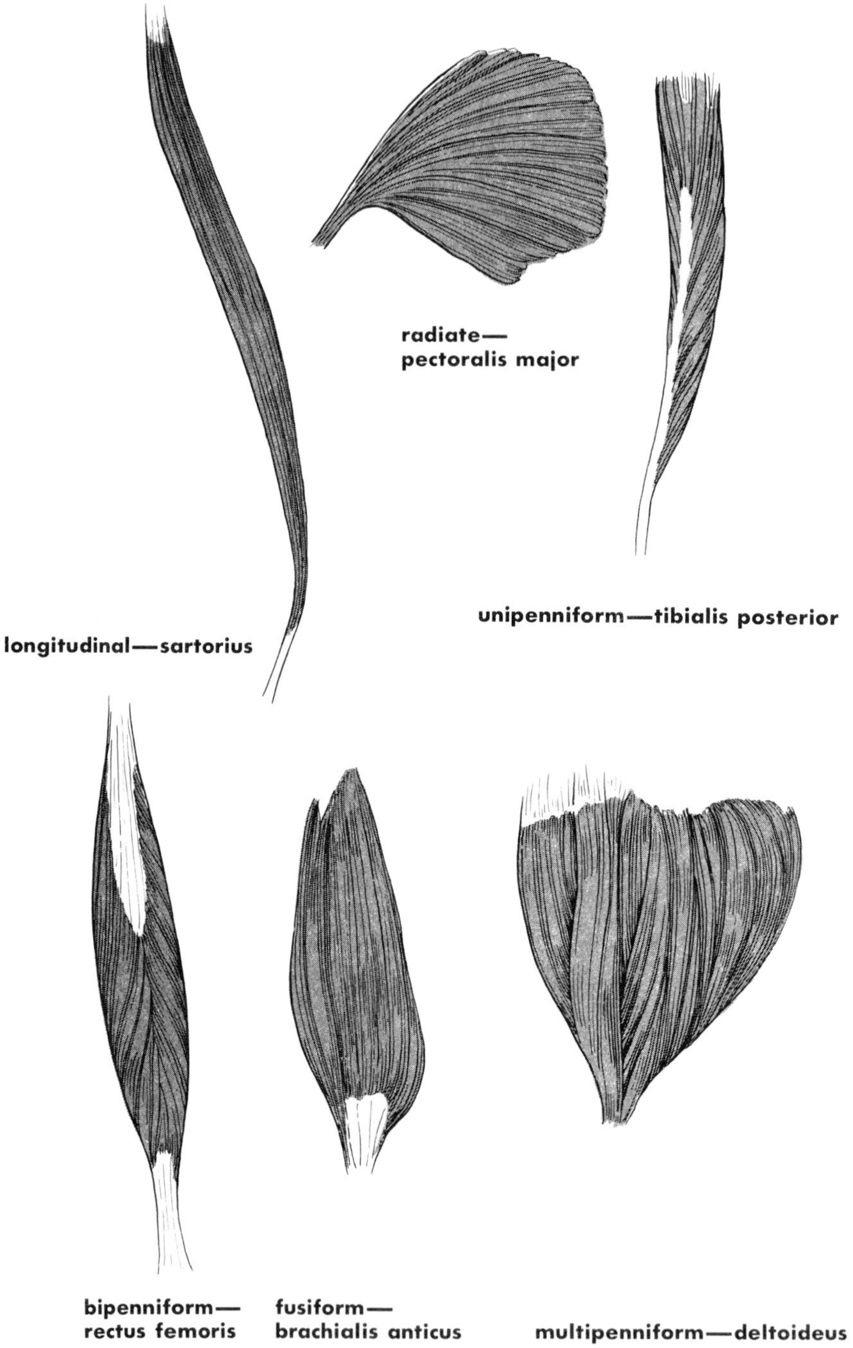

Fig. 1–4. Examples of pinnate fiber arrangements. (From Crouch, J.E. *Functional Human Anatomy*, 4th Ed. Courtesy of Lea & Febiger, 1985.)

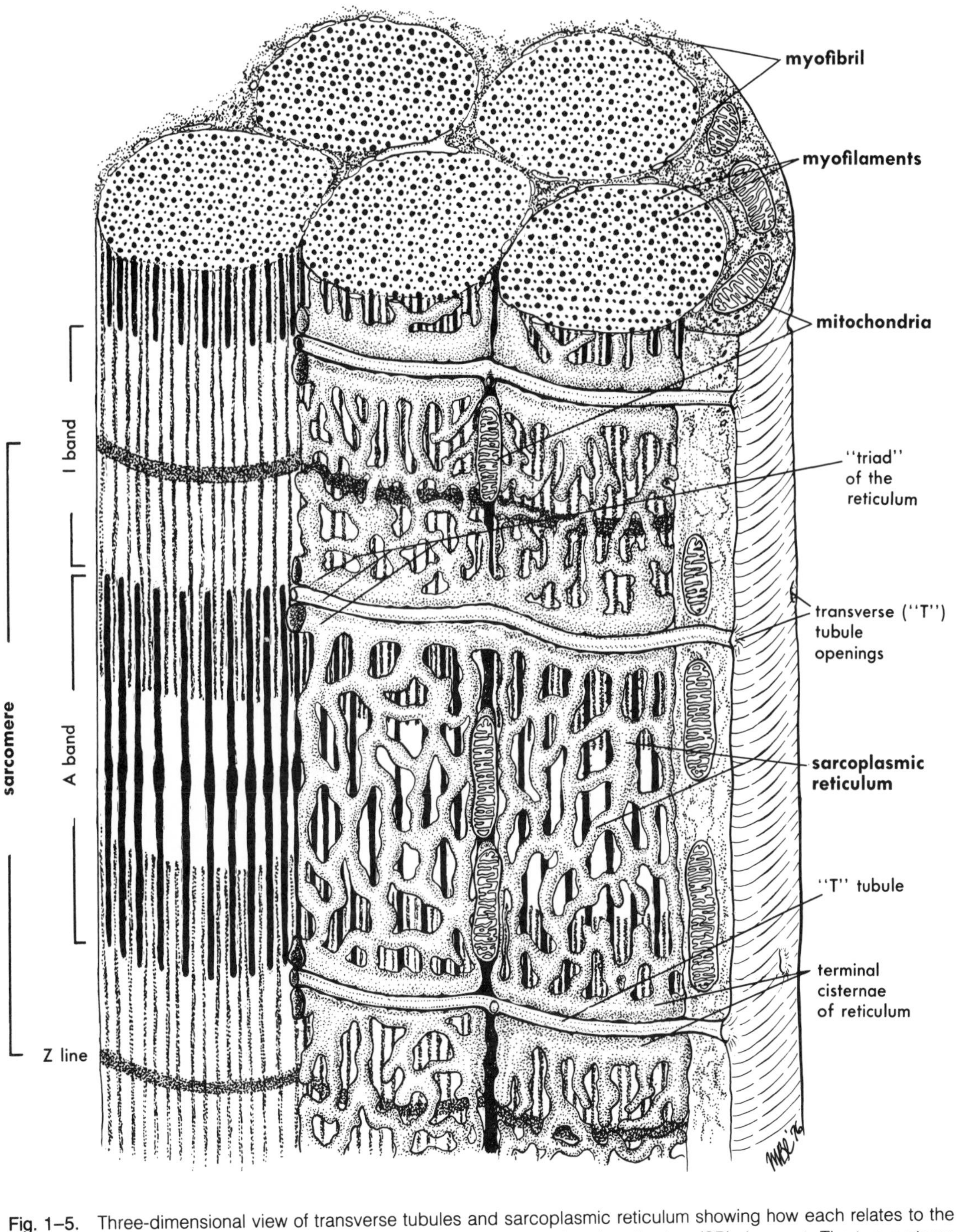

Fig. 1–5. Three-dimensional view of transverse tubules and sarcoplasmic reticulum showing how each relates to the other. The T-tubules open to the fiber's exterior, whereas the sarcoplasmic reticulum (SR) does not. The two systems are involved in the triggering and release of calcium ions in the cell. (From Crouch, J.E. *Functional Human Anatomy*, 4th Ed. Courtesy of Lea & Febiger, 1985.)

mammalian cardiac muscle, they are large and located at the Z-line (see next section).

ULTRASTRUCTURE OF SKELETAL MUSCLE

When a section of skeletal muscle is removed from the body, sliced into thin sections, and viewed under a light microscope, a repeating pattern of light and dark areas is seen (Fig. 1–6). This pattern is the basis of the term "striated muscle." The dark and light portions of the pattern represent the optical characteristics of the contractile proteins within the muscle cell. These proteins are called "myofibrils," and are made up of smaller protein strands called actin and myosin. The actin and myosin strands lie in a regular pattern, in which the two kinds of protein strands overlap each other. In fact, it is this overlapping that allows the proteins to hook on to each other and pull, which is the essential mechanism of muscle contraction, as shall be seen in the next section.

Actin fibers are thin proteins, and light passes through them easily. Myosin fibers, on the other hand, are dense and appear dark through the microscope. The darkest part of the pattern occurs where both actin and myosin overlap each other; the lightest is where only actin exists. The central part of the myosin strand is usually free from actin and appears slightly lighter than the places where both actin and myosin are absorbing light. Thus, the myosin band or dark band is not of uniform darkness, but rather is dark on both ends and a little lighter in the center. For this reason, it was named the *anisotropic* band (*an*—negative prefix, *iso*—the same, and *tropic*—consistency), meaning that it was not all the same consistency. This name is abbreviated the A band. The lighter area in the center where the actin does not overlap is called the H zone (see Fig. 1–6).

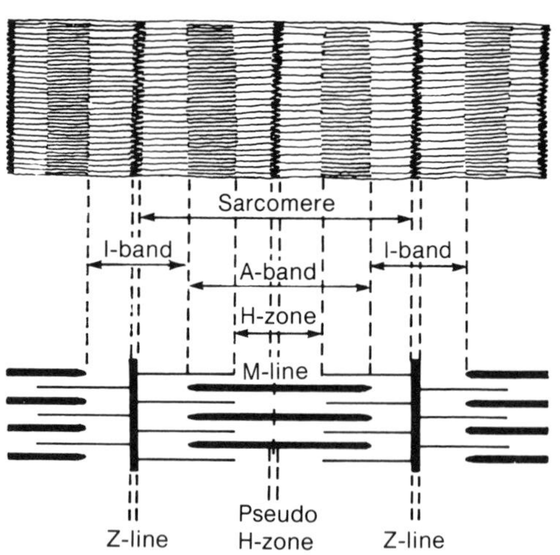

Fig. 1–6. Longitudinal section of striated muscle, together with a diagram showing the overlap of filaments that give rise to the band pattern. (From Stracher, A. *Muscle and Nonmuscle Motility.* Courtesy of Academic Press, 1983.)

In contrast to the anisotropic band is the *isotropic* band, where there are only actin filaments. These areas are uniformly light in color, and hence were given that name. Their name too, is usually abbreviated and is called the I band.

Both the actin and myosin filaments are anchored in their respective places by dense proteins that block more light than the myosin strands. These anchoring areas appear as stripes or lines through the microscope. *Z-line* is the name given to the proteins which anchor the actin strands at their extremes. These lines divide the myofibril into its perfectly repeated patterns, and the area in between two Z lines is called a *sarcomere.* The proteins that anchor the myosin strands are near the center of the sarcomere, and are called *M lines* because they anchor myosin.

When a muscle cell is viewed in cross-section, there is a hexagonal arrangement of actin filaments surrounding each myosin filament. This arrangement gives stability to the system and allows each actin to be held in place and acted upon by three different myosins. Notice in Figure 1–7 that cross-sectional cuts at the H-zone show only myosin filaments, while cuts at the I-band show only actin filaments. Both filaments are present when cuts are made in the darker portion of the A-band (Fig. 1–7).

As a muscle contracts, actin filaments are levered past the myosin filaments until they completely overlap. This phenomenon was first discovered by H.E. Huxley and is referred to as the *Huxley sliding filament theory of contraction.* During contraction, the Z-lines pull closer together, and the lighter I bands

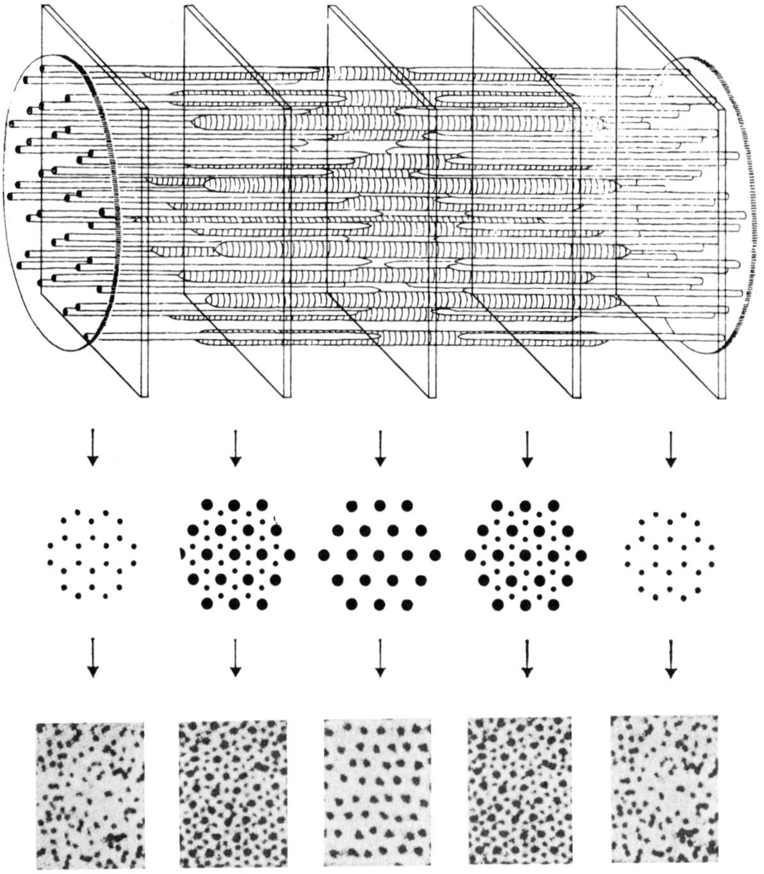

Fig. 1–7. Transverse sections through a three-dimensional array of filaments in vertebrate striated muscle (top) show how the thick and thin filaments are arranged in a hexagonal pattern (middle). At bottom are electron micrographs of the corresponding sections. (From Huxley, H.E.: The Contraction of Muscle. Sci Am. *199*:67, 1958.)

and H-zones compress as more filaments move in to fill the open space (Fig. 1–8).

During contraction, the length of the individual A bands remains constant, because the A bands consist primarily of the thick myosin filaments which do not move. However, both the I band and the H-zone will get smaller when the muscle contracts because the actin filaments are pulled into the myosin as the muscle shortens. It is important to note that the distance from the end of one H-zone through the Z-line to the edge of the next H-zone remains the same because the actin filaments stay the same length. All the changes are related to the interdigitation of the two sets of filaments as they slide past each other.

CONTRACTILE PROTEINS

Much is known concerning the composition of the actin and myosin filaments, and this knowledge is helpful to the understanding of the contractile process. A *myosin molecule* looks like a thin rod with two "heads" or *crossbridges* on one end and the other end extending away like a tail. The molecules are arranged in the thick filament so that the heads point toward the two ends and the tails toward the middle. The body of the myosin filament is composed of the "tails" of the myosin molecule and the heads or crossbridges are the "levering arms" that pull actin into the myosin during contraction (Fig. 1–9).

The actin filament is composed of three different proteins; globular actin (G-actin), troponin, and tropomyosin.

The G-actin protein molecule forms the basic structure of the actin filament, which is composed of hundreds of these small spherical particles arranged in a helix, resembling two strings of beads wrapped around each other (Fig. 1–10). Each spherical bead has a recognizable active site which binds with specific active sites on the cross-bridge of the myosin molecule. The other two proteins, *troponin* and *tropomyosin* lie in the groove formed by the helix of the actin and regulate muscle contraction. Tropomyosin molecules form a

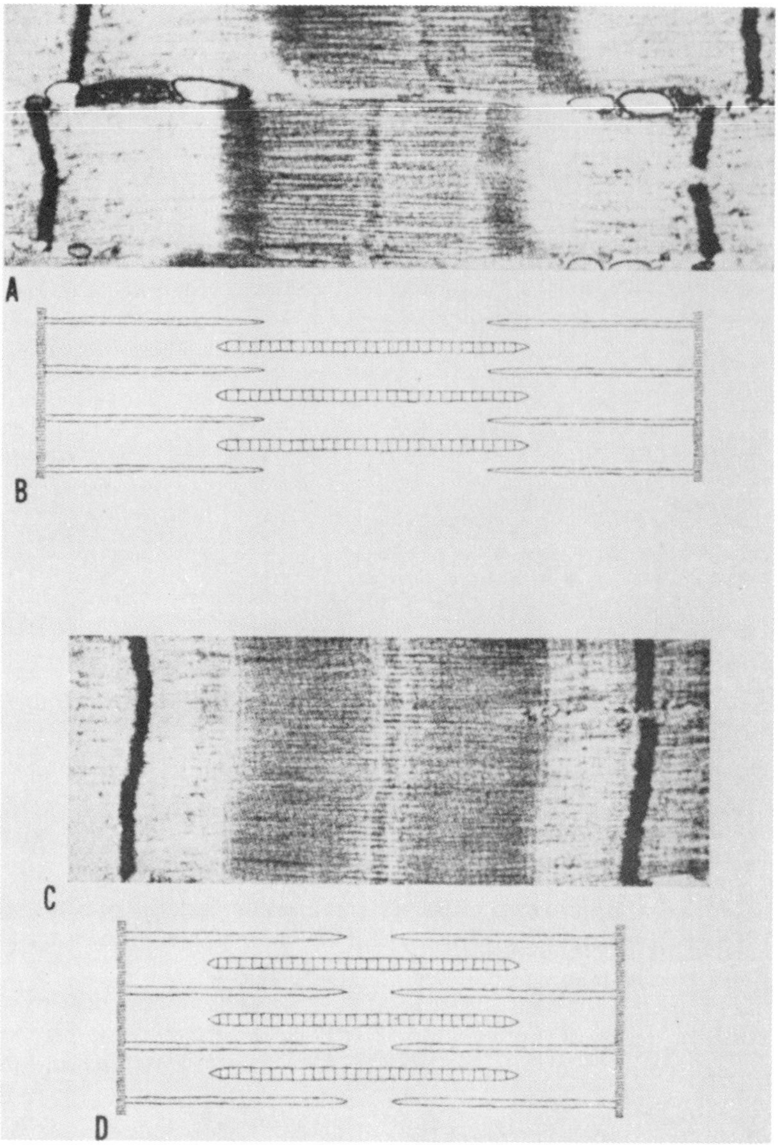

Fig. 1–8. *A and C.* Longitudinal section of a muscle fixed during isometric contraction at two different lengths, examined under an electron microscope. The drawing of the position of the actin filaments during the longer *(B)* and shorter *(D)* lengths shows clearly how the actin filaments "slide" into the myosin filaments. (From Huxley, H.E.: The Contraction of Muscle. Sci Am. *199*:67, 1958.)

long thin thread on the surface of the actin strand that provides rigidity to the actin structure, and prevents contraction from occurring by covering the active sites on the actin. Troponin molecules are more globular than tropomyosin molecules and sit on the tropomyosin molecules a short distance from one end. Note that the thin tropomyosin molecule extends over *seven* actin molecules with one troponin molecule on the end. Each filament of actin contains 300 to 400 actin molecules and about 40 to 60 tropomyosins.

TRIGGERING OF CONTRACTION

Muscle contraction is triggered by an electrical impulse flowing down a motor neuron to the individual muscle cells. When this impulse reaches the muscle cell, it sets up an electrical charge on the sarcolemma (cell membrane) covering the cell, and this electrical charge is transmitted into the cell via the T-tubule system (see Chapter 2 for further information concerning the flow of an impulse and cell membrane mechanics). The

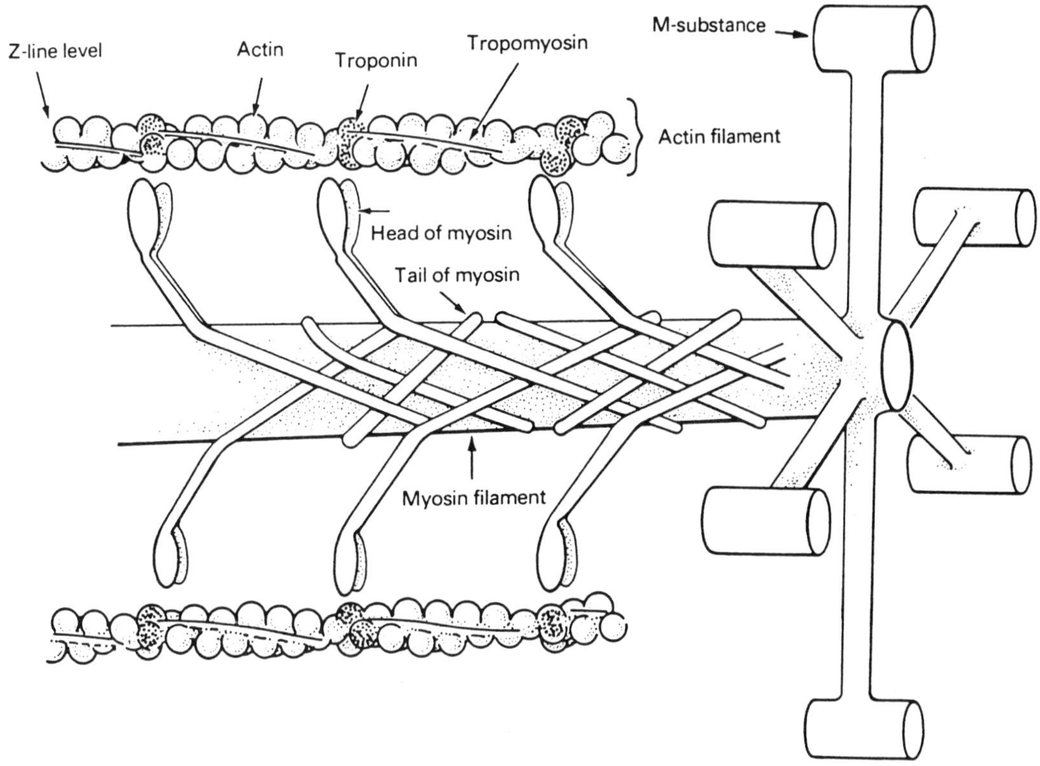

Fig. 1–9. Schematic drawing showing the arrangement of the myosin molecules that form the myosin filament and their relationship to other structural and contractible elements in the cell. (From Edington, D.W., and Edgerton, R.E. *Biology of Physical Activity.* Courtesy of Dee Edington.)

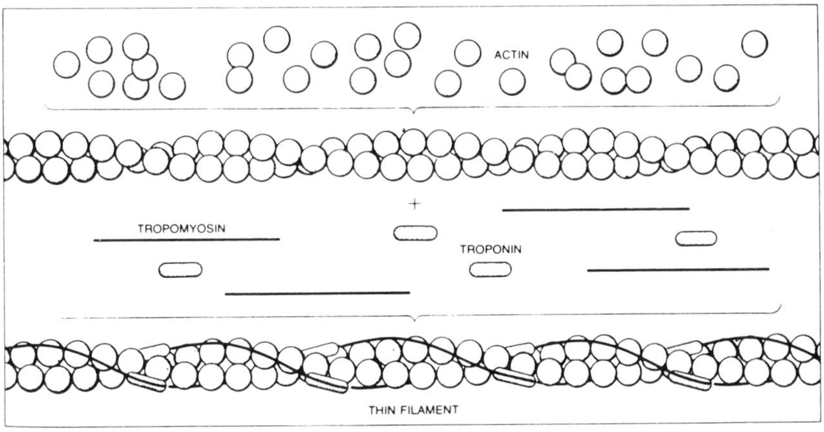

Fig. 1–10. Schematic drawing of the actin filament. The thin filament is an assembly of actin, tropomyosin, and troponin molecules. The actins (present in the largest amount) are small spherical molecules that are linked to form a double helix. Tropomyosin (a long thin molecule) forms a continuous strand that sits on the string of actins alongside each groove of the double helix. A globular troponin molecule is affixed near one end of each tropomyosin. One tropomyosin extends over seven actin molecules and there are 300 to 400 actin in the micron-long filament. (From Murray and Weber: The Cooperative Action of Muscle Proteins. Sci Am. *230*:61, 1974.)

movement of the electrical impulse down the T-tubule releases calcium ions from their storage sites in the terminal cisternae or lateral sacs. These calcium ions move into the muscle and bind directly onto the troponin complex causing troponin to physically "twist" the tropomyosin strand away from the active site it covers on the actin filament. The active sites are then exposed to the charged heads of the myosin. Although the myosin heads are fairly stable in their resting condition, they quickly bind to the actin molecule when the active sites are uncovered.

The energy needed for a muscle to contract is provided by the breakdown of a high energy molecule called *ATP*. This ATP molecule is thought to be bound to a particular site on the surface of the myosin heads. Almost all of the myosin heads have an ATP molecule bound to them, "charging" them in preparation for the contraction. These charged heads are unable to couple with the actin molecules until calcium has effectively uncovered the active sites. In fact, the presence of ATP on the myosin cross-bridge actually inhibits any interaction of these two proteins. But once the myosin heads couple with the actin molecule forming an *actomyosin complex,* energy from ATP is released and a conformational change in the cross-bridges pulls the actin molecules toward the center of the cell (Fig. 1–11).

Since the cross-bridges of the myosin filament are oriented opposite to each other, the individual actin filaments are pulled toward the center, shortening the sarcomere. The force of contraction is not produced by all the cross-bridges attaching and swiveling at the same time, but is produced by asynchronous power strokes by numerous cross-bridges.

MOVEMENT OF THE MYOSIN

The energy for contraction comes from adenosine triphosphate (ATP), which is produced by metabolic processes (see Chapter 3) and is stored on the myosin cross-bridges prior to contraction. Also on the cross-bridge (near the actin binding site) is the enzyme *adenosine triphosphatase (ATPase).* When calcium attaches to the troponin molecule exposing the actin "active site," ATPase is activated to break down ATP which provides the energy for shortening the muscle (contraction). The speed of this reaction and the amount of energy released by it are linearly related to the amount of ATPase available. Not surprisingly, fast, powerful fast-twitch (FT) muscle fibers have more ATPase than slow, more endurance oriented slow-twitch (ST) fibers.

As long as Ca^{++} and ATPase are present in the muscle, cross-bridges will *attach* to the active site on the actin molecule and *swivel* to pull the actin towards the center of the sarcomere.

However, since most muscles shorten from a fixed end, the cross-bridges on the fixed side

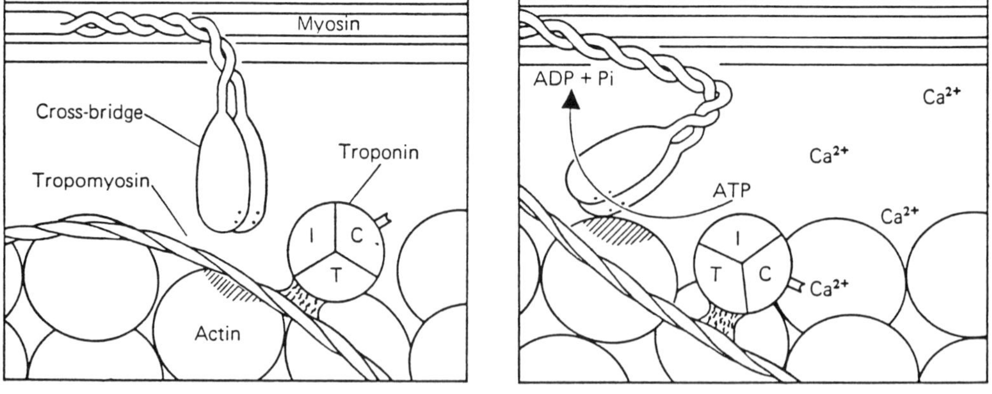

Fig. 1–11. Schematics of the charged myosin head inhibited from attaching to the actin binding sites and the initiation of muscle contraction by Ca^{++}. After Ca^{++} attaches to troponin, the binding sites are exposed and the crossbridges can pull the actin filaments toward each other, shortening the muscle. (Modified from Katz, A.M. Congestive heart failure. N. Engl. J. Med. *293*:1184, 1975.)

of the sarcomere pull the M-line towards the fixed end while the cross-bridges on the moveable end pull the actin towards the M-line (center).

The final stage of contraction, involving the detachment of the cross-bridges, is reached only after a new ATP molecule has bound to the myosin head of the cross-bridge. When this occurs, the cross-bridge will release the actin and swivel back to its original position for another cycle. A single cycle can occur 25 to 50 times per second. The attachment and detachment of the individual cross-bridges at different intervals produces a smooth contraction.

RELAXATION

When the signal from the motor neuron ceases, calcium is quickly removed to the storage vesicles by a calcium "pump" situated in the membrane of the sarcoplasmic reticulum. This pump is an "active" process that removes Ca^{++} rapidly but requires energy in the form of ATP to work. When calcium is removed, the muscle relaxes.

If for some reason, a muscle is contracted but no ATP molecule is available to release the actin-myosin complex, a *rigor complex* is formed that will detach only by having a new ATP molecule bind to it. This is the basis of *rigor mortis*, which affects muscles after the death of the organism because the supply of ATP is exhausted after about 6 to 8 hours.

A summary of the contraction and relaxation is illustrated in Figure 1–12.

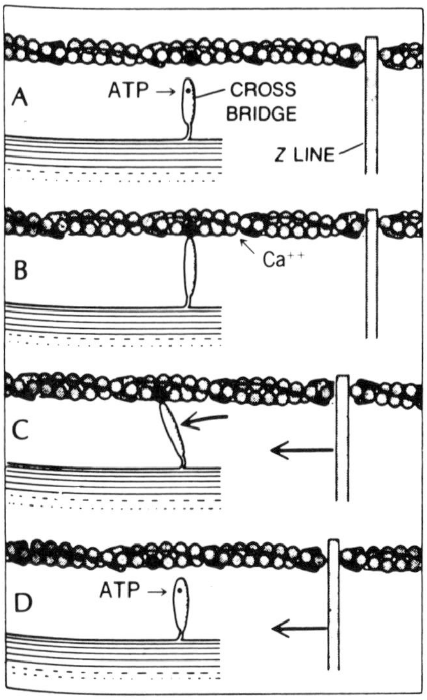

Fig. 1–12. At rest *(A)* the attachment sites for the cross-bridges are blocked by tropomyosin. Attachment of Ca^{++} to troponin (dark structures) moves the troponin-tropomyosin so that the cross-bridges can attach to the actin molecule *(B)*, followed by the hydrolysis of ATP and a power stroke *(C)*. Detachment of the cross-bridges from actin *(D)* allows the contraction cycle to be repeated. (After Murray and Weber: The Cooperative Action of Muscle Proteins. Sci. Am. *230*:61, 1974.)

CONTRACTION PROCESS—OTHER THEORIES

It must be pointed out that the mechanisms of explaining muscle contraction are theories rather than facts, and that the explanation of contraction outlined in the previous pages is just one theory among many. Two other interesting theories of muscle contraction that have been proposed are discussed briefly below:

Theory 1 : In this theory, the myosin head contains an ATP molecule but is already bent backward in a position considered its resting state. ATP is first broken down, causing the myosin to swivel forward (an unstable configuration), and then attaches to the actin filament. The creation of an actomyosin complex provides the impetus for the myosin to swivel backward, pulling with it the actin filament, until the myosin reaches its resting bent position. Available ATP circulating in the sarcoplasm then attaches to the head of the myosin, releasing the ADP and causing detachment from the actin. The cycle continues as long as Ca^{++} ions and ATP are both present. The main difference between this theory and the one previously discussed is that work is done *after* energy is released.

Theory 2 (Fig. 1–13): The *electrostatic* theory of contraction states that no cross-bridge attachment takes place, but instead that the myosin molecules acting as charged capacitors set up an electrical field in the sarcoplasm around the actin which draws the actin in, much like a plunger through a solenoid. Release of

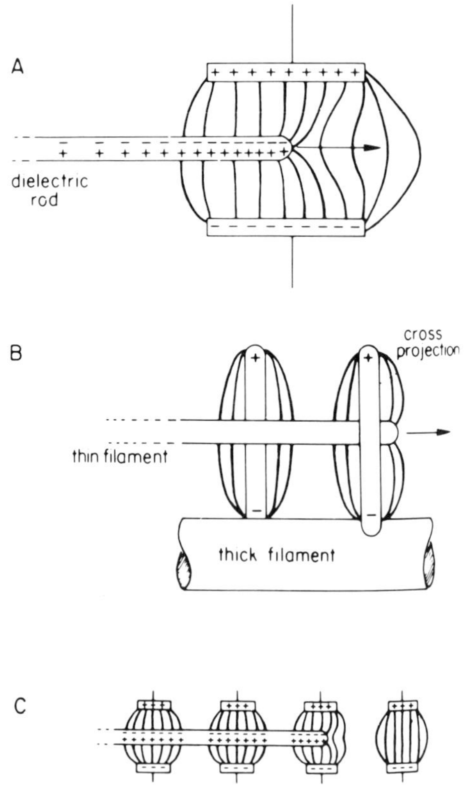

Fig. 1–13. Mechanism of force generation proposed by the electrostatic theory. The principle is that the myosin is like a dielectric rod suspended in the field of capacitors (actin). The charge is set up by the splitting of ATP. (From Noble, M.I.M., and Pollack, G.H.: Molecular Mechanisms of Contraction. Circ. Res. *40*:333, 1977. By permission of the American Heart Association, Inc.)

Ca^{++} activates the ATPase which splits ATP to set up the electrical charge. The electrical potential of the contraction is proportional to the amount of calcium released.

HOW MUSCLES ARE ORGANIZED

Earlier it was learned that skeletal muscles require a signal from the nervous system to contract. In the body, these signals are sent down large neurons called *motor neurons* that originate in the anterior portion of the spinal cord. The motor neuron and all of the muscle fibers (cells) it innervates is called a *motor unit.* The motor unit is the functional unit for neural control of motor activity and has several important characteristics. First, motor units vary in the number of muscle fibers according to the degree of control needed for that unit. For example, motor units to muscles involved with fine motor movements (such as the hands) have only a small number of muscle fibers per motor neuron. However, units in large muscles such as the quadriceps may contain 1000 or more muscle fibers per neuron. Second, all of the muscle cells in a motor unit will have the same biochemical and physiologic properties. Motor units (and therefore skeletal muscle fibers) can be classified into a general category of "fast" or "slow" based on twitch response time or speed of contraction. They can also be classified metabolically in terms of the metabolic characteristics of the individual muscle fibers contained in them. The metabolic classifications are as follows: (1) Type I, slow oxidative (SO), (2) Type IIa, fast-oxidative glycolytic (FOG), and (3) Type IIb, fast glycolytic (FG).

Type I (SO)

Typically, the distance runner has a high proportion of the type I, slow oxidative "red" fibers because they are so well adapted for aerobic or endurance type work. They are innervated by smaller, slower neurons that are easily stimulated, but the twitch response is slow. They have a high mitochondrial content and are often identified with a stain that reacts with an oxidative enzyme or enzyme complex. They also have a high level of myoglobin, a substance that helps oxygen get to the mitochondria (and contributes to the red color of these fibers). This biochemical set-up gives type I fibers the ability to resist fatigue for long periods of time.

Type IIa (FOG)

Type IIa fibers, although red and fatigue resistant, are categorized as "fast twitch" fibers because the speed of contraction (twitch response) is faster, and the neurons that fire these fibers are larger and more difficult to fire than the type I neurons. This fiber type could be especially important for athletes in middle-distance events that require both speed and endurance.

Type IIb (FG)

Sprinters, jumpers, and other "power" athletes have a high percentage of type IIb fibers. These fibers have little oxidative capacity and therefore fatigue rather rapidly. They are innervated with large, high threshold neurons, and have a fast twitch response time. Speed of contraction is indicated best by a stain for myofibrillar ATPase. Type IIb fibers show much of this substance. They also stain high for anaerobic metabolic pathway enzymes, but show very little mitochondrial or oxidative enzyme content. They also have more sarcoplasmic reticulum than slow-twitch fibers to aid in the movement of calcium into and out of the muscle. Table 1–1 shows the various properties and differences among the different fiber types, which are shown in Figure 1–14. Many of the metabolic differences will be clearer after studying Chapter 3.

OBTAINING A MUSCLE SAMPLE

Obtaining a muscle tissue for enzymatic and staining procedures is a painless and rather simple process. However, since the biopsy procedure is minor surgery, precautions must be taken to ensure that all instruments are sterile. The biopsy needle, a hollow needle approximately the width of pencil lead, has a tip designed to shear a small portion of muscle tissue (Fig. 1–15). To obtain the muscle sample, the needle is inserted through a small incision in the skin into the belly of the muscle. The muscle is pulled into the needle by suction and snipped off at the tip. To preserve enzyme activity, the muscle tissue is immediately frozen in liquid nitrogen. Thin sections (10 μm thick) of tissue are later shaved off using a cryostat, and mounted for individual staining. Sections cut in series from the same muscle can be stained with different stains to differentiate the different fiber types.

CAN MUSCLE FIBER TYPES BE CHANGED?

Some studies have shown that prolonged treadmill running can result in as much as a 2-fold increase in the oxidative capacity of mixed skeletal muscle in rodents. Other studies have shown that training increases the endurance capacity of human muscle as well. Although there seems to be agreement that endurance training increases the endurance capability of any muscle, and that power training increases the power potential of muscle, there is still some controversy regarding whether there can be an actual change in muscle fiber types. Some researchers have reported changes in the *subtypes* of fast twitch fibers (types IIa and IIb). It is clear that type IIa are more aerobic than type IIb. With training, the type IIb fibers begin to take on the characteristics of the type IIa fibers. Although the significance of these changes is not

Table 1–1. Comparison of the Various Fiber Types

	Fiber Type		
Quality Compared	*Type I*	*Type IIa*	*Type IIb*
Other names	slow red slow oxidative oxidative	fast red fast-oxidative glycolytic	fast white fast glycolytic
Properties			
speed of contraction	slow	fast	fast
resistance to fatigue	high	high	low
glycogen content	low	high	high
diameter	small	large	large
force production	low	moderate	high
Structural Differences			
mitochondria	high	high	low
capillary density	high	high	low
sarco reticulum	low	high	hgh
Enzymatic Differences			
Myosin ATPase	low	high	high
Glycolytic capacity	low	high	high
Glyogenolytic cap	low	high	high
myoglobin content	high	low	low
Troponin affinity for Ca^{++}	low	high	high
Order of recruit	1	2	3

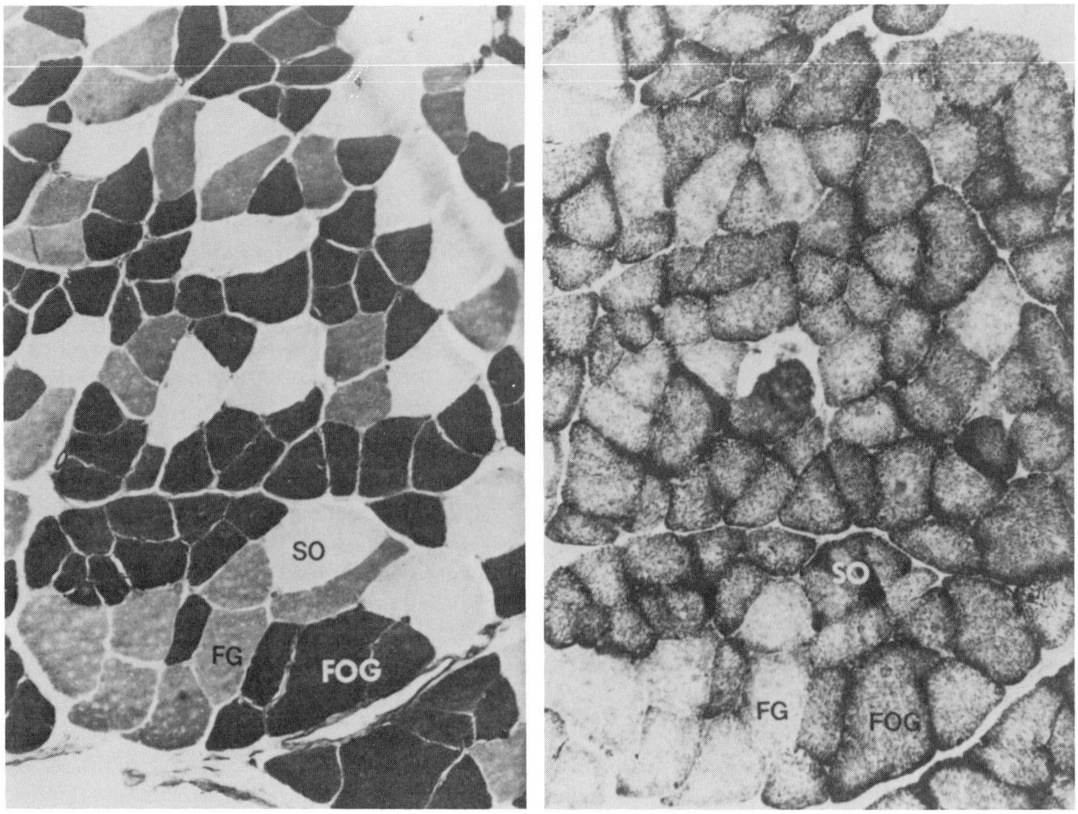

Fig. 1–14. *A.* Muscle fibers stained with myofibrillatory ATPase stain. The darkness of this stain relates to pH changes in the fibers, but clearly shows the three fiber types which are indicated as SO, FG, and FOG. *B.* A nearby section of the same muscle stained for an oxidative enzyme (succinic dehydrogenase). (Photomicrographs by P. Watt of Muscle Research Unit, University of Hull, England. *In Handbook of Physiology,* edited by Peachy, L.D. Courtesy of Oxford University Press, 1983.)

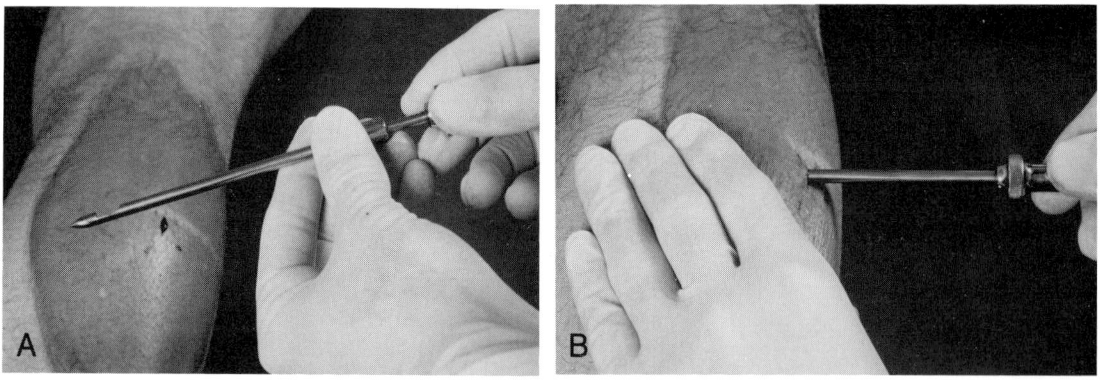

Fig. 1–15. *A.* A muscle biopsy of the gastrocnemius showing muscle preparation and a standard muscle biopsy needle. *B.* Needle inserted to obtain a sample.

known, it may explain why there are so few type IIb fibers in the leg muscles of highly-trained distance runners.

Other researchers have reported fast-to-slow fiber type transformation when fast fibers were innervated with slow fiber neurons or when fast fibers were stimulated electrically (via implanted electrodes) with a frequency pattern which is normally delivered to a slow-twitch muscle. In time, the fast fibers changed and became true type I fibers not only in metabolic properties, but also in the Ca^{++} handling systems and the myofibrillar protein structure. These changes come about slowly and sequentially, but they do seem to occur given enough time. These same changes were seen in another study as a result of the increased contractile activity as in endurance training. Although the changes occurred much more slowly than with chronic stimulation, they did occur, but only with a long-term, high-intensity running program.

Although the final answer to fiber type transformations is still not available, there is at least some evidence that muscle is an extremely adaptable tissue and may change to meet the needs of the organism.

HOW FIBER TYPES AFFECT PERFORMANCE

On average, leg muscle contains about half type I (slow, oxidative) fibers, about 25% type IIa (fast, oxidative, glycolytic) fibers, and about 25% type IIb (fast, glycolytic) fibers. Some outstanding athletes have a much higher percentage of whichever fiber type would be advantageous to their event. For instance, studies of elite male and female distance runners show that some have calf muscles composed of more than 90% ST (type I) fibers. In contrast, some sprinters were found to have as much as 92% type FT (type II) fibers. Many outstanding world-class athletes are endowed with a greater proportion of one muscle fiber type or another.

The question is, what is the role of genetics in determining the potential to be a world-class athlete. Earlier studies have shown little evidence that the percentage of ST or FT change appreciably following only a few months of training. More recent evidence suggests the possibility of fiber type change with high volume of training. However, the percentage of change may be much too small to make enough difference in sports that require a high percentage of one fiber type or another. That is to say, it would be unlikely that a sprinter's fiber type could be converted to that of a long-distance runner. Because of this, it could be concluded that genetics do play a fairly important role in certain types of athletic events. In fact, some Soviet bloc countries do fiber-typing on young athletes to determine which has a genetic predisposition for certain activities.

Fortunately, there are many sports that seem to have no prerequisite in terms of a given fiber type for success. Elite cyclists have about 55 to 45% ST vs. FT, and weight lifters are also near the norm. Many other sports (golf, volleyball, tennis) have champions with nearly equal amounts of ST and FT fibers. It is clear that muscle fiber type is only one of the factors related to potential for athletic success (Fig. 1–16).

RECRUITMENT

Because muscle fibers are classified as "fast" or "slow," there is a tendency to think that slow fibers are used for slow work and fast fibers for fast work. It is true that slow fibers are used most often for slow, postural-type activity. However, recruitment of muscle fibers is not so simple as this. The general rule is that the smaller the cell body of the motor unit neuron, the easier it is to fire (Fig. 1–17). This means that slow (type 1) fibers are probably used more often because their neurons are smaller and easier to fire. However, muscle fiber recruitment is more dependent on the *force* or *resistance* than on the speed of movement. For example, lifting a light weight rapidly will probably recruit slow fibers as well as will cycling at a high rate with low resistance. Heavy resistance lifting or pedaling slowly with heavy resistance while cycling will recruit both fast and slow twitch fibers.

Recruitment of motor units is also important in the *gradation* of muscle strength. Since motor units are "all or none," that is, they either fire all of their fibers or none of their fibers, the best way to increase the force of

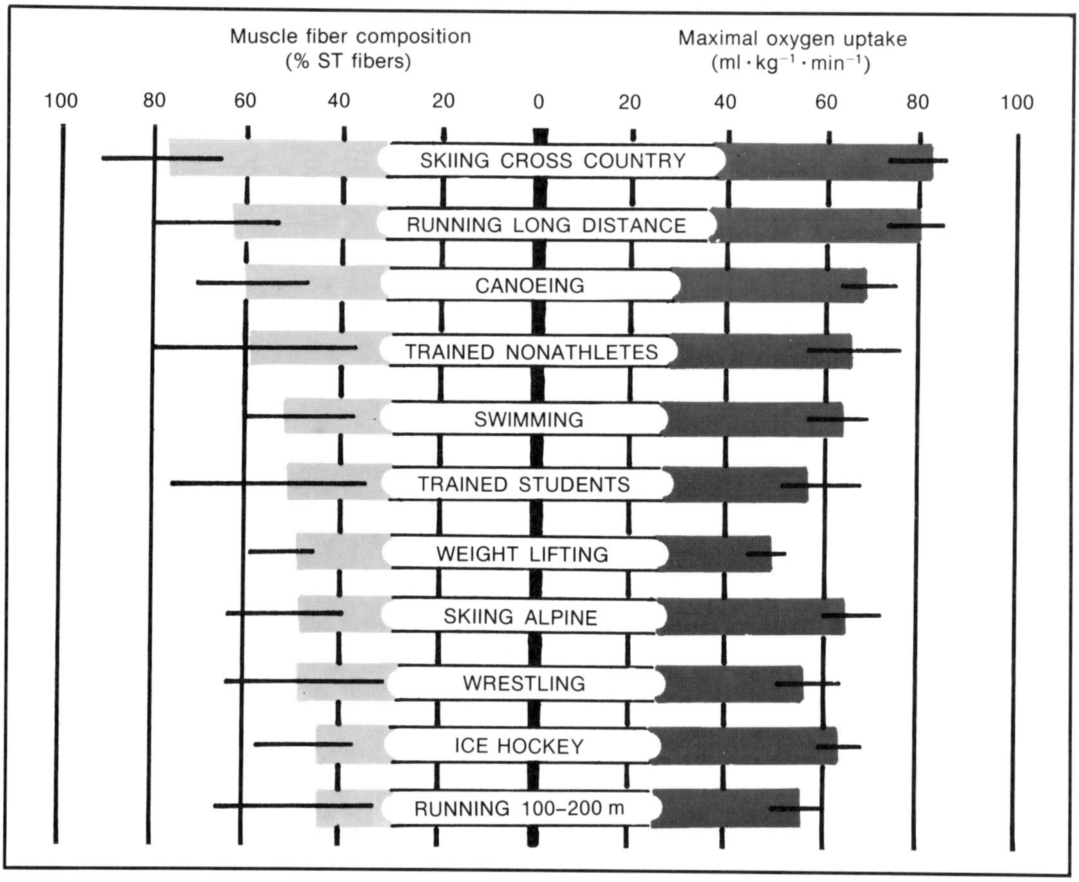

Fig. 1–16. Muscle fiber composition (percentage of slow-twitch muscles on left side) and maximal oxygen uptake or aerobic endurance (right side) in athletes representing different sports. The dark horizontal bar denotes the range. (From McArdle, W.D., Katch, F.I., and Katch, V.L. *Exercise Physiology*, 2nd Ed. Courtesy of Lea & Febiger, 1986.)

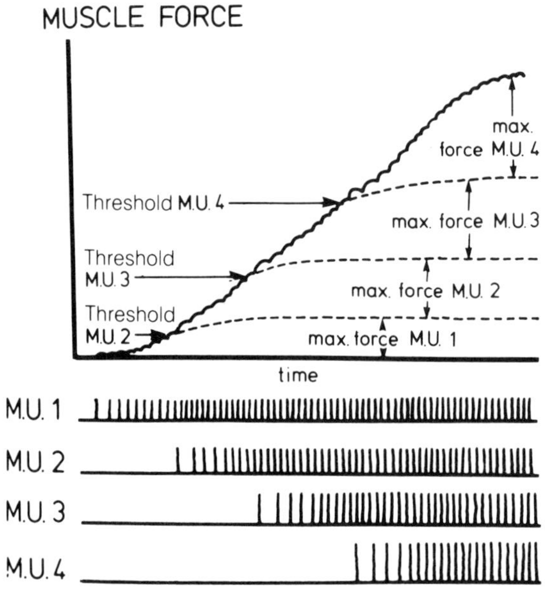

Fig. 1–17. Illustration of size principle of recruitment of motor units. Smaller motor units are recruited first; successively larger units begin firing at increasing tension levels. In all cases the newly recruited unit fires at a base frequency, then increases to a maximum. M.U. = motor unit. (From Astrand, P.O., and Rodahl, K. *Textbook of Work Physiology: Physiological Basis of Exercises*, 2nd Ed. Courtesy of McGraw Hill, 1986.)

contraction is to increase the number of motor units fired. Lifting a piece of chalk would require only a few motor units (and probably those with the smallest, most easily fired motor neuron). With a moderate weight, the number of motor units is increased. With an extremely heavy weight, the maximum number of motor units that can be fired will be fired. Most people cannot fire all of their motor units unless extremely excited or frightened. Strength training helps increase the efficiency of the recruitment process, allowing more motor units to be consciously used.

Another way to increase or decrease the force of contraction is to increase or decrease the frequency of firing to the motor unit. When motor neurons fire at higher rates (about 30/sec with slow fibers and 120/sec with fast), the muscle tension increases to levels above the single twitch level for two reasons; (1) the connective tissue is shortened and the slack is taken out, and (2) there is more time for calcium release from the lateral sacs and this increases the possibility of actin-myosin interaction.

TYPES OF CONTRACTIONS

Concentric Contractions

When muscles develop enough tension to exceed the resistance, the muscles shorten and the body segment moves (Fig. 1–18A). The muscles are then said to have contracted *concentrically* (this is a form of isotonic or dynamic contraction). For example, in a pull-up the biceps brachii and other muscles contract, causing the elbows to bend and draw the shoulders closer to the hands. In vigorous motor movements, such as in athletics, most of the apparent contractions are *concentric*, but many of the less-apparent contractions are either eccentric or static in nature.

Eccentric Contractions

A muscle contracts *eccentrically* when the resistance it experiences exceeds the force (Fig. 1–18B), thus causing the muscle to lengthen instead of shorten (this also is a form of isotonic contraction). Eccentric contractions are demonstrated by moving slowly from a standing to a squatting position. To allow this movement, the leg extensor muscles must lengthen while contracting (applying tension) to control the body's weight. Eccentric contraction is also demonstrated in the actions of the biceps when the body is lowered from a pull-up position, and in the actions of the triceps in lowering the body from the push-up position.

In all eccentric contractions, the movement is directly opposite the action ordinarily assigned to the muscle. In lowering from the pull-up the movement is elbow extension, but

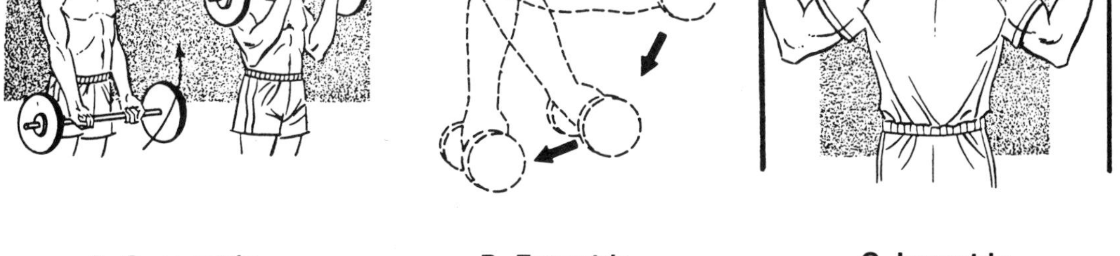

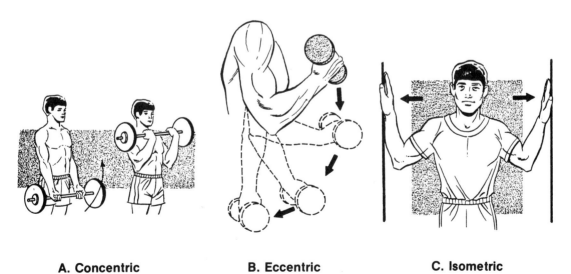

A. Concentric **B. Eccentric** **C. Isometric**

Fig. 1–18. Examples of concentric, eccentric, and isometric contractions. (From McArdle, W.D., Katch, F.I., and Katch, V.L. *Exercise Physiology*, 2nd Ed. Courtesy of Lea & Febiger, 1986.)

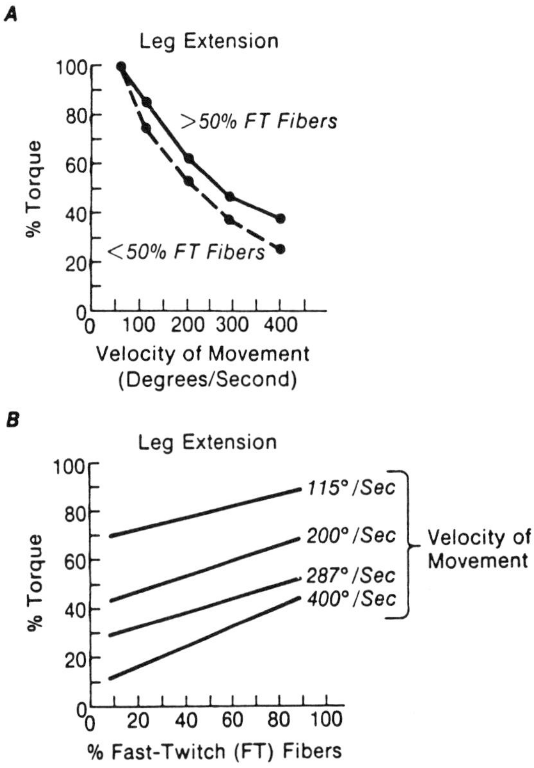

Fig. 1–19. Muscle force-velocity relationships. *A.* The peak torque (force) generated by a muscle decreases with increasing velocities of movement, i.e., the greatest torque is produced at the slowest speeds of movement. *B.* At any given velocity of movement, the torque produced becomes greater as the percentage of distribution of fast-twitch (FT) fibers in the muscle grows. The data were obtained during leg extension movements. (From Mathews, D.K., and Fox, E.L. *Physiological Basis of Physical Education and Athletics,* 2nd Ed. Courtesy of W.B. Saunders Co., 1976.)

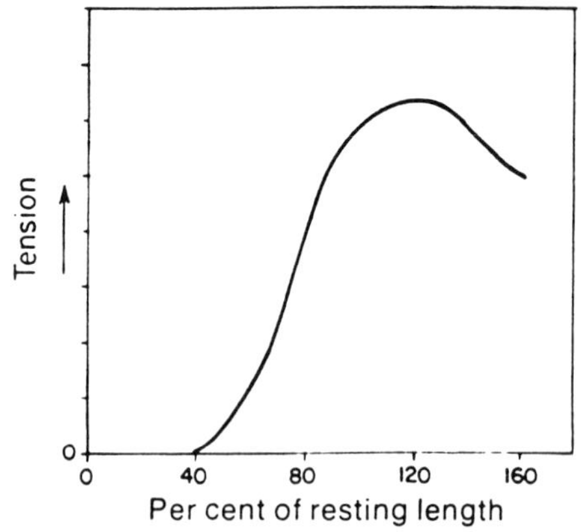

Fig. 1–20. Length-tension relationship in skeletal muscles. (From Jensen, C.R., and Fisher, A.G. *Scientific Basis of Athletic Conditioning,* 2nd Ed. Courtesy of Lea & Febiger, 1979.)

the active muscles are the elbow flexors. Eccentric contractions are common in wrestling and football, in which force applied by the opponent often causes muscles to lengthen while in contraction, and in gymnastics, in which the body, in arm-supported positions, is often lowered slowly. When the body lands, or when a heavy object is received, the muscles contract *eccentrically* to absorb the shock of the force. It should be noted that the lengthening of a muscle in a relaxed condition (no tension) owing to contraction of opposite muscles is not considered to be an eccentric contraction.

Isometric Contractions

A muscle contracts isometrically when it attempts to shorten (applies tension) but does not overcome the resistance; therefore, shortening of the muscle and movement of the body segment fail to occur (Fig. 1–18C). Isometric contraction occurs when a person pushes or pulls against a fixed object, or when the muscular tension equals the opposing force. Such *isometric* contractions are used frequently in stabilizing the body or portions of the body during performance.

EFFECT OF SPEED OF CONTRACTION AND LENGTH OF MUSCLE ON TENSION

It is generally known that as the speed of shortening increases, the tension exerted by a muscle decreases. This can be explained by assuming that there is only a certain period of time available for a cross-bridge to become attached as the actin filaments slide past. Therefore, as the speed of contraction increases, the number of effective cross-bridges formed would decrease, decreasing overall tension. Note also that muscles with more FT fibers produce more tension at any speed (Fig. 1–19).

The amount of tension a muscle can exert is also related to the length of the muscle as it contracts. This phenomenon can be explained by referring to the principles of contraction discussed previously. A shortened muscle loses tension because of the bare-zone (the H zone) in the center of the myosin filament. This area may be devoid of cross-bridges. No tension would be applied to the actin filament pulled into this area as the muscle shortens. Conversely, a muscle that is lengthened to such a point that the overlap between actin and myosin is reduced would also decrease the number of cross-bridge attachments, and a decreased tension would result. The length-tension relationship of skeletal muscle is illustrated in Figure 1–20. Luckily, the length of the muscle is usually related to the mechanical advantage of the joint so that the force at the end of the lever arm is fairly constant through the full range of motion.

SELECTED READINGS

Adelstein, R.S., and E. Eisenberg: Regulation and Kinetics of the Actin-Myosin-ATP Interaction. Ann. Rev. Biochem. *49*:921–956, 1980.

Baldwin, K.M., Winder, W.W., Terjung, R.L., et al.: Glycolytic enzyme in different types of skeletal muscle: Adaptation to exercise. Am. J. Physiol. *225(4)*:962–966, 1973.

Sjostrom, M., Angquist, K., Bylund, A., et al.: Morphometric analyses of Human Muscle Fiber Types. Muscle & Nerve, *5*:538–553, 1982.

Baldwin, K.M., et al.: Glycolytic enzyme in different types of skeletal muscle: Adaptation to exercise. Am. J. Physiol. *225*(4):962–966, 1973.

C. Cohen: The protein switch of muscle contraction. Sci. Am. *233*(5):70–85, 1979.

Costill, D.I., Daniels, J., Evans, W., et al.: Skeletal muscle enzymes and fiber composition in male and female track athletes. J. Appl. Physiol. *40*(2):149–154, 1976.

Costill, D.L., et al.: Adaptation in skeletal muscle following strength training. J. Appl. Physiol. *46*:96–99, 1979.

Coyle, E.F., et al.: Skeletal muscle fiber characteristics of world class shot-putters. Res. Quart. *49*:278–284, 1978.

Curtin, N.A., and R.C. Woledge: Energy changes and muscular contraction. Physiol. Reviews *558*:690–761, 1978.

Davies, R.E.: A molecular theory of contraction: calcium-dependent contractions with hydrogen bond formation plus ATP-dependent extension of part of the myosin-actin crossbridges. Nature, *199*:1068–1074, 1963.

Elder, C.G.B., Bradbury, K., and Roberts, R.: Variability of fiber type distributions within human muscles. J. Appl. Physiol. Respirat. Environ. Exercise Physiol. *53*(6):1473–1480, 1982.

Gans, C.: Fiber Architecture and Muscle Function. Ex. and Sp. Sc. Reviews, *10*:160–207, 1982.

Garrett, W.E., et al.: Ultrastructural difference in human skeletal muscle fiber types. Orthop. Clin. No. Am. *14*(2):4113–4125, Apr. 1983.

Gollnick, P.D., Armstrong, R.B., Saltin, B., et al.: Effect of training on enzyme activity and fiber composition of human skeletal muscle. J. Appl. Physiol. *39*(1):109–111, 1973.

Gollnick, P.D., et al.: Enzyme activity and fiber composition in skeletal muscle of untrained and trained men. J. Appl. Physiol. *333*(3):312–319, 1972.

Gollnick, P.D., and Hodgson, D.R.: The Identification of Fiber Types in Skeletal Muscle: A Continual Dilemma. ESSR, Vol. 14, ASSM, 1986.

Gonyea, W.J.: Role of exercise in inducing increases in skeletal muscle fiber number. J. Appl. Physiol.: Respir. Environ. Exercise Physiol. *48*(3):421–426, 1980.

Huxley, A.F.: Muscular Contraction. J. Physiol. *243*:1–43, 1974.

Jolesky, F., and F.A. Sreter.: Development, Innervation, Activity-Pattern Induced Changes in Skeletal Muscle. Ann. Rev. Physiol. *43*:531–552, 1981.

Kanekisa, H., et al.: Effect of isometric and isokinetics muscle training on static strength and dynamic power. Eur. J. Appl. Physiol. *50*(3):365–371, 1983.

Lexell, J., Henriksson-Larsen, K., Winbald, B., et al.: Distribution of Different Fiber Types in Human Skeletal Muscles: Effects of Aging Studied in Whole Muscle Cross Sections. Muscle and Nerve, *6*:588–595, 1983.

MacDougall, J.D., Sale, D.G., Moroy, J.R., et al.: Mitochondrial volume density in human skeletal muscle following heavy resistance training. Med. Sci. Sports Exercise *11*(2):163–166, 1979.

Murray, J.M., and A. Weber. The cooperative action of muscle proteins. Sci. Amer. *230*:58–71, 1974.

Newham, D.J., et al.: Ultrastructural changes after concentric and eccentric contractions of human muscle. J. Neurol. Sci. *61(1)*:109–122, 1983.

Noble, M.I.M., and G.H. Pollack. Molecular Mechanisms of Contraction. Circ.Res. *40(4)*:333–342, 1977.

Peachy, Lee D.: Skeletal muscle. Section 10. Handbook of Physiology, American Physiological Society, 1983.

Pette, D.: Activity-induced fast and slow transitions in mammalian muscle. Med. Sci. Sp. & Ex. *16*:6, 517–528, 1984.

Pette, D., and Vrbova, G.: Invited Review: Neural Control of Phenotypic Expression in Mammalian Muscle Fibers. Muscle and Nerve *8*:676–689, Oct. 1985.

Porter, K.R., and C. Franzini-Armstrong. The Sarcoplasmic Reticulum. Sci. Amer., March, 1965.

Salleo, A., Anatasi, G., LaSpade, G., et al.: New muscle fiber production during compensatory hypertrophy. Med. Sci. Sports Exercise *12*(4):268–273, 1980.

Schantz, P., et al.: Increases in myofibrillar ATPase intermediate human skeletal muscle fibers in response to endurance training. Muscle and Nerve *6*(8):553–556, 1983.

Schantz, P., et al.: Muscle fiber type distribution, muscle, cross-sectional area, and maximal voluntary strength in humans. Acta Physiol. Scand. *117*(2):219–226, 1983.

Smith, M.J.: Muscle fiber types: Their relationship to athletic training and rehabilitation. Orthop. Clin. No. Am. *14*(2):403–411, 1983.

Sug, H., and G.H. Pollack: *Crossbridge Mechanism in Muscle Contraction.* Baltimore: University Park Press, 1979.

Thorstensson, A.: Muscle strength, fiber types, and enzyme activities in man. Acta Physiol. Scand. *443* (suppl):1–45, 1976.

Watt, P.W., et al.: Changes in fiber type composition in growing muscle as a result of dynamic exercise and static overload. Muscle and Nerve 7(1):50–53, 1984.

2

Nervous System

We have learned that skeletal muscle contracts only when triggered by a signal from the nervous system. This signal arrives at the muscle by way of a *motor neuron* which originates from the anterior horn of the spinal cord. Whether the motor neuron fires (and thus the muscle contracts) depends on integrated analysis of bits of information from memory circuits, sensory organs, and higher centers of control since movement is a complex result of many different controls. The purpose of this section is to help the student understand the complexity of movement by discussing the various factors that affect its neural control.

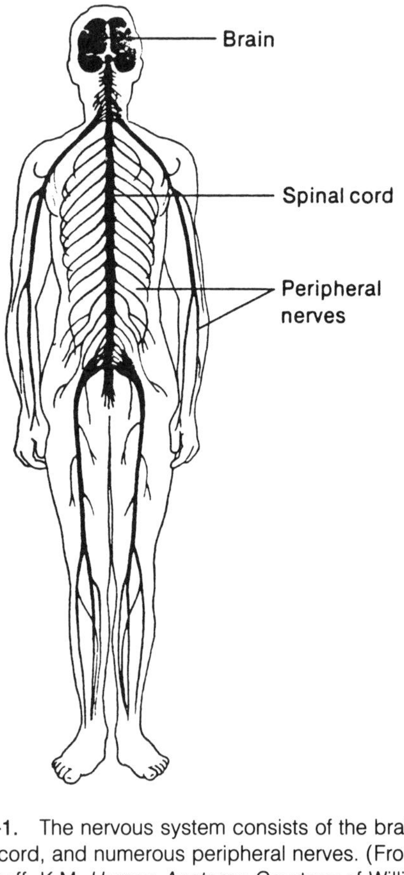

Fig. 2–1. The nervous system consists of the brain, the spinal cord, and numerous peripheral nerves. (From Van De Graaff, K.M. *Human Anatomy.* Courtesy of William C. Brown, 1984.)

ORGANIZATION OF THE NERVOUS SYSTEM

The nervous system is critical to the study of exercise physiology. Without it no activity can take place. It is within the central nervous system that thousands of bits of information from various receptor organs are integrated with whatever movement pattern or physical response of the body is desired.

Anatomically, the nervous system consists of the brain, spinal cord, and peripheral nerves (Fig. 2–1) and is sometimes divided into the central nervous system (CNS) and the peripheral nervous system (PNS). The CNS is made up of the brain and spinal cord, and the PNS includes all the other nerve tissues in the voluntary system.

The nervous system can also be divided into two divisions: *sensory and motor.* The sensory division processes information from the various sensory receptors of the body and either reacts immediately or stores the information for use in determining the body's reaction to some future stimulus. Information from receptors in the deep structures of the body, from the surface of the body, or from visual and auditory input enters the nervous system through the spinal nerves and is conducted to virtually every level of the CNS (Fig. 2–2A).

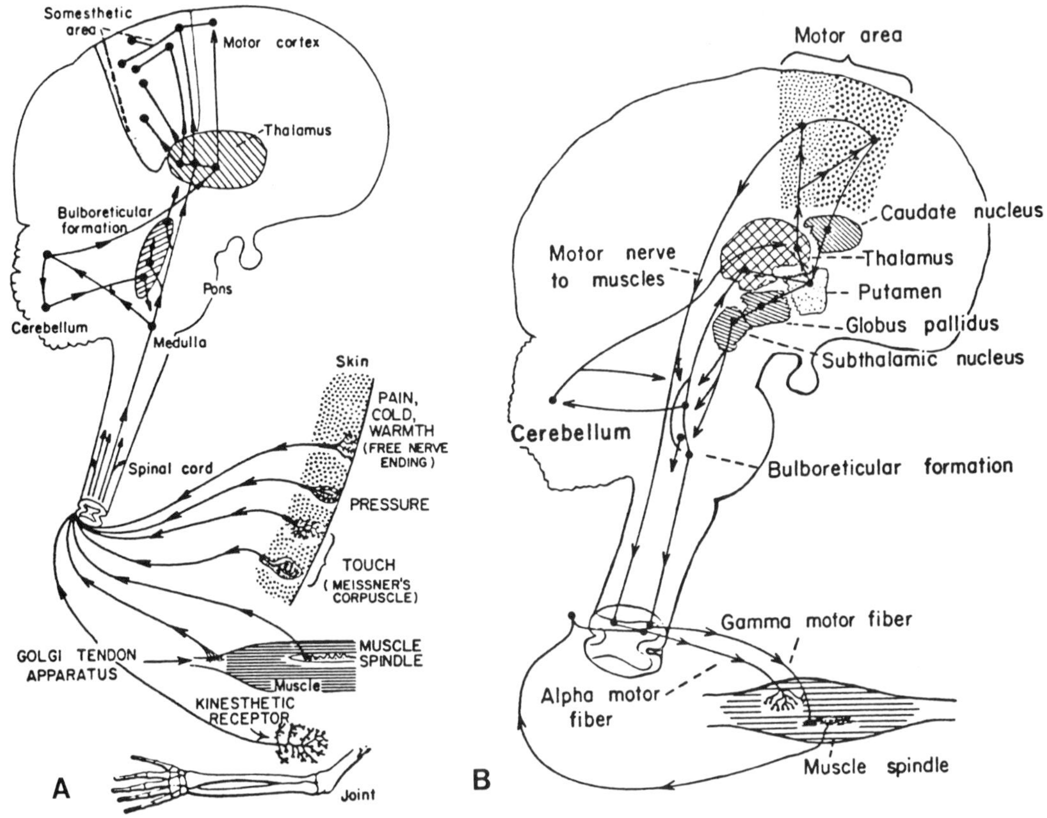

Fig. 2–2. *A and B.* The somatic (sensory) and motor axes of the nervous system. (From Guyton, A.C. *Human Physiology and Mechanism of Disease,* 4th Ed. Courtesy of W.B. Saunders Co., 1987.)

The motor division is responsible for controlling skeletal muscle contractions, and does this from several different levels of the CNS—the lower regions are usually more concerned with autonomic, reflex responses of the body to sensory stimuli and the higher regions with the more deliberate movements related to conscious control such as learning skills and performing new tasks. Figure 2–2B shows the complexity of the stimuli traveling to muscles from the motor axis in the CNS.

LEVELS OF NERVOUS SYSTEM FUNCTIONS

It is postulated that the nervous system inherited specific characteristics from early stages of evolutionary development so that the spinal cord, midbrain, and higher centers all serve widely different functions.

Spinal Cord Functions

Most spinal cord functions are reflex in nature and occur almost instantaneously in response to sensory signals. Responses usually occur at the same segment of the cord at which the sensory signal enters or in a nearby segment, and include such reflexes as the stretch and withdrawal reflex. If the brain is removed from animals that have spinal cords, many of these animals can still stand, make walking or running movements, scratch and empty the bladder. Obviously, many automatically controlled activities occur at the spinal level with the brain playing only a modifying role.

Midbrain

Most of the subconscious physiologic control functions such as blood pressure, respiration, feeding, salivation, certain coordinated movements of the eyes, sexual excitement, and reactions of pleasure occur in the midbrain area. These activities are often critical to the maintenance of life and operate at a subconscious level.

Higher Brain Levels

Since many of the intrinsic life support processes of the body are controlled at lower levels, it seems obvious that higher centers are important for processes such as thinking, memory, learned motor control, etc. Interestingly, more than 75% of all neuronal cell bodies are found in these higher regions and it is here that memories of past experiences and patterns of complex motor response called *engrams* are stored and can be recorded to perform the intricate movement patterns associated with athletic events.

Of course, some areas of the cerebral cortex are not concerned with sensory or motor activity, but are used for the more abstract processes we call thinking, but even these areas have direct neural contact with the lower areas of the brain to help control the subconscious actions of the body.

NEURONS

Cells in the nervous system are called *neurons.* Because of their special duties in transmitting information, their structure is unique. A typical vertebrate neuron has a *cell body* containing the nucleus and various organelles, *dendrites* which receive signals from the environment and from the end terminals of other neurons, and *axons,* which transmit signals through small terminal endings or foot processes. Neurons exhibit the properties of *excitability* and *conductivity.* When a cell is excitable, it has the ability to respond to a stimulus, and if it passes that response to another cell, it exhibits conductivity.

There are essentially three types of neurons that govern motor activity: *motor neurons, sensory neurons,* and *interneurons.*

Motor Neurons

A typical motor neuron is shown in Figure 2–3A. The cell body is located in the anterior horn of the spinal cord and the axon carries information through the terminal branches to all the muscle fibers it innervates.

Motor neurons have thousands of small synaptic knobs on the surface of their dendrites and cell bodies (see Fig. 2–8). These knobs are the terminal ends of nerve fibrils from many other neurons that are seeking to either excite or inhibit the motor neuron. The axons of motor neurons are also insulated by a special cell called a *Schwann cell* that completely encompasses the axon in a thick *myelin sheath.* The sheath is interrupted at regular intervals so that the nervous impulse can depolarize the membrane of the axon at points called *nodes of Ranvier.* Conduction down myelinated fibers is called *saltatory conduction* and is advantageous because the speed of conduction is increased dramatically with a concomitant decrease in the energy cost (Fig. 2–3B).

Sensory Neurons

These neurons pass information to the CNS from the periphery of the body. Information passes up the dendrite (which is the longest part in sensory neurons) to the cell body, located in the dorsal root ganglion, and into the spinal cord (Fig. 2–3C). Once in the spinal cord, information may be passed up the cord to higher centers, or be passed directly to a motor neuron to cause a reflex contraction.

Interneurons

All sensory and motor nerve cells in the body can be classified functionally as *excitatory* neurons. However, in the gray matter of the spinal cord, there are short neurons, called *interneurons,* which can either be excitatory or inhibitory. When excited, some of these neurons secrete a chemical that excites other nerve cells by depolarizing their membranes. Others inhibit nerve cell transmission by hyperpolarizing cell membranes. The importance of an interneuron system which can inhibit as well as excite is that information from other areas can be modified to suit the needs of the organism, by either passing it along the pathways or by stopping it from being transmitted. For example, the inhibition or blocking of nerve impulses to antagonistic muscles is of utmost importance in the efficiency and speed of any movement.

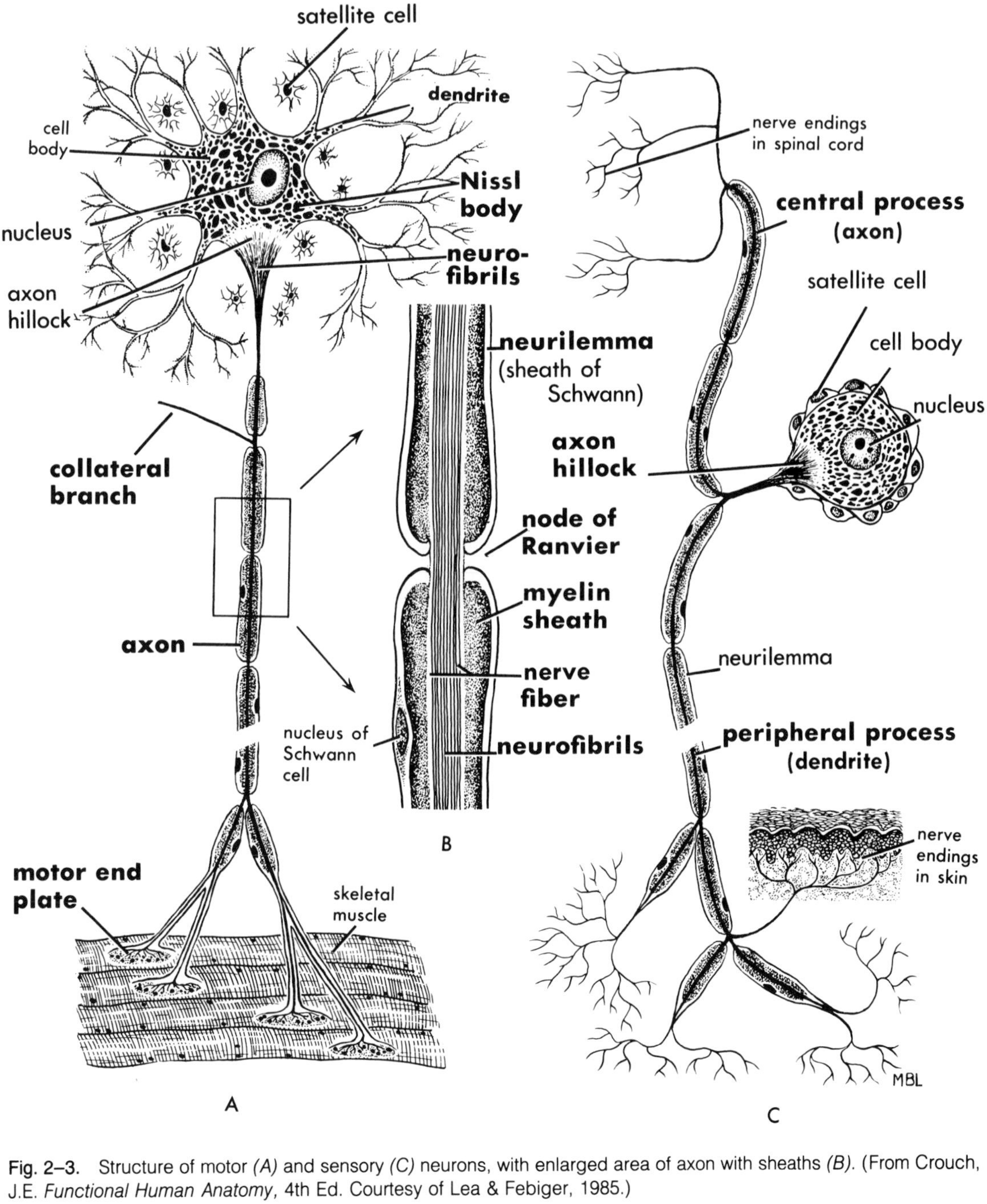

Fig. 2–3. Structure of motor *(A)* and sensory *(C)* neurons, with enlarged area of axon with sheaths *(B)*. (From Crouch, J.E. *Functional Human Anatomy,* 4th Ed. Courtesy of Lea & Febiger, 1985.)

SPINAL NERVES

Millions of motor neuron axons and sensory neuron dendrites are packaged together to form the *spinal nerves.* These nerve bundles are held together by a series of connective tissues called the endoneurium, perineurium, and epineurium (*neurium* means nerve). These connective tissues resemble the connective tissues that surround and hold muscle fibers together. There is a tendency to confuse the term "nerve" with "neuron" or "nerve fiber." Remember, neurons are the basic functional units of the nervous system and include axon cell bodies (soma) and dendrites. Nerves are groups of neurons or nerve fibers which function much like a cross-country telephone cable, with messages traveling both ways in the communication process (Fig. 2–4).

ESTABLISHING A MEMBRANE POTENTIAL

All cells have cell membranes which act as barriers, selecting what substances enter and exit the cell. Cell membranes are composed of a lipid matrix and globular proteins of various sizes which "float" in the lipid bilayer much as a buoy floats in the sea (Fig. 2–5).

Cell membranes have electrical charges or potentials across them. This means that the sum of the electric charges on the chemicals inside the cell is different from the sum of the charges on the chemicals outside the cell. The cell membranes of nerve and muscle cells are also able to "depolarize" and "repolarize" by changing the concentrations of charged particles inside and outside the cell, and are thus able to transmit electrical impulses which are later translated into messages and bodily movements. This property is known as "excitability."

There are two properties of nerve cell membranes, that allow them to be excitable. They are (1) the sodium-potassium (Na^+-K^+) pump, and (2) selective permeability of the cell membrane. These two properties will be examined in more detail below.

1. *The Na^+-K^+ pump.* The Na^+-K^+ pump is an active transport mechanism which pumps Na^+ ions out of the cell and K^+ ions in. Active transport means that the ion being pumped moves against a concentration gradient (as opposed to diffusion, where the ion goes with the gradient). It also means that the process requires energy. Since both ions pumped are positive, pumping a Na^+ in and a K^+ out would not by itself, create a membrane potential.

2. *Selective permeability of the cell membrane.* The key to creating a membrane potential is that the membrane is about 50 times more permeable to K^+ than Na^+. This means that K^+ can move back out of the membrane with relative ease, but Na^+ cannot get back in eas-

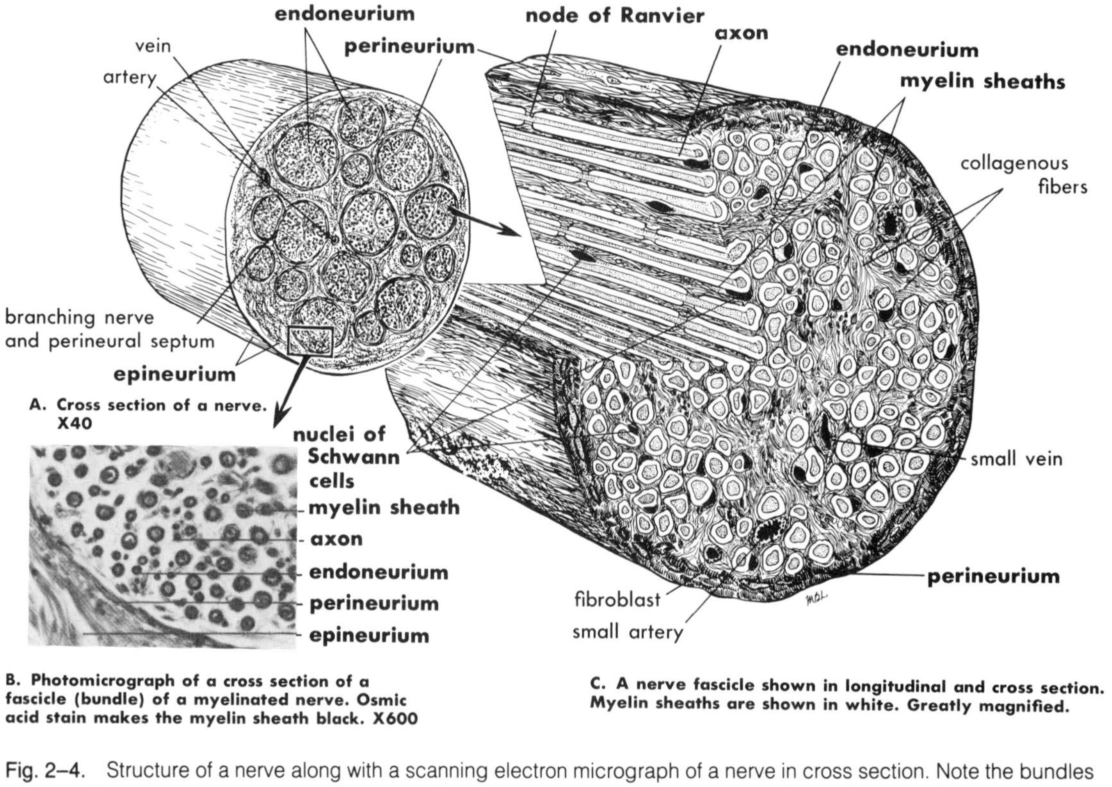

Fig. 2–4. Structure of a nerve along with a scanning electron micrograph of a nerve in cross section. Note the bundles of nerve fibers. (From Crouch, J.E. *Functional Human Anatomy*, 4th Ed. Courtesy of Lea & Febiger, 1985.)

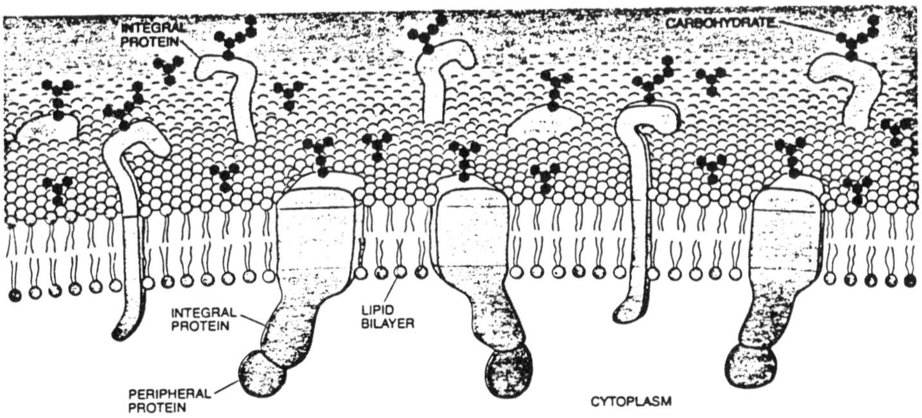

Fig. 2–5. Cell membrane is composed mainly of a lipid bilayer with large numbers of integral and peripheral protein molecules floating in the bilayer. (From Guyton, A.C. *Human Physiology and Mechanism of Disease,* 4th Ed. Courtesy of W.B. Saunders Co., 1987.)

ily. As the membranes pump Na^+ and K^+, two factors begin to play a role; the concentration gradient and the electro-chemical gradient. Since the pump increases the concentration of K^+ inside the cell, more of the K^+ molecules go back outside, even though the outside has a positive charge. The membrane *resting potential* occurs when all of the ions involved reach a homeostatic condition with the pump working.

Intracellular proteins (with a negative charge) are unable to leave the cell by any means, and Cl^- ions leave the cell only by diffusion. Thus, their movement across the cell membrane is governed solely by its concentration gradient.

With the above players and rules in mind, it is a simple matter to envision how a membrane potential is set-up. It happens as follows: the Na^+ and K^+ pump begins to work, sending Na^+ ions out of the cell and K^+ ions into the cell. This creates increasing concentrations of each ion on one side of the membrane. Since the membrane is much more permeable to K^+, it begins to move back out of the cell because of the concentration gradient which makes the outside more positive than the inside. This repels the Cl^- ion and causes it to exit the cell by diffusion. Its exodus is initially quite rapid, but slows as its concentration outside the cell increases. The Na^+-K^+ pump continues to pump, but of course K^+ will be able to leave the cell by diffusion with relative ease. The build-up of Cl^- ions outside the cell draws the K^+ out of the cell, but the slowed exodus of the Cl^- ions, together with the increasing concentration of K^+ ions outside the cell moderates their diffusion. In this fashion, the charges eventually reach and maintain equilibrium across the cell membrane, and the charge difference thus arrives at what is called the net membrane potential (Fig. 2–6).

The resting membrane potential for mammalian nerve and muscle cells is between −70 and −100 mV. As long as the membrane is undisturbed, the pump will continue to keep this small charge at the expense of ATP produced in nearby mitochondria.

Nernst Equation. The magnitude of the membrane potential can be determined using the Nernst equation:

$$\text{EMF (in millivolts)} = -61 \log \frac{[\text{Conc. Inside}]}{[\text{Conc. Outside}]}$$

This formula can be used to explain how a concentration of a diffusible ion that is greater on one side of the membrane than the other can cause a membrane potential. For potassium (K^+), the concentration inside the cell is about 140 mEq/l and outside the cell is about 4 mEq/l. Therefore:

$$\begin{aligned} \text{EMF} &= -61 \log \frac{[140 \text{ mEq/l}]}{[4 \text{ mEq/l}]} \\ &= -61 \log 35 \\ &= -91 \text{ mV} \end{aligned}$$

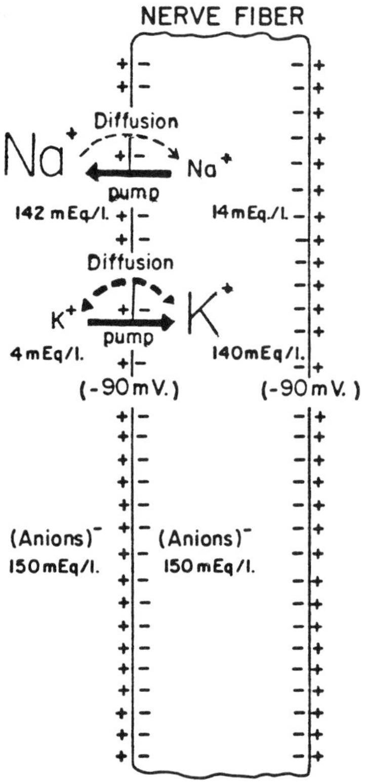

Fig. 2–6. Establishment of a membrane potential in the normal resting nerve fiber is created by developing a concentration gradient of Na^+ and K^+ ions on opposing sides of the membrane. The dashed arrows represent diffusion, and the solid arrows represent active transport. (From Guyton, A.C. *Human Physiology and Mechanism of Disease*, 4th Ed. Courtesy of W.B. Saunders Co., 1987.)

This calculated value is very near the normal resting potential of 60 to 100 mV. The actual negative potential inside the cell is probably 20 mV less than that calculated (about −70 mV) because of the K^+ pump which actually works against the natural outward movement of K^+. The calculated Nernst potential for Na^+ is:

$$\text{EMF} = -61 \log \frac{[14 \text{ mEq/l}]}{[140 \text{ mEq/l}]}$$

$$= +61 \text{ mV}$$

This value is not only positive, but very near the actual reverse potential experienced by the membrane when it is depolarized. During depolarization, the membrane is about 30 times as permeable to Na^+ as it is to K^+ and the Nernst equation is based on the results of a *diffusible ion* with different concentrations on each side of the membrane.

EXCITATION—INHIBITION

A membrane with a *resting membrane potential* is now ready to transmit nerve impulses, which is how information is transmitted from one area of the nervous system to another. This transmission occurs because of the *action or spike potential* (Fig. 2–7).

The action potential is most often elicited by the release of a chemical transmitter substance from a synapse, but can be caused by anything that increases the membranes permeability to Na^+ (see transmitter substances, p 35). When the transmitter chemical is secreted onto the membrane, Na^+ begins to leak into the cell and the membrane potential moves toward *threshold.* The threshold is that point at which the membrane will proceed to depolarize and carry an impulse.

Once threshold is reached, however, complete depolarization occurs. It is in this sense that depolarization is considered an "all-or-none" process. Sodium and potassium probably diffuse through specific pores or channels that are guarded by gates that can open or close. At rest the Na^+ gate is quite closed, but the K^+ channel is partially open. During depolarization, the Na^+ gate opens wide and the permeability increases about 5000-fold for just an instant. This results in a rapid movement of Na^+ that causes the "spike" (depolarization) seen in Figure 2–7. Once depolarized, the Na^+ channels close, the K^+ channels open, and K^+ flows rapidly back out of the cell causing the membrane to repolarize. The portion of the spike above the 0 volt line is sometimes called the *reverse potential.*

Luckily, the quantity of ions involved in the depolarization-repolarization process is extremely slight, allowing the process to be repeated many times, even if too little time is allowed for the Na^+-K^+ pump to reestablish normal values. Even poisoning the pump will have little effect on the membranes ability to react until literally thousands of signals have been sent.

In muscle cells, the action potential triggers the contraction mechanisms causing muscle fibers to contract. In nerve cells, the action

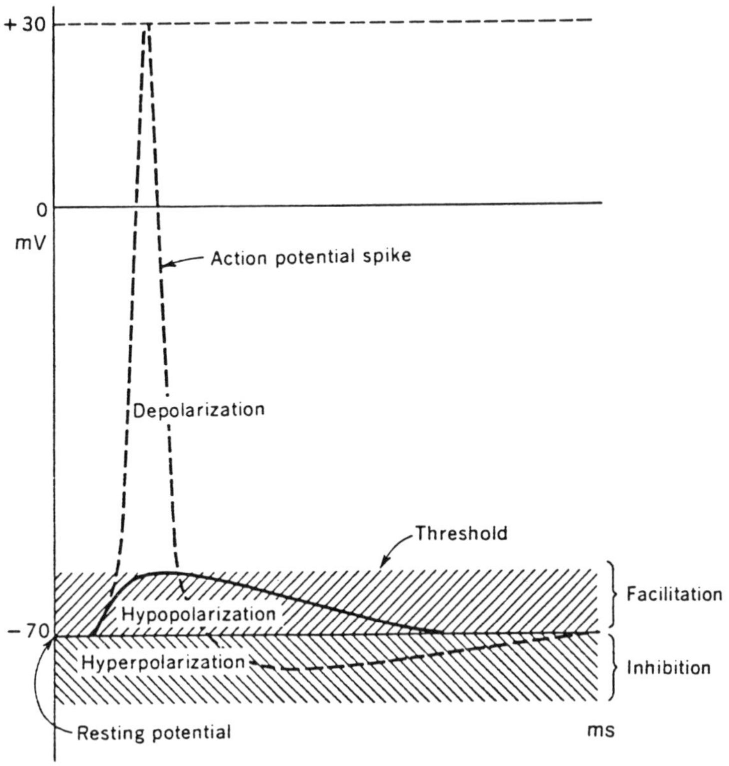

Fig. 2–7. Summary of the terminology used to describe electrical activity in a nerve cell under various conditions. (From Astrand, P.O., and Rodahl, K. *Textbook of Work Physiology. Physiological Basis of Exercises,* 2nd Ed. Courtesy of McGraw Hill, 1986.)

potential causes a propagation impulse to travel down the nerve cell transmitting information to other body parts. Apparently, the action potential at a particular point along the membrane causes an increased permeability to sodium in adjacent sections of the membrane, and the action potential spreads in all directions like circles in water caused by a thrown rock. This transmission of the depolarization process along a nerve or muscle fiber is called an impulse. This "wave" of depolarization over the entire membrane of the axon is relatively slow and quite costly in metabolic terms because the entire membrane must be restored by the Na^+-K^+ pump. Conduction of a myelinated axon (saltatory conduction) is less costly and much more rapid (up to 120 meters/sec), because only the bare areas of the axon need to undergo depolarization and subsequent restoration by the Na^+-K^+ pumps.

Signals that are not large enough to open the Na^+ gates (i.e., do not cause the membrane to reach threshold), are said to be *subliminal.* However, these stimuli do *facilitate* the membrane, causing it to move toward the threshold or firing point. Such a subthreshold stimulus can also be called an *excitatory postsynaptic potential* or *EPSP.* Within a few milliseconds of the arrival of an EPSP, the Na^+-K^+ pump will restore the membrane potential to its normal level, and another EPSP will merely repeat the local *hypopolarization.* If a new stimulus arrives before the effects of the first subliminal stimulus are restored, the two will be additive and the two or maybe a 3rd or 4th stimulus will depolarize the membrane to threshold, and it will fire. The fact that a series of subliminal signals received by the membrane in rapid succession will cause the membrane to reach threshold is referred to as *temporal summation.* If several nerve endings close to each other release EPSPs (or facilitating signals) at the same time, the membrane may also fire due to *spatial summation.*

In any case, if the sum of the signals is

enough to elicit an action potential, the magnitude of this spike is independent of the strength of the signal and is "all-or-none"—that is, the membrane either fires (if it reaches threshold) or it does not.

During the spike potential, the nerve is in a *refractory period* and cannot be stimulated until it becomes fairly negative again. Of course, this limits how rapidly a neuron can be fired, but large myelinated neurons can be fired about 1000 times per second.

Some chemical transmitters actually open the K^+ gates wider and allow greater diffusion of K^+ out of the cell (and Cl^- into the cell). This *hyperpolarizes* the membrane and causes the resting membrane potential to be *farther* from the threshold. A stimulus that carries this action is an *inhibitory postsynaptic potential* (IPSP). *With IPSP,* an excitatory stimulus that would normally fire the neuron may be now too small to reach threshold. This is referred to as *inhibition* of transmission. Inhibition occurs only in the spinal cord and only as the result of small connective spinal neurons called *interneurons.* All transmission pathway neurons (including peripheral afferent and efferent neurons) are excitatory. So, too, are many interneurons.

NEURAL JUNCTIONS (SYNAPSES)

The nervous system is made up of millions of separate neurons that must transfer information to other neurons for proper function to occur. Each of these neurons transfers information to other neurons by way of a neural junction called a *synapse.* A motor neuron may have thousands of synapses on its soma and dendrites (mostly on the dendrites) with the terminal ends of neurons from many different areas. Usually not more than a few are from any one neuron. Many of these synapses are *excitatory* and secrete chemicals that open the Na^+ gates; others are *inhibitory* and secrete chemicals that open K^+ and Cl^- gates. Other neurons throughout the nervous system may look different from a motor neuron in terms of size, length of the axon, and the number of synaptic knobs or endings attached to their dendrites, but all receive information from many other sources through the synapses or nerve junctions that impinge upon them. Most synapses resemble small oval knobs that are separated from their attachment site by a *synaptic cleft* (Fig. 2–8).

Each synaptic knob contains *synaptic vesicles* filled with chemical transmitters, and mitochondria to provide energy for the synthesis of these transmitter substances. The amount of stored transmitter substance is small and must be rapidly synthesized or transmission would last only a short time.

Calcium appears to play a role in the release of the transmitter substance, since the number of vesicles which release their chemical is decreased when the quantity of extracellular Ca^{++} is reduced. It has been postulated that an action potential on the membrane near the synapse causes a small amount of Ca^{++} to move into the knob, attracting the vesicles to the membrane and causing them to release their transmitter substance. New chemicals are probably produced in the cytoplasm of the synaptic knob and transported into the vesicles to be stored until needed. The membrane of the *postsynaptic* neuron (onto which the transmitter substance is released) has specific receptor molecules (probably proteins) that bind the transmitter substance and respond by changing their shape or activity so that the desired activity (excitatory or inhibition) occurs in the cell. Interestingly, the same transmitter substance may cause either excitation or inhibition depending upon the nature of the receptor in the postsynaptic membrane. For instance, norepinephrine causes inhibition in some CNS sites, but is excitatory at most other neural junctions. There is also a difference in the response time of different transmitter substances, some may affect the neuron for only a few milliseconds and others for as long as 200 to 300 msec.

Transmitter substances can also affect the rate of firing of neurons or the neuron's sensitivity to other transmitter substances (modulators). In any case, it is clear that motor activity is influenced by the *sum* of all the neuronal activity which occurs in the system and reacts for the best good of the organism which would not be possible without a complex system of synapses between all of the neurons in the system.

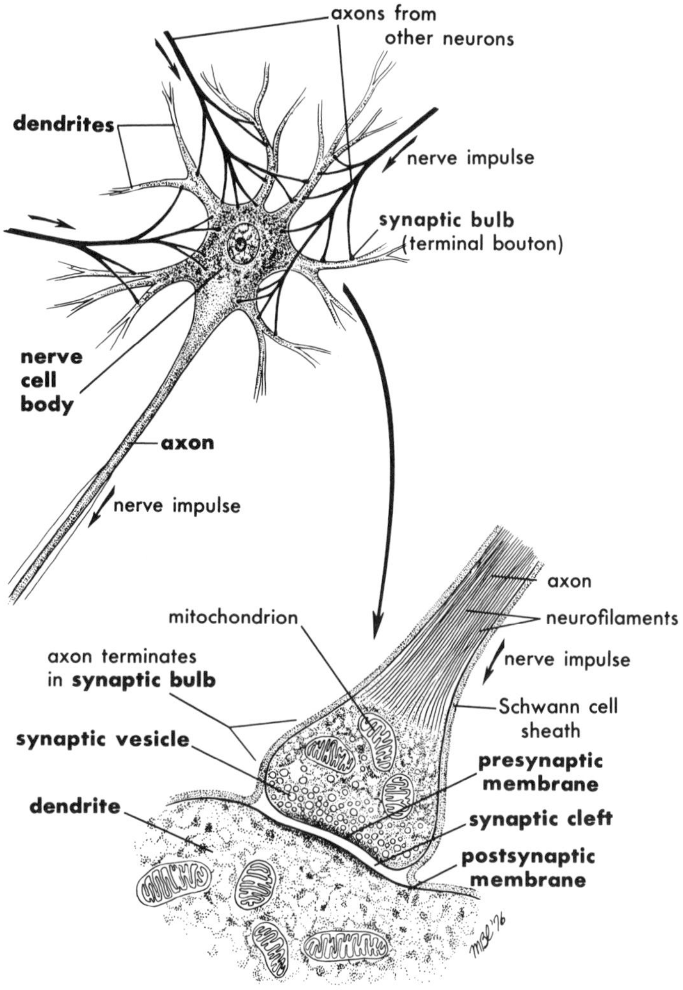

Fig. 2–8. The synapse is the relay point where information is conveyed by chemical transmission from neuron to neuron. Note both the synaptic vesicles filled with a chemical transmitter substance and the mitochondria, which provide energy for the synthesis of the transmitter. Separating the two membranes is a small gap or synaptic cleft. (From Crouch, J.E. *Functional Human Anatomy,* 4th Ed. Courtesy of Lea & Febiger, 1985.)

PROCESSING INFORMATION

The stimulation of a single excitatory synaptic knob almost never stimulates a postsynaptic neuron. Instead, a large number of knobs must fire on the same neuron simultaneously, (spatial summation) or a few knobs must fire in rapid succession (temporal summation) to bring the membrane to threshold. This system maximizes the input potential from many different neurons for action to occur. The nervous system is made up of literally hundreds of separate *neuronal pools* in order to process information effectively. Figure 2–9A shows one way these pools may be organized to accomplish proper information processing. Note that the input fibers (afferent) on the cleft divide many times to reach output fibers (efferent) over a large area of the pool. Most of the input fibers are clustered near the center of the field, with fewer neurons by the outer edges. For example, if depolarization (threshold) were to occur when six synaptic knobs discharged a signal down fiber (1) it would always cause fiber (a) to fire, but would not fire fibers (b) and (c). In the same way, fiber (2) will always fire fiber (d) but not fibers (b) and (c). If both (1) and (2) fire simultaneously, (a) and (d) will be depolarized as usual, as will fiber (c). Fiber (b) will

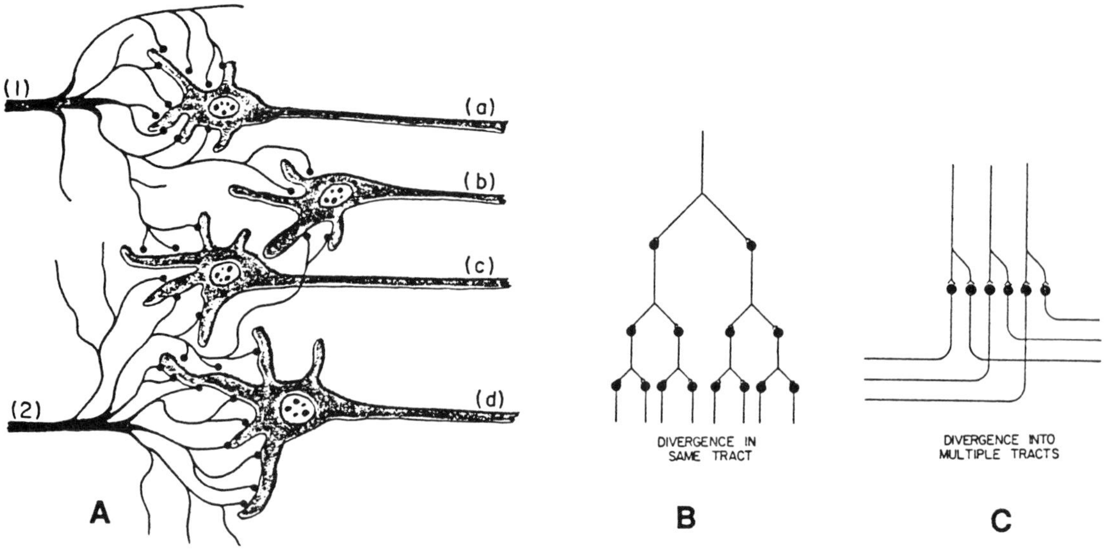

Fig. 2–9. *A–C.* Illustration of the basic arrangement of a neuronal pool where the neural pathways can "diverge" to amplify a signal, or diverge into several tracts to transmit the signal to other areas of the nervous system. (From Guyton, A.C. *Human Physiology and Mechanism of Disease,* 4th Ed. Courtesy of W.B. Saunders Co., 1987.)

be facilitated, and could be fired more easily by synaptic knobs from another neuron. One of the fibers in the pool could be inhibitory and when fired, could cause inhibition of a signal at its termination.

The term *convergence* refers to the control of a single neuron by fibers from another single neuron or by fibers of several different neurons. For instance, a motor neuron receives direct signals from peripheral sensory nerves entering the cord, from small interneurons that are stimulated by peripheral receptors, and by spinal fibers passing from one segment of the cord to another. Convergence thus allows summation (and inhibition) from many different sources and helps the CNS sort through the various information and pass on only that which matters.

Divergence is the process of stimulating multiple output fibers from a single input fiber. This system tends to amplify a signal through various levels (Fig. 2–9B). For instance, a single pyramidal cell in the motor cortex can stimulate several hundred interneurons, which in turn can stimulate a like number of motor neurons, which may result in the contraction of 4 to 5 times as many muscle fibers. Divergence can also occur into several different neuron pools (Fig. 2–9C). For example, sensory information traveling up the spinal cord diverges into the cerebellum, passing through the lower regions of the brain and into the cerebral cortex. Each of these areas may also pass information along to other tracts.

The nervous system can do more than just pass information along using convergent or divergent pathways. It is also capable of prolonging a signal using several different mechanisms. First, the postsynaptic membrane potential of a motor neuron lasts about 15 msec. As long as this lasts, it can excite the neuron extending this discharge to the motor unit for that entire period. *After discharge* circuits are also available. Some use a complex series of neurons to delay signals until the more directly routed ones have fired so that signals continue to reach the output neurons for a period of time after the initial discharge.

KNOWN TRANSMITTER SUBSTANCES

There are many known transmitter substances throughout the body, each with its own actions (excitation or inhibition) and duration of stimulation. Some substances have different effects in different areas depending on the type of receptor involved. The duration of response also varies widely depending on location and transmitter substance. The most common substances are listed below:

Acetylcholine (Ach). Ach is one of the well-studied transmitter substances. It is usually excitatory. However, in the parasympathetic system it inhibits the heart, slowing rate and decreasing force of contraction. Nerve membrane receptors that are sensitive to acetylcholine are referred to as cholinergic or parasympathetic receptors.

Norepinephrine (Norepi). One of the "fight-or-flight" chemicals, norepinephrine causes an increased readiness for action when secreted by the sympathetic nervous system. Norepinephrine is also a transmitter in some of the areas of the brain.

Epinephrine (Epi). The primary source of Epi in the body is the adrenal gland. However, certain neurons secrete epinephrine, but only in small amounts. In general, the action of Epi parallels that of norepinephrine.

Dopamine. Most often found at synapses in the brain and spinal cord—usually acts as an inhibitor. Also acts as a precursor of Epi and Norepi.

Gamma Aminobutyric Acid (GABA). Secreted by nerve endings in many areas of the brain and spinal cord. It is believed to always be inhibitory.

Serotonin. Secreted by nuclei that originate in the brain stem and project into many areas of the CNS. Serotonin acts as an inhibitor of pain pathways in the spinal cord, and is involved with mood changes and sleep.

Glutamic Acid. Probably secreted by synapses in at least some of the sensory pathways. Always excitatory.

MYONEURAL JUNCTIONS

The junction between the endings of motor neurons and the muscle fibers they innervate is quite similar to the synapse. Each motor neuron branches many times and stimulates from several to hundreds of muscle fibers to form its motor unit.

However, there is usually only one junction per muscle fiber, as opposed to the thousands of synapses on the motor neuron. Note the *subneural clefts* (or folds) under the synaptic knob. These folds greatly increase the area upon which the transmitter substance can act. Numerous mitochondria produce energy for the production of the transmitter substance *acetylcholine (Ach)* which excites the muscle fiber. No inhibitory signals are formed at this level. When a motor neuron fires, all of the muscle fibers it innervates contract. A chemical called *cholinesterase* is also found on the subneural clefts. Cholinesterase destroys the effect of Ach within a very short time, preventing constant excitation (Fig. 2–10).

SENSORY RECEPTORS

Muscle Spindle

Input to the CNS comes from many different sensory regions that detect such stimuli as touch, sound, light, cold, stretch, and body position. In terms of activity, one of the most important sensory organs is the *stretch receptor* or *muscle spindle.*

Muscle spindles are located at regular intervals in the muscle bed to help the body detect changes in muscle fiber length and their rate of change. Figure 2–11 shows the organization of the muscle spindle. Each spindle contains from 3 to 10 small *intrafusal* fibers which are diffeent from regular muscle fibers in that the *central* region has few or no actin and myosin filaments and is therefore unable to contract. The ends of the fibers do contract and are innervated by a neuron that is somewhat smaller than the regular motor neurons that form motor units. These smaller neurons are called "gamma" motor neurons and they connect directly into the contractile portion of the small intrafusal fibers of the muscle spindle. The central portion of the intrafusal muscle fibers (noncontractile) are surrounded by sensory neurons called *primary endings* (sometimes referred to as annulospiral endings) and *secondary endings* (sometimes called flowerspray endings).

Both endings are stimulated by stretching the central region of the intrafusal fibers, and the number of impulses increases directly in proportion to the degree of stretch. The primary endings exhibit a strong *dynamic* response to any change in length of the spindle. A rapid increase in length causes a large increase in the number of impulses, but only while the length is actually increasing. On the

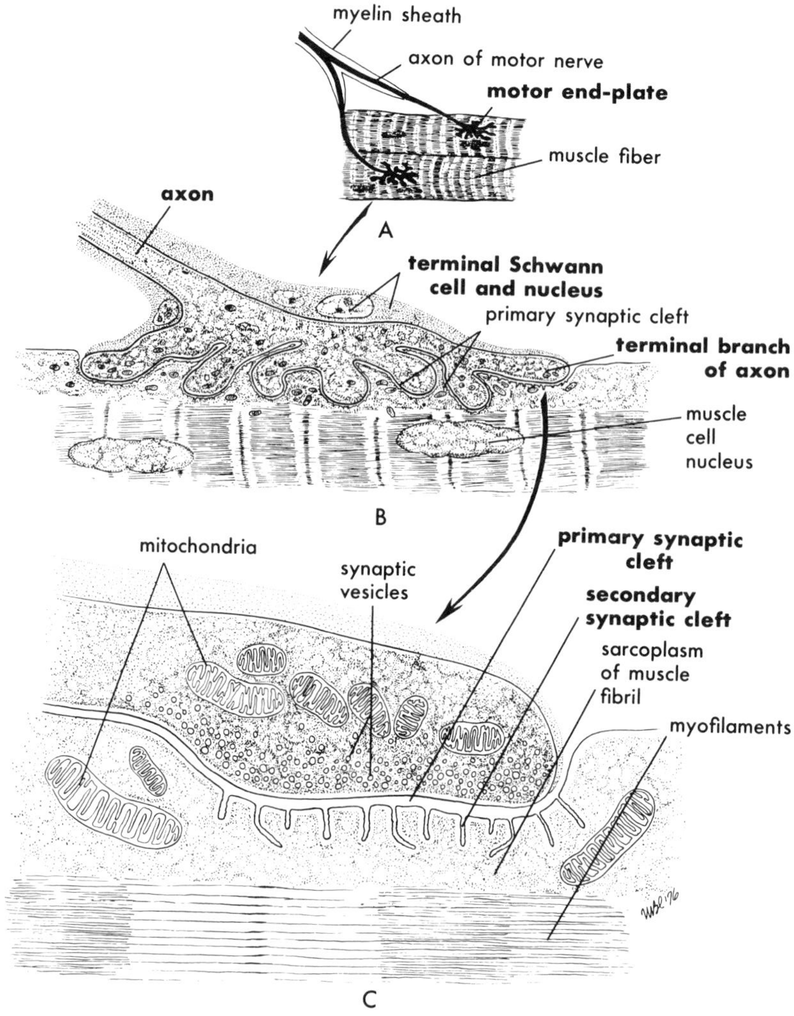

Fig. 2–10. *A.* Myoneural junction or motor end-plate. *B.* One motor end-plate greatly enlarged. *C.* One terminal branch of an axon greatly enlarged to show in detail the structures involved in activating a muscle. (From Crouch, J.E. *Functional Human Anatomy*, 4th Ed. Courtesy of Lea & Febiger, 1985.)

other hand, the secondary endings fire as long as stretch is maintained. This is called the *static response* of the spindle.

The muscle spindle sends its signal *directly* to the regular motor neurons near the spindle through a monosynaptic reflex arc. In effect, the muscle spindle acts to compare the length of the intrafusal fibers (in the muscle spindle) to the extrafusal fibers (the regular muscle), helping maintain the status quo of muscle length. The simple knee-jerk reflex is an example of the muscle spindle in action. Hitting the tendon stretches the spindle which sends a signal to contract the muscles around the stretched spindle to bring it back to its prestretched size (Fig. 2–12).

The spindle also helps to increase contractile force when a heavy load is added, and to decrease force if the load is removed (load reflex). It also uses a process called signal averaging to dampen uneven signals from the CNS, ensuring smooth movement of body parts.

The *gamma efferent system* signals to the contractile part of the intrafusal fibers are also important to the contractile process in muscle. At least 30% of all motor neurons are gamma neurons (neurons to muscle spindles). When signals are sent to muscles through the alpha motor neurons, the gamma system is also stimulated, so that intrafusal fibers contract and shorten the spindles at the same time as

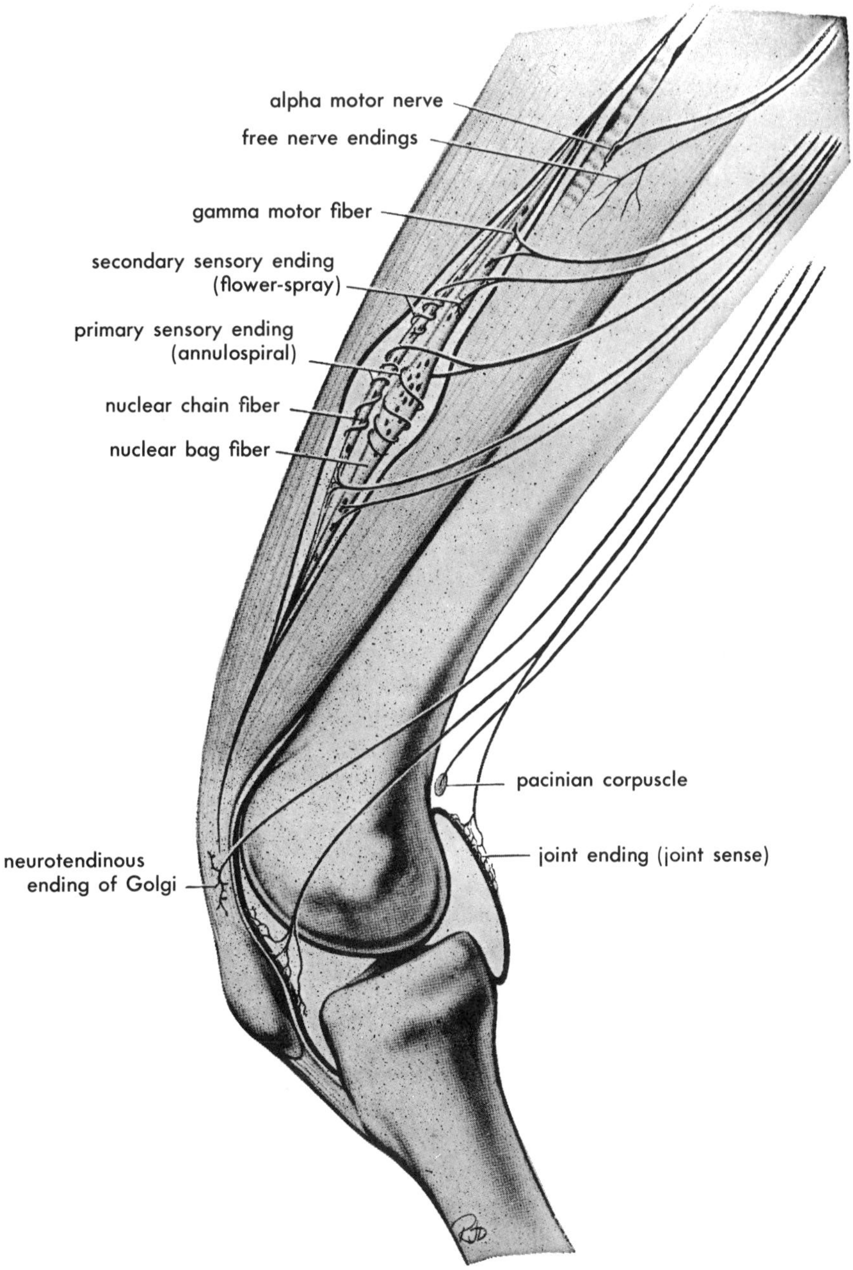

Fig. 2–11. Nerve endings in voluntary muscles, tendons, and joints. The muscle spindle is disproportionately large and shows only two intrafusal fibers: one nucleus bag (found in slow fiber types) and one nuclear chain (found in fast fiber types). (From Nobach, C.R., and Demarest, R. *The Human Nervous System: Basic Principles of Neurobiology*, 3rd Ed. Courtesy of McGraw-Hill, 1985.)

the muscle shortens. This keeps the muscle spindles from opposing muscle contraction. This also enables the spindle to maintain the proper length for maximal efficiency regardless of muscle length. Gamma neurons can also be used to initiate movement using gamma loop feedback control. This is used to make fine, carefully controlled movements to predetermined positions.

Golgi Tendon Organs

Golgi tendon organs help protect tendons from injury by detecting tension in the tendons. There are usually about 10 to 15 muscle fibers connected in series to each golgi tendon organ, and the signals from the tendon organs are passed to the spinal cord where they excite *inhibitory* interneurons. These, in turn,

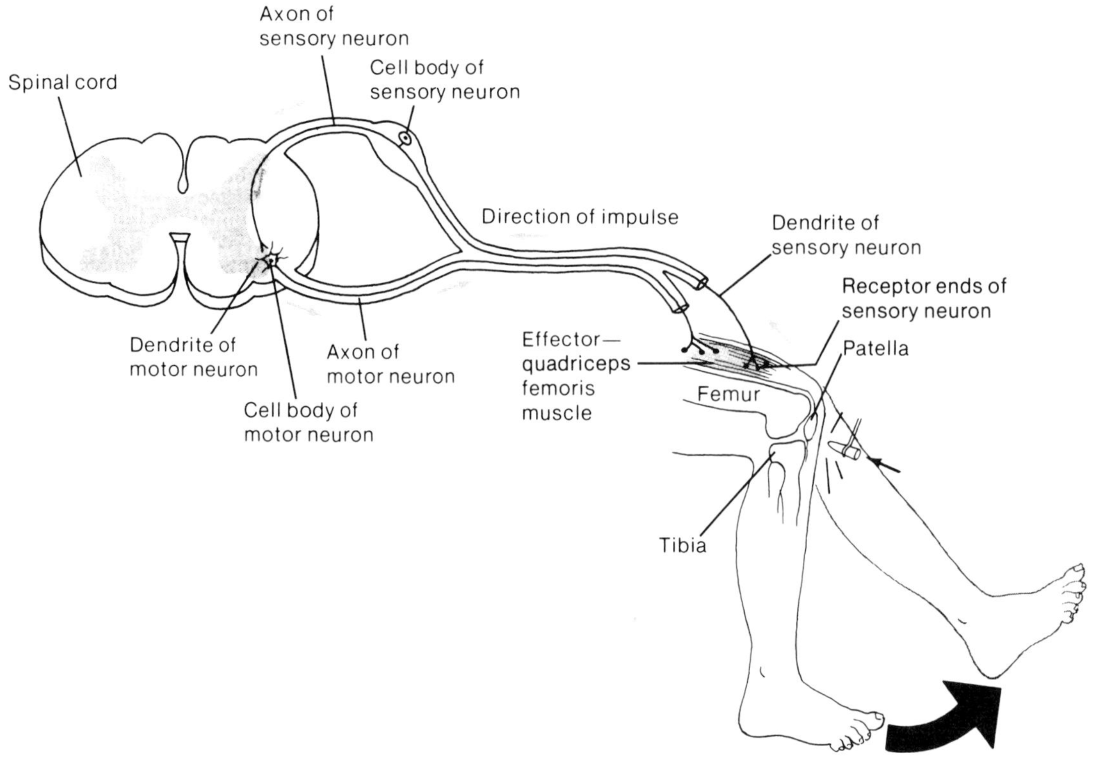

Fig. 2–12. The knee-jerk reflex. (From Van De Graaff, K.M. *Human Anatomy.* Courtesy of William C. Brown, 1984.)

inhibit the alpha motor neuron to that muscle. Extremely high tension can cause a sudden relaxation of the muscle involved (the lengthening reaction). This reaction occurs to protect the muscle or the attachment from tearing (Fig. 2–11).

The muscle tendon organ can probably also operate to help control muscle tension. If tension is too high, inhibition can decrease it to a more nominal level; if too low, a lack of inhibition allows the alpha motor neuron to be more easily activated.

Pacinian Corpuscles

Pacinian corpuscles are a type of mechanoreceptor that have been carefully studied. Understanding how they function aids in understanding how the body interprets positional changes. As movement of the body part occurs, pacinian corpuscles are deformed by an overlying tendon or other structure, causing a local current flow that tells the CNS about the movement. As with many other receptors, the pacinian corpuscle adapts after a short period of time (within a few hundredths of a second). This adaptation occurs because the fluid within the distorted corpuscle redistributes itself so that pressure on the central nerve is equalized. When the pressure that caused this initial distortion is reversed, the reverse event occurs, and a new signal is generated until the fluid redistributes itself again. The central nerve will eventually accommodate, so that even continual pressure on the nerve will yield a decreasing activity level. Pacinian corpuscles are "rate" (or phase) receptors, and they, together with other receptors located in or near the joint capsules, help the nervous system stay ahead of rapid movements such as running. Obviously, pacinian corpuscles are effective in transmitting information about rapid changes in body position, but not as good at detecting changes that remain constant (Fig. 2–11).

Some receptors (so called *tonic* receptors) continue to send impulses to the brain for long periods of time. For instance, joint capsule receptors keep the body informed of joint position, and muscle spindles and golgi tendon organs allow the body to know the status of muscle contraction and load, respectively. Other tonic receptors are pain receptors, baroreceptors, chemoreceptors, and tactile receptors such as Ruggini endings and Merkel's discs (Fig. 2–13).

MOTOR CONTROL

Much of the activity of the nervous system is stimulated by sensory information coming from receptors throughout the body. This information may cause an immediate reaction at the spindle level (e.g., knee-jerk reflex), or its memory may be stored in the brain and used later in the processing of information in response to some new activity.

Voluntary control of motor activity occurs in the higher regions of the CNS and involves primarily the cerebral cortex, the basal ganglia, and the cerebellum.

The Cerebral Cortex

Most of the cranial cavity is occupied by the largest section of the brain called the cerebrum. The surface area of the cerebrum is called the cortex (cerebral cortex) and is the seat of voluntary movement. The cortex is responsible for consciousness, perception, memory (including the majorities of movement patterns), interpretation, and reasoning. A combination of these functions results in what is known as judgment. The exact response of the body to specific motor stimuli is probably based upon the success or failure of similar actions in the past. The more extensive and well-established its store of memories, the faster and more accurate will be its responses in terms of muscular actions. Children should probably be provided many opportunities for a variety of basic movement patterns before their interests become too specialized. Otherwise, overall skill development may be limited.

The two most important parts of the cerebral cortex are the *motor cortex* (or pyramidal cortex) and the *premotor cortex* (or extrapyramidal cortex). The motor cortex is located just anterior to the central sulcus (a notch or break in the cortex dividing the front from the back) (Fig. 2–14). This area gets its name from the way it functions in terms of motor control and because of the giant *Bentz* or *pyramidal* cells that originate from this area. Axons from these cells form pyramidal tracts that pass downward through the brain stem, cross to the opposite side, and descend in the *lateral corticospinal tracts*. Most of these tracts end on interneurons, many of which carry information to still other interneurons before finally exciting the motor neurons. Stimulat-

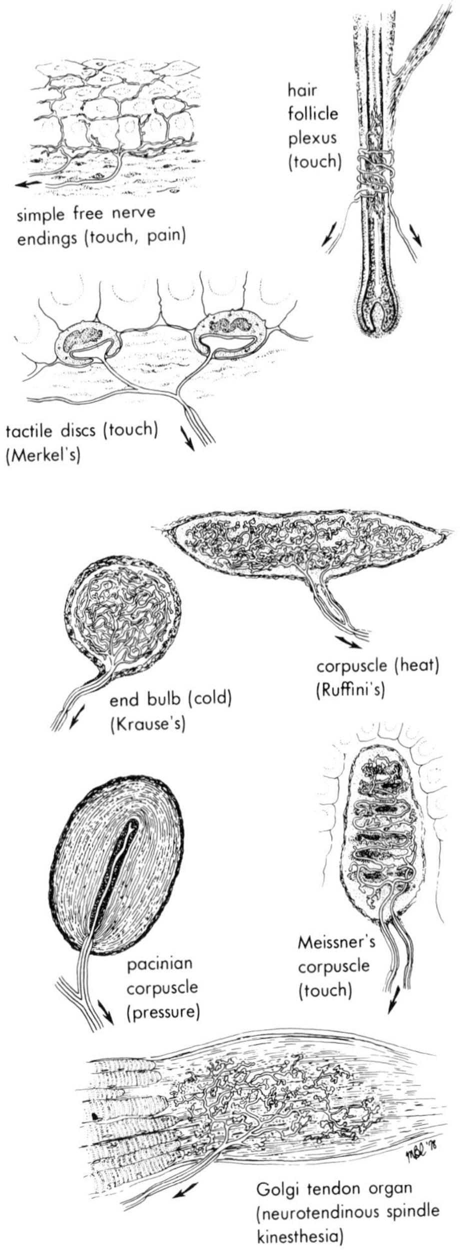

Fig. 2–13. Examples of different types of sensory receptors. (From Crouch, J.E. *Functional Human Anatomy,* 4th Ed. Courtesy of Lea & Febiger, 1985.)

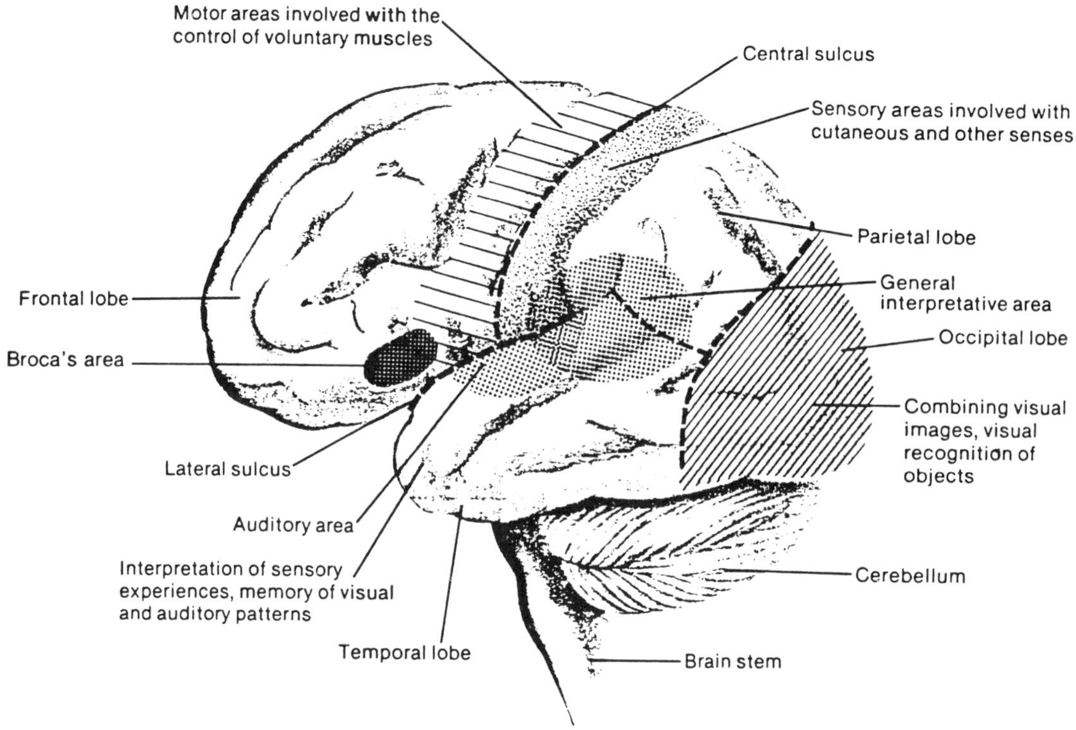

Fig. 2–14. Lobes of the left cerebral hemisphere showing both motor and sensory cortex. (From Van De Graaff, K.M. *Human Anatomy.* Courtesy of William C. Brown, 1984.)

ing neurons in certain areas of the motor cortex causes rather discrete movements in very specific muscles of the finger and thumb region. In other areas, stimulation causes small *groups* of muscles to respond. Many stroke victims (with motor cortex injury) and animals with small portions of the motor cortex removed can still perform gross postural and limb function movements, but lose fine motor control.

Electrical stimulation in the area of the cortex one to three centimeters anterior to the motor cortex often elicits complete contractions of muscle groups. This area, sometimes called the *premotor cortex* or *extrapyramidal cortex,* also has diffuse connections with other important areas of the brain. The final major pathway for transmission of extrapyramidal signals is the reticular spinal tract from which information is relayed to the motor neuron via interneurons. It is thought that the extrapyramidal area may be associated with control of coordinated movements which involve many muscles simultaneously because damage to this area often results in loss of certain coordinated skills such as speech, eye and hand movements, and some learned skills. This area is also connected to other areas of the brain known to be involved in the coordination of motor output. Interestingly, injury to this area gives rise to muscle rigidity. This is because the extrapyramidal tract transmits inhibitory signals through areas of the midbrain to modulate the activity of the pyramidal tracts. This accounts for the bent limbs so commonly seen in stroke patients.

Spinal reflexes and movement patterns are also involved along with signals from the higher centers. For instance, when the brain signals a muscle to contract, it is not necessary for it to inhibit the antagonistic muscle—it is inhibited by *reciprocal inhibition* at the spinal cord. Other cord reflex mechanisms can also be activated by the brain with very simple signals. Of course, the cord reflexes can also be inhibited so that they do not interfere with patterns of activity generated within the brain itself.

Basal Ganglia

The basal ganglia constitute the central gray matter of the cerebrum and are composed of several important neural junctions. Although the anatomy of the basal ganglia is poorly understood, its role in movement is known to be important. Numerous nerve pathways pass into this area from the extrapyramidal area and many other short neuronal connections exist among the various structures of the ganglia. This area also sends many neurons into the lower brain stem to complete the circuit from the extrapyramidal or *motor association area* and the reticulospinal tracts.

In animals, the basal ganglia are highly developed and perform essentially the same function as the motor cortex does in man. Therefore, removing the cortex removes only the fine motor functions, allowing them to walk, eat, fight, etc. In humans, injury to the cortex destroys the coordinated movement of the body, allowing a crude walk, some balance, and other subconscious movements. However, injury to the basal ganglia (particularly the caudate nuclei) almost totally paralyzes the opposite side of the body and results in muscular rigidity throughout the body.

Cerebellum

Early research involving the cerebellum was disappointing because electrical stimulation of this area failed to elicit either sensation or movement. However, removal of the cerebellum caused major movement problems. The reason for its importance is that it *monitors* movement and compares what really happens to what was *supposed* to happen and makes corrections in this system.

Intuitively, it would seem that if the cerebellum is to make corrections, it should receive input from both peripheral receptors and cerebral motor areas, and this, indeed, turns out to be the case. The cerebellum receives peripheral information from muscle spindles, golgi tendon organs, pacinian corpuscles, and other receptors in the skin and joints that tell the cerebellum the status of muscle contraction, tension on tendons, body position, and forces acting on the body surface. This information reaches the cerebellum via ventral and dorsal spinocerebellar tracts (Fig. 2–15), where it is processed and used to correct movement to coincide with the information regarding discrete movement patterns from the motor areas of the brain.

Figure 2–15 shows a schematic diagram of the pathways involved in cerebellar control of voluntary movement. Note that signals which activate muscles also activate the cerebellum. After the signals from the periphery and those from the motor cortex are compared, every signal is sent to the motor cortex to correct any deviation from normal using this complex feedback circuit. The cerebellum also "dampens" the pendulum-like movements of the limbs to keep them from overshooting. It also works to predict not only future positions of the various body parts, but also the rate of progress of the body as it relates to other objects. Monkeys with the visual portion of the cerebellum removed will actually walk into walls because they are unable to predict their approach to the wall.

Sensory Area of the Brain

Much of the activity of the nervous system is stimulated by sensory activity at various levels. The sensory area of the cortex is located just posterior to the central sulcus (Fig. 2–14). The effects of repeated motor activity are thought to cause "memory" or "sensory" engrams to be formed. This takes place primarily in the sensory and sensory association

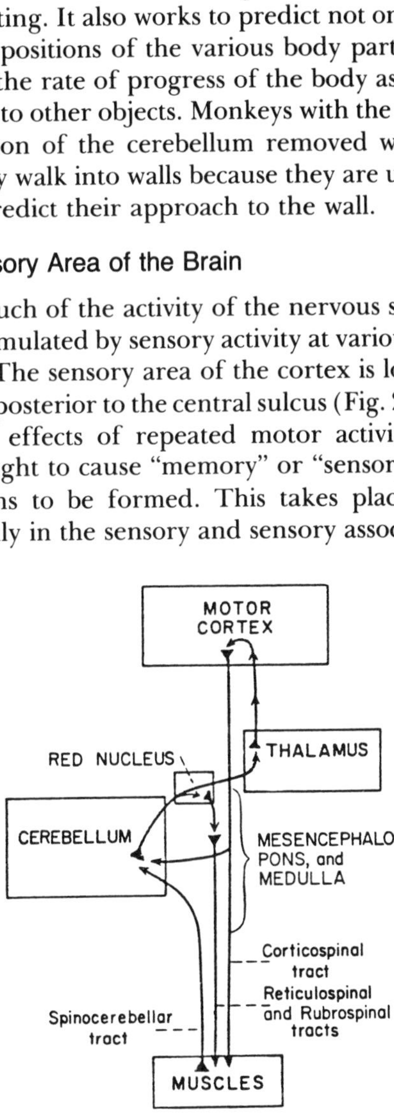

Fig. 2–15. Pathways for cerebellar control of voluntary movements. (From Guyton, A.C. *Human Physiology and Mechanism of Disease*, 4th Ed. Courtesy of W.B. Saunders Co., 1987.)

areas of the cortex. When a person wishes to perform an activity, he calls forth the engram, and the engram sets the motor pathways into action to reproduce the stored sensory pattern. Feedback pathways to modify engram activity arise from proprioreceptors and pass to the sensory areas of the cerebral cortex and travel to the motor cortex as well as through the cerebellar feedback system. In this case, the motor cortex is not the controller, but merely follows the corrected pattern from the sensory areas.

OTHER AREAS OF THE BRAIN

The interior of the cerebrum (just below the cortex) is composed mostly of white matter which links the cerebrum to all the levels of the spinal cord. This white matter (because of myelination) provides fast and often direct impulse conduction from the higher centers to the various junctions in the spinal cord. The nerve fibers composing the white matter are bundled together into *nerve tracts*. The afferent (sensory) bundles are ascending tracts and transmit sensory impulses to the sensory cortex. The efferent (motor) bundles are descending tracts which conduct impulses from the highest centers to the motor neurons as described above.

In addition to the white matter in the interior of the cerebrum, several clusters of gray matter, called nuclei, are present. Little is known about the functions of some of these clusters. However, the largest and probably the most important to motor movement is the *thalamus*. The thalamus serves as an important relay center for both motor and sensory impulses. It also has extensive connections with the cortex.

The *brain stem* is the direct connection between the brain and the spinal cord, and thus impulses pass through it in both directions. The functions of the brain stem are more directly concerned with autonomic responses than with responses involving the voluntary nervous system. Part of the stem (the medulla and the pons) governs the rates of respiration and heart beat (Fig. 2–16).

Thus, motor activity is influenced by the sum of all of the information reaching the motor neurons from both the higher center

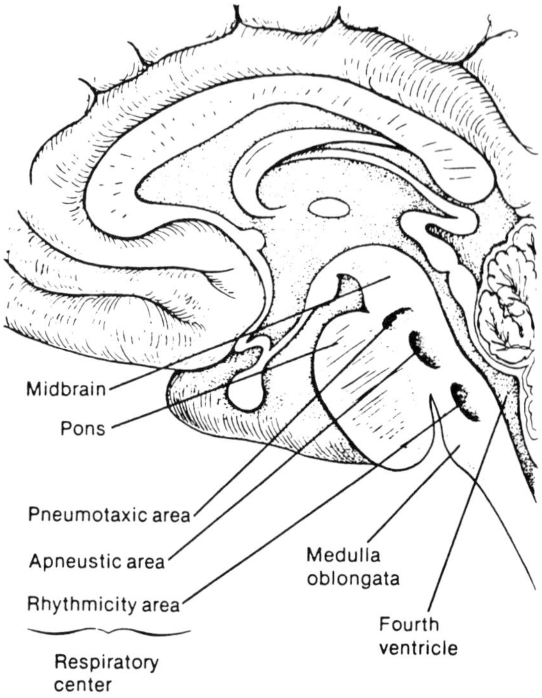

Fig. 2–16. Nuclei within the pons and the medulla oblongata constitute the respiratory center. (From Van De Graaff, K.M. *Human Anatomy*. Courtesy of William C. Brown, 1984.)

and the sensory organs. The descending impulses from the higher center of the brain, including those voluntarily evoked, are modified on the basis of information from the receptor organs because of the many possible alternatives available through the synaptic system of interneurons within the spinal cord. This coordination of motor information makes possible the movement pattern associated with athletic performance.

NERVE FIBER SIZE

Some signals need to be transmitted to the muscle rapidly if they are to be of much use. With other information, there is no hurry at all (e.g. an aching pain from a sprained ankle). Conduction velocity is related mostly to fiber size: the larger the fiber, the faster the conduction velocity. Figure 2–17 shows nerve fiber classification based on size (diameter and length) and conduction velocity. Type A fibers (both alpha and gamma) are typical myelinated fibers of spinal nerves: Type C, small unmyelinated low-velocity fibers. Type C fi-

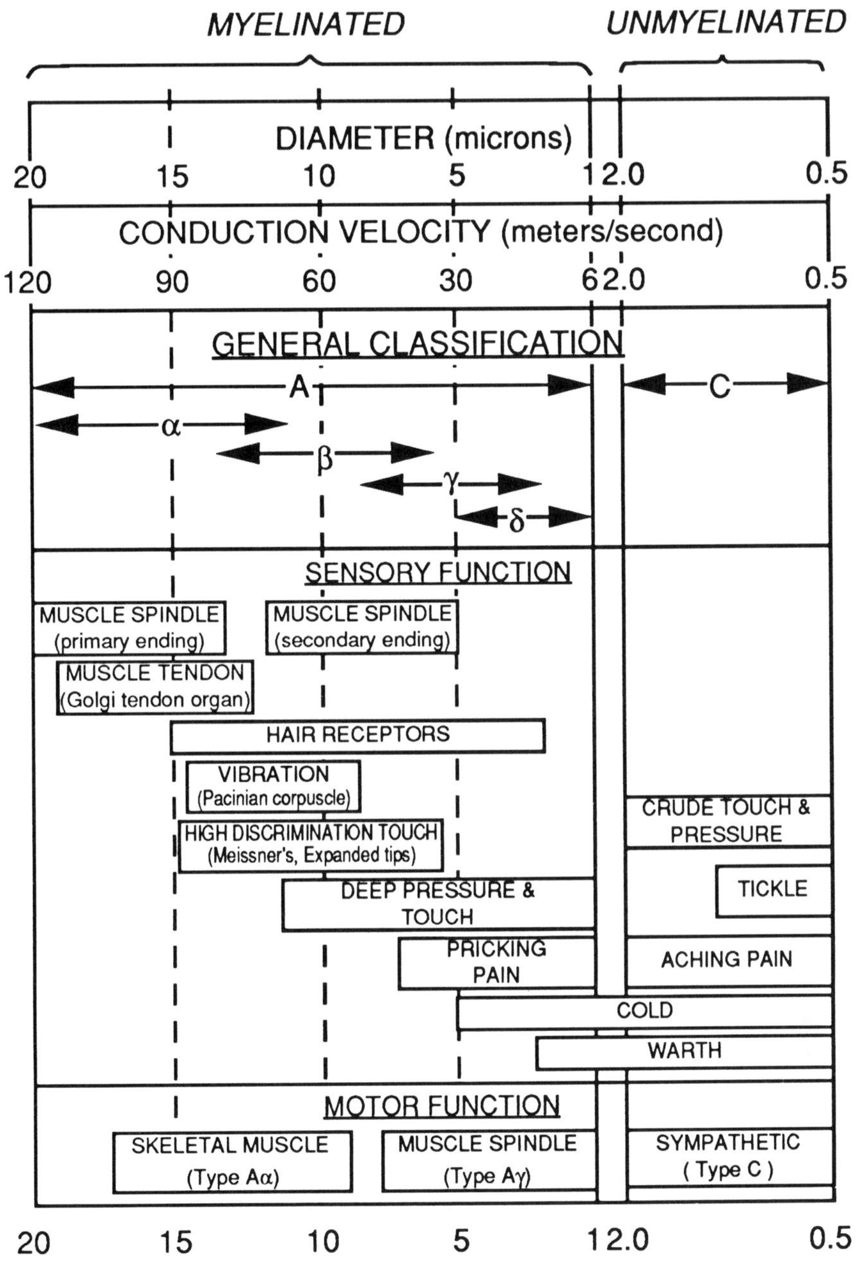

Fig. 2–17. Physiologic classification and functions of nerve fibers. (Modified from Guyton, A.C. *Human Physiology and Mechanism of Disease,* 4th Ed. Courtesy of W.B. Saunders Co., 1987.)

bers constitute more than half of all sensory fibers in peripheral nerves, and all of the postganglionic fibers of the autonomic nervous system.

Note that Type A or myelinated fibers range in diameter from 2 to 20 microns, and as a result have a higher conduction velocity (from 6 to 120 meters per second). The unmyelinated nerve fibers (Type C) measure from 0.5 to 2 microns and have a slower conduction velocity of 0.5 to 2 m/sec.

Note also that the functions of the body that require fast reaction times (such as reflex arcs, golgi tendon organs, etc.) are endowed with large diameter myelinated nerve fibers, whereas crude touch, pressure and pain receptors are transmitted by Type C fibers.

Nerve fiber size also plays a role in the func-

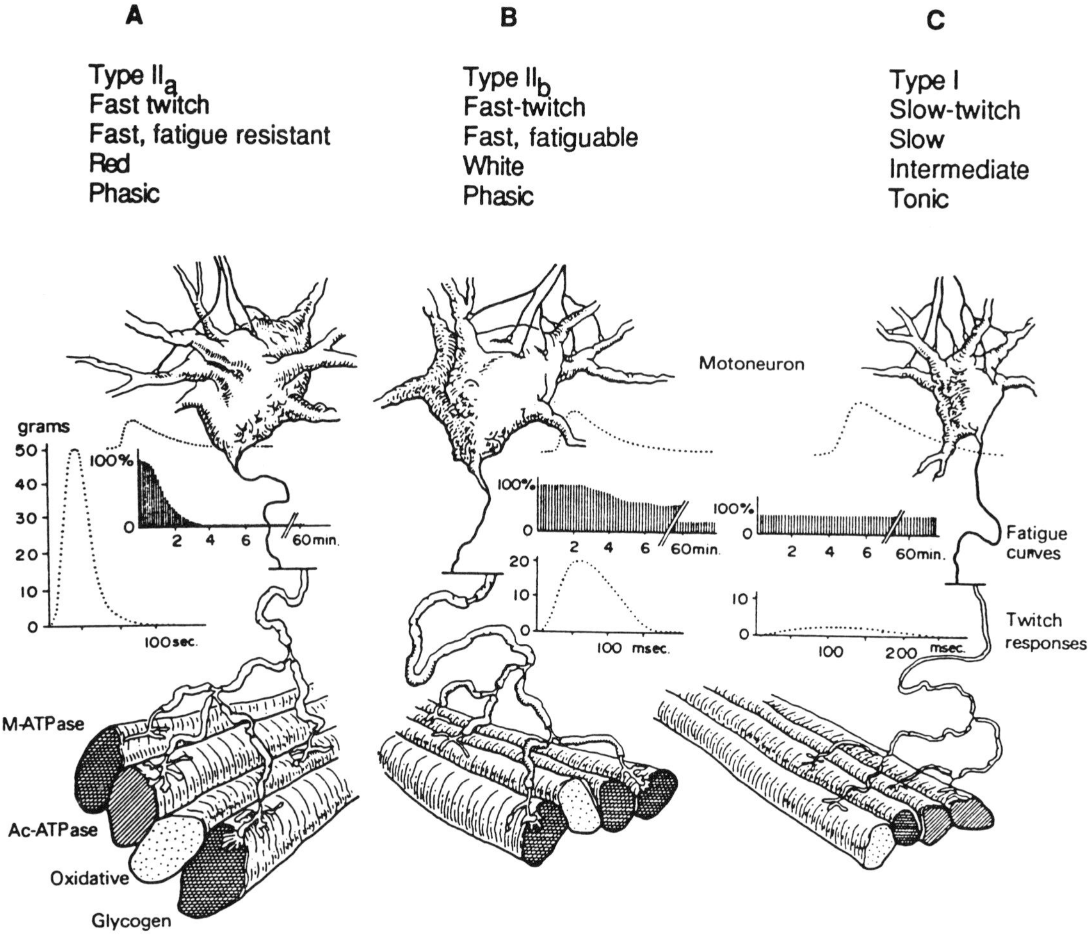

Fig. 2–18. *A–C.* Motor units containing mostly Type I fibers are innervated with smaller, more easily tired motor neurons. Motor units with Type II fibers produce more force, but are not so easily tired and they fatigue more easily. (From Edington, D.W., and Edgerton, R.E. *Biology of Physical Activity.* Courtesy of Houghton Mifflin Co., 1986.)

tion of motor units. Motor units containing mostly type I fibers have smaller motor neurons that are more easily fired (Fig. 2–18). These motor units are *tonic* (slow and continuous) and support much of the normal daily activity of the body. Motor neurons innervating type II motor units are larger, faster, and more difficult to fire. When they do fire, there is a fast twitch response time, but because of the biochemical properties of the muscle fibers, these motor units are more fatiguable (see fatigue curves, Figure 2–18). Type II motor units also contract with more force, but are more phasic (fire rapidly, but with short bursts) than type I motor units.

AUTONOMIC NERVOUS SYSTEM

The automatic control of various body functions is under the control of the autonomic nervous system which plays a major role in the regulation of circulatory functions (heart rate, blood pressure, blood vessel control, etc.), and so-called visceral functions (body temperature, intestinal motility, secretions, etc.). It is activated by centers located in the spinal cord, brain stem, and hypothalamus, sometimes by means of *autonomic reflexes*—a reaction to signals sent by peripheral nerve receptors.

There are two major divisions of the autonomic nervous system, the *sympathetic* and the *parasympathetic* (Fig. 2–19).

Generally, the sympathetic system is related to "fight-or-flight" responses. It increases the effectiveness of the heart as a pump, constricts blood vessels in non-critical areas while relaxing those in the muscle being used, increases blood pressure, releases glucose from

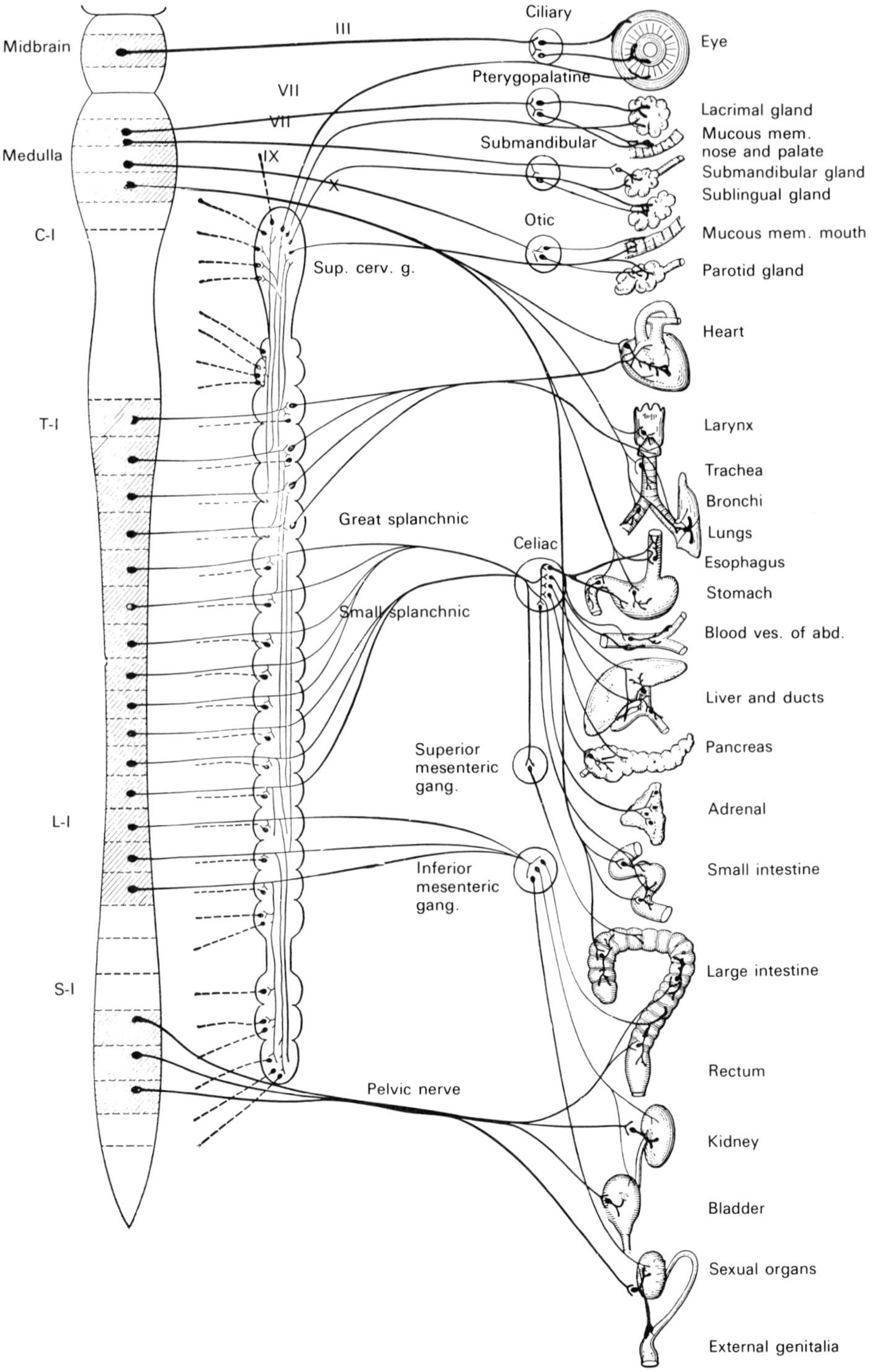

Fig. 2–19. The parasympathetic and sympathetic nervous systems. (From Clemente, C.D. *Gray's Anatomy of the Human Body,* 30th Ed. Courtesy of Lea & Febiger, 1985.)

Table 2–1. Autonomic Effects on Various Organs of the Body. (Adapted from A.C. Guyton, p. 442. Reproduced with permission of publisher)

Organ	*Effect of Sympathetic Stimulation*	*Effect of Parasympathetic Stimulation*
Eye: Pupil	Dilated	Contracted
Ciliary muscle	None	Excited
Glands: Nasal, Lacrimal, Parotid, Submaxillary, Gastric, Pancreatic	Vasoconstriction	Stimulation of thin, copious secretion containing many enzymes
Sweat glands	Copious sweating (cholinergic)	None
Apocrine glands	Thick, odoriferous secretion	None
Heart: Muscle	Increased rate Increased force of beat	Slowed rate Decreased force of atrial beat
Coronaries	Vasodilated	Constricted
Lungs: Bronchi	Dilated	Constricted
Blood vessels	Mildly constricted	None
Gut: Lumen	Decreased peristalsis and tone	Increased peristalsis and tone
Sphincter	Increased tone	Decreased tone
Liver	Glucose released	None
Gallbladder and bile ducts	Inhibited	Excited
Kidney	Decreased output	None
Ureter	Inhibited	Excited
Bladder: Detrusor	Inhibited	Excited
Trigone	Excited	Inhibited
Penis	Ejaculation	Erection
Systemic blood vessels:		
Abdominal	Constricted	None
Muscle	Constricted (adrenergic) Dilated (cholinergic)	None
Skin	Constricted (adrenergic) Dilated (cholinergic)	Dilated
Blood: Coagulation	Increased	None
Glucose	Increased	None
Basal metabolism	Increased up to 150%	None
Adrenal cortical secretion	Increased	None
Mental activity	Increased	None
Piloerector muscles	Excited	None

the liver (to increase the amount of circulating blood sugar), increases glycogenolysis in muscle (see Chapter 3), and increases muscle strength (Table 2–1 shows a complete listing of effects).

The sympathetic nervous system is composed of a pre-ganglionic fiber (that is, a fiber that proceeds to a synapse *outside* of the CNS) whose cell body or soma lies in the spinal cord. The axon of this neuron passes through the anterior root of the spinal cord in the spinal nerve. After several centimeters, the axon leaves the nerve and passes to a ganglion of the sympathetic chain. Here it synapses with one of the post-ganglionic fibers of the sympathetic chain or continues back into the spinal nerve and proceeds to an outlying ganglion to connect to a post-ganglionic fiber. In either case, the post-ganglionic fiber then goes to its destination in one of the organs. The post-ganglionic fibers usually pass back into a spinal nerve at some level to continue their journey.

Certain sympathetic preganglionic fibers pass directly into the *adrenal medulla* without synapsing. Stimulation of the adrenal medulla causes the same effects as direct sympathetic stimulation except that, because the effector chemicals (epinephrine and norepinephrine) are blood borne, the effects last about 10 times as long. In addition, the effects also occur in tissues that are not directly innervated. This system also acts as a stand-by, for use if something happens to the nervous system itself.

The parasympathetic system is sometimes called the "feed and breed" system because of its effects on the body relating to these functions. However, it does have a major role in the control of resting heart rate. Increased tone of the parasympathetic system is thought to be the cause of the low resting heart rate associated with endurance training.

About 75% of parasympathetic fibers are contained in the *vagus nerves,* which serve the entire thoracic and abdominal regions. The parasympathetic nervous system also has pre- and post-ganglionic fibers, but the pre-ganglionic fibers in this system usually pass directly to the organs, where they synapse with the post-ganglionic fibers in the walls of the organs themselves.

The pre-ganglionic fibers of both the sympathetic and parasympathetic nervous systems secrete acetylcholine (ACh), and are therefore called *cholinergic.* Once secreted by the nerve ending, ACh is broken down by the enzyme *cholinesterase* (just as in myoneuronal junctions). Therefore, the action of ACh lasts only a few seconds or less. The post-ganglionic fibers of the parasympathetic nervous system also secrete ACh. However, most post-ganglionic fibers of the sympathetic system secrete norepinephrine (Norepi) and are classified as *adrenergic.* Norepi is removed from the secretory site by being "pumped" back into the nerve ending by an active transport mechanism or by simple diffusion away from the receptor site. These processes also occur in only a few seconds. The norepinephrine and epinephrine secreted by the adrenal medulla, however, remain very active for 10 to 30 seconds and have some activity for several minutes.

SELECTED READINGS

Axelrod, J.: Neurotransmitters. Sci. Amer. June 1974.

Carew, T.J.: Spinal Cord I: Muscle and muscle receptors. In Kandel, E.R. and J.H. Schantz (eds). *Principles of Neural Science.* New York: Elsevier/North Holland, 1981, pp. 284–292.

Evarts, E.V.: Brain mechanisms of movement. Sci. Amer. Sept. 1979.

Guyton, A.C.: *Textbook of Medical Physiology.* 6th ed., Philadelphia: W.B. Saunders Co., 1981.

Guyton, A.C.: *Human Physiology and Mechanism of Discussion.* 3 ed., Philadelphia: W.B. Saunders Co., 1982.

Halater, Z.: *The Mechanoreceptors of the Mammalian Skin.* New York: Springer-Verlag, 1975.

Hunt, C.C., and S.W. Kaffler: Stretch receptors discharge during muscle contraction. J. Appl. Physiol. *113*:298–315, 1951.

Kandel, E.R.: Small systems of neurons. Sci. Amer. Sept. 1979.

Katz, B: *Nerve, Muscle and Synapse.* New York: McGraw-Hill, 1966.

McGrea, D.: Spinal Cord Recruiting and Motor Reflexes. In Ranfolf, K. (ed.), *Exercise and Sports Sciences, Rev., 14*:105–141, ACSM, 1986.

Merton, P.A.: How we control the contraction of our muscles. Sci. Amer. *226*:30–37, 1972.

Morell, P., and Norton, A.T.: Myelin. Sci. Amer. 1980.

Noback, C.T., and Denauert, R.: *The Human Nervous System.* 3rd ed. New York: McGraw-Hill, 1980.

Norton, W.J.H., and Feirtag, M.: The organization of the brain. Sci. Amer. August, 1977.

Pearson, K.: The control of walking. Sci. Amer. *235*:72–86, 1976.

Precht, W.: Vestibular mechanism. Amer. Rev. Neurosci. 2:265, 1979.

Sale, D.G. Influence of Exercise and Training on Motor Units Activation. In Pandorf, K.B. (ed), ESSR, Vol. 15, ACSM, 1987.

Shepard, G.M.: Microcircuits in the nervous system. Sci. Amer. *238*(2):92, 1978.

Singer, S.J.: Architecture and topography of biological membranes. In *Cell Membrane, Biochemistry, Cell Biology, and Pathology.* G. Weissman and R. Clairborne (eds.). New York: H.P. Publishing Co., Inc., 1975.

Stevens, C.F.: The Neuron. Sci. Amer. *241*(3):54, 1978.

Uttley, A.M.: *Information Transmission in the Nervous System.* New York: Academic Press, 1979.

3

Metabolism

Remember from Chapters 1 and 2 that muscles need both a signal from the nervous system and energy to contract. Although low to moderate activity is seldom a problem in terms of energy supply, athletes who produce the most energy often win their event. One of the major goals of most conditioning programs is to increase the energy production capability of the athlete. The purpose of this chapter is to discuss energy and the energy producing systems so that the reader will understand how to best use and train these systems for maximum performance.

ENERGY

All energy as we know it originates from the sun. As the sun loses mass, in accordance with Einstein's formula $E = mc^2$, energy reaches the earth at the rate of 2×10^{13} kilocalories per second, and is stored in many different forms (chemical, electrical, mechanical, and thermal energy). Plants use this energy to convert 6 water (H_2O) molecules and 6 carbon dioxide (CO_2) molecules to glucose ($C_6H_{12}O_6$) while giving off oxygen as a by-product *(photosynthesis)* (Fig. 3–1). This process takes two compounds (H_2O and CO_2) whose chemical bonds contain little transferable energy and converts them to carbohydrates (CHO) molecules with high levels of free energy contained within their chemical bonds. Carbohydrates are then eaten by animals, digested, absorbed through the cells of the intestinal tract, and used for energy to power muscular contractions or to be stored as fat for later use (Fig. 3–2).

In the body, the food we eat is processed by cells to provide energy in the form of ATP for muscular contraction.

Organisms exist because they are able to take energy from their environment and use it to drive life-sustaining processes, and do so by obeying the first and second law of thermodynamics. The *first law of thermodynamics* states that energy can neither be created nor destroyed, but can only be converted from one form to another (e.g., the sun's radiant energy is converted into plant CHO). This law is sometimes referred to as the law of conservation of energy. The *second law of thermodynamics* (law of entropy) states that the universe seeks a state of randomness or entropy. This means that a structured molecule containing high levels of free energy will readily release its energy.

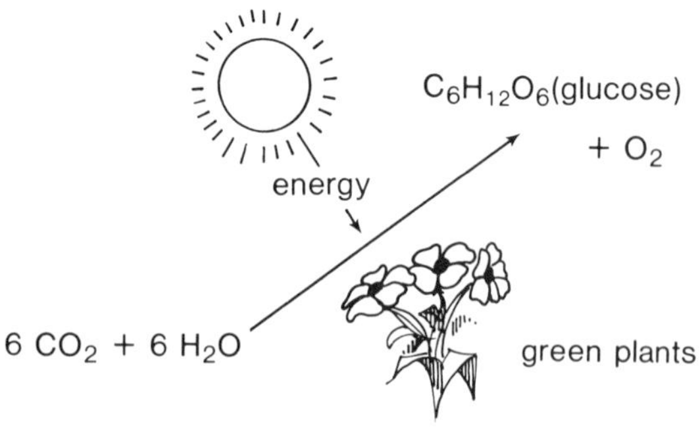

Fig. 3–1. Simplified diagram of photosynthesis. Some of the sun's radiant energy is captured by plants and used to produce glucose from carbon dioxide and water. Glucose has a higher free energy content than the initial reactants.

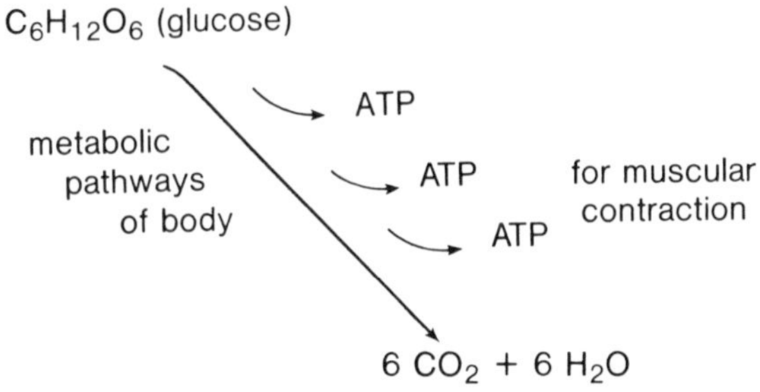

Fig. 3–2. Because glucose contains more free energy from carbon dioxide and water, glucose can be broken down stepwise within the muscle to provide energy for muscular contraction in the form of ATP.

THE METABOLIC PATHWAYS—OVERVIEW

Cells have complex ways of processing the digested products of ingested food to produce energy. These small pieces of carbohydrates, fats, and proteins are processed through the cell's metabolic pathways until all that is left is water and carbon dioxide. As these food molecules are degraded in the metabolic pathways, energy is released *(entropy)*.

The cell is able to harness much of this energy, but a vast amount is lost as heat. These processes are collectively known as *cellular respiration* (Fig. 3–3). The term *respiration* refers to chemical reactions within a cell that liberate energy. Interestingly, glucose can release a small amount of energy even in the absence of oxygen, a process called *anaerobic respiration.* A greater release of energy occurs when sufficient oxygen is available to serve as the final electron acceptor, a process known as *aerobic respiration.*

Since the energy released from the metabolic pathways cannot be used directly, it is "captured" in the basic energy molecule of the cell, called adenosine triphosphate (ATP). Although ATP is not the only energy-carrying molecule in the body, it is the primary energy molecule and is often called the "energy currency" of the body. ATP consists of three main subunits: adenine, a ribose sugar, and three phosphate radicals (Fig. 3–4).

The bonds between the phosphate units are high energy bonds and contain about eight Kcal each. Since there is always a resting supply of ATP in the cell, these bonds can be broken rapidly to supply the immediate need for energy to use in the muscular contraction, as shown by the reaction below:

$$ATP + H_2O \xrightarrow{\text{ATPase}} ADP + P_i + \text{energy}$$

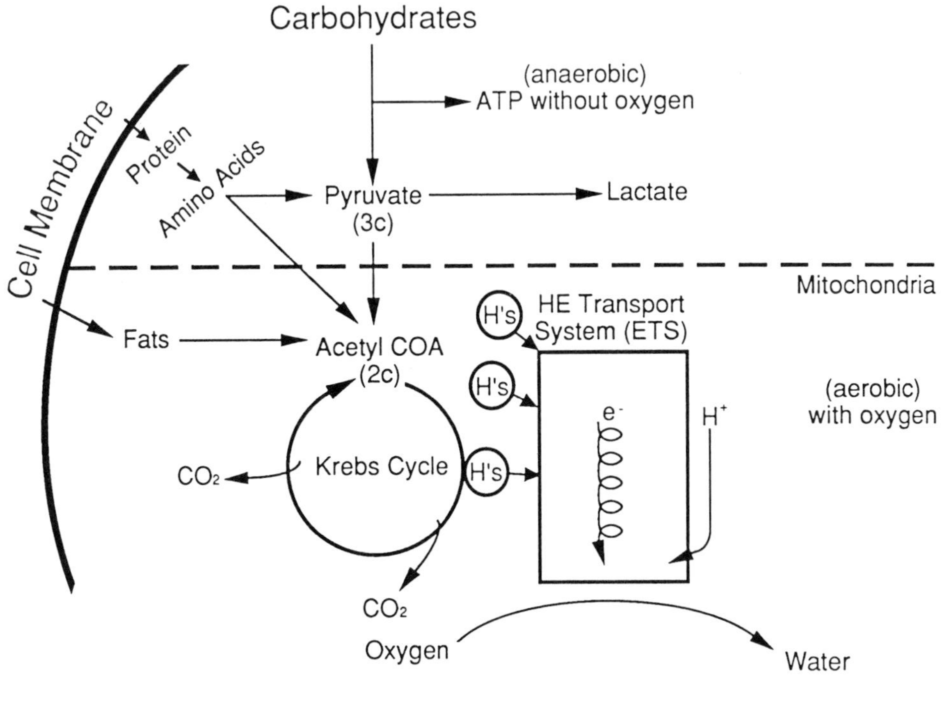

Fig. 3–3. Schematic diagram showing energy liberation and transfer in the living cell.

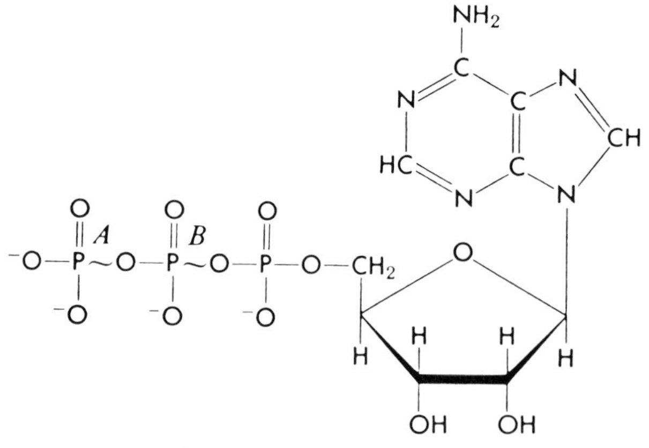

Adenosine triphosphate (ATP)

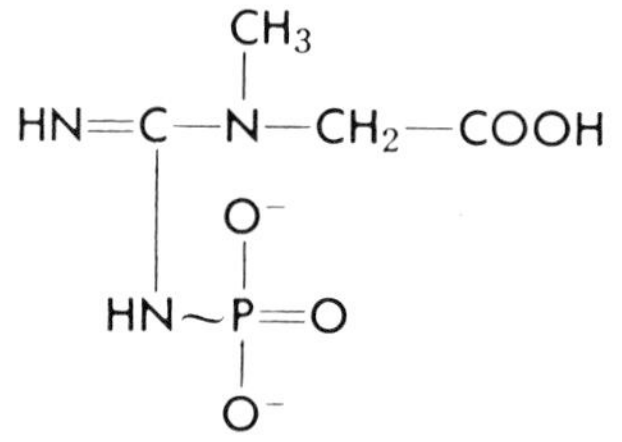

Creatine phosphate (CP)

Fig. 3–4. Structure of an ATP molecule. The wavy lines connecting the last two phosphates represent high-energy chemical bonds from which energy can be released quickly. (From Jensen, C.R., and Fisher, A.G. *Scientific Basis of Athletic Conditioning,* 2nd Ed. Courtesy of Lea & Febiger, 1979.)

Another important energy molecule is *creatine phosphate (CP),* whose bond energy is even higher than that of ATP. However, CP cannot be used directly as an energy source to power muscular contraction. When immediate energy is needed, ATP is broken down to ADP to supply that energy need and is then restored very rapidly by CP under the influence of creatine kinase according to the reaction below:

$$\text{CP} + \text{ADP} \xrightarrow{\text{creatine kinase}} \text{ATP} + \text{C}$$

Even though the concentration of CP is greater than that of ATP, the combined energy available during such work from both molecules will last only a few seconds (10 to 15). After the work has terminated, CP is resynthesized using a reverse process, being fueled by new ATP created during oxidative metabolism. Because of the role of CP in keeping energy in the form of ATP available, it is sometimes called an "ATP sparer."

$$\text{ATP} + \text{C} \longleftrightarrow \text{CP} + \text{ADP}$$

ATP for rapid use can also be generated directly from two ADP molecules under the influence of adenylate kinase:

$$\text{ADP} + \text{ADP} \xrightarrow{\text{adenylate kinase}} \text{ATP} + \text{AMP}$$

If energy is needed for high work levels lasting longer than 10 to 15 seconds, glucose must be processed anaerobically by the glycolytic pathway. Using this pathway, ATP is created, but lactic acid is also produced. This source of energy can last up to about one minute at maximum effort. Longer duration work bouts require a decrease in intensity and the use of oxidative pathways, where both sugars and fats are processed.

CYCLIC AMP

Besides ADP and AMP, ATP is converted to another important messenger molecule called *cyclic AMP* (abbreviated *cAMP*). The binding of such hormones as epinephrine to the cell membrane activates the enzyme *adenyl cyclase,* responsible for catalyzing adenosine triphosphate (ATP) into cAMP. As a result, the intracellular concentration of cAMP is increased. This increased level of cAMP sets off a series or cascade of reactions that activates a previously inactive *protein kinase.* The active protein kinase catalyzes the attachment of phosphates to different enzymes in the cell. For example, the addition of a phosphate group to inactive phosphorylase kinase activates this enzyme, which in turn activates the previously inactive glycogen phosphorylase which promotes the breakdown of glycogen to glucose-1-p. Activation of protein kinase has the oposite effect on glycogen storage because it inactivates glycogen synthetase (Fig. 3–5). Although cAMP is not a major energy-carrying molecule in the body, it is a very important *second messenger,* whose cascade reaction controls glycogen synthesis and breakdown, the rate of glycolysis, and many other metabolic functions.

ENZYMES

It should be pointed out that the splitting of the ATP bonds to release energy, the formation of cAMP, and every other chemical reaction in the body are accelerated by *enzymes.* In fact, reactions catalyzed by enzymes can occur 1,000,000 or more times faster than if the two reacting molecules randomly interact. The mechanisms by which enzymes operate are still not totally understood. Each enzyme is specific, meaning that it reacts with only the substrate or reactant for which it was designed. The substrate attaches to a specific site on the enzyme called the *active site.* The combined substrate and enzyme is referred to as an *enzyme-substrate complex.* Two ways that substrates fit into the active sites of enzymes are shown in Figure 3–6.

The body contains thousands of enzymes which can be classified according to the reactions they trigger: *dehydrogenases* remove hydrogen atoms from substrates; *hydrolases* promote hydrolysis reactions (breaking apart of molecules with water); *phosphatases* catalyze the removal of phosphate groups; *kinases* help

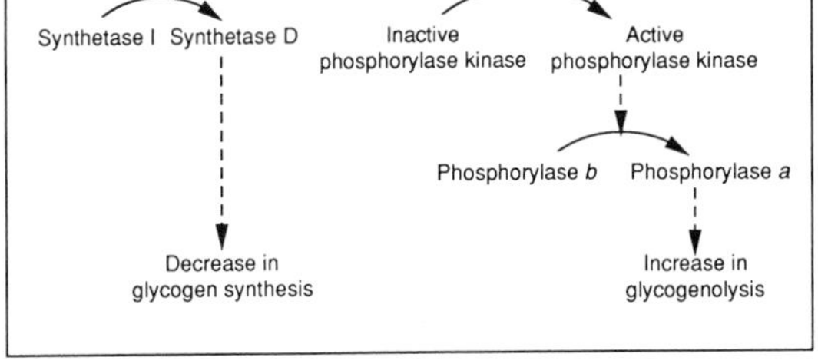

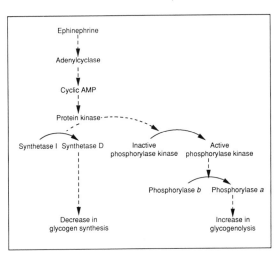

Fig. 3–5. An increase in the intracellular concentration of cAMP promotes the breakdown of glycogen and inhibits glycogen syntheses.

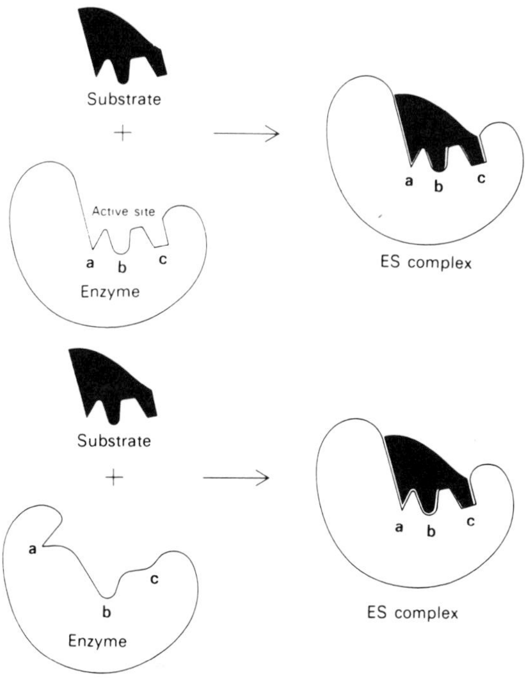

Fig. 3–6. *A.* In the lock-and-key model, the active site of the enzyme is by itself complimentary in shape to the substrate. *B.* In the induced-fit model, the active site becomes complimentary in shape only after the substrate is bound. (From Stryer, L. *Biochemistry.* Courtesy of W.H. Freeman, 1975.)

transfer phosphate groups; and *isomerases* help rearrange the molecule into a structural isomer. You will notice that with few exceptions, enzymes are distinguished by the suffix *-ase*. The names of most enzymes will specify the substrate that is acted upon and the category or activity of the enzyme. For example, lactate dehydrogenase (an enzyme in glycolysis) acts on the substrate pyruvate to form lactate and glycogen synthetase helps produce glycogen from pieces of sugar.

COFACTORS AND COENZYMES

Many enzymes are inactive, or unable to catalyze a reaction unless modified by smaller organic molecules called *cofactors*. For example, some enzymes have active sites that are morphologically unsuited for a substrate unless a cofactor alters its shape first. Cofactors include such ions as calcium (Ca^{++}), magnesium (Mg^{++}), copper (Cu^{++}), and zinc (Zn^{++}).

Coenzymes are molecules that help transport hydrogen atoms and other small molecules from one enzyme to another. The most common coenzymes are Coenzyme A which carries small 2-carbon molecules from glycolysis to the Krebs cycle, or from beta-oxidation to the Krebs, and NAD and FAD, which both carry hydrogen atoms from place to place in the metabolic pathways.

The amount of energy needed to initiate a chemical reaction is termed its *energy of activation*. In the laboratory, adding heat is one way of transferring activation energy to make the reaction go faster. In the body, a catalyst is used to lower the activation energy so that the speed of the reaction is increased (Fig. 3–7).

None of the enzymatic reactions that occur in the metabolic pathways of the body happens independently; but are, in fact, linked in a specific series of reactions. The initial substrate (such as glucose) is broken down to a number of intermediate molecules before the final product is formed. The enzymes in the metabolic pathway cooperate so that the product of one enzyme is the substrate for the next enzyme. The site at which the substrate is broken down is controlled by the amount of substrate available to the enzyme, and by the concentration of each enzyme. It is possible that if one enzyme is in substantially lower concentration than its neighboring enzyme, it would end up controlling the overall rate of the entire metabolic pathway. The slowest step in the reaction pathway is sometimes referred to as the "rate-limiting" step, because the entire series of reactions can proceed only as quickly as its slowest step. Some pathways can be switched on or off, or controlled by hormones released in the blood or by the accumulation of the final product (Fig. 3–8).

CARBOHYDRATE METABOLISM

From 40 to 70% of the calories ingested in the diet are from carbohydrates. These carbohydrates, from foods such as fruits, vegetables, beans, and grains begin digestion in the mouth by an enzyme called ptyalin which hydrolyzes starches into maltose. They pass through the stomach with little change, but are attacked in the small intestine by pancreatic *amylases,* which break them into the monosaccharides *glucose, fructose,* and *galactose*. These small sugars are absorbed through the walls of the small intestine into the portal blood and carried to the liver, where fructose and galactose are converted to glucose. Some of the glucose is stored as *glycogen* to be used later as blood sugar levels begin to fall between meals. The rest of it is carried to the muscle (and other) cells of the body to be used as a substrate for producing ATP for muscle contraction and other functions or to be stored as muscle glycogen. As the blood glucose levels rise after a meal, the pancreas increases its secretion of insulin, because insulin is required for the transport of glucose into muscle, fat and other tissues.

Immediately upon entering liver or muscle cells, glucose is converted to glucose-6-phosphate (a process called phosphorylation) by adding a phosphate molecule onto the sugar molecule at the 6th carbon. This process is reversible in the liver because sugars must be released from the liver to help maintain proper blood sugar levels. In muscle cells, the phosphorylation process is irreversible and the glucose molecule can never be released back into the circulation. Once sugar (glucose)

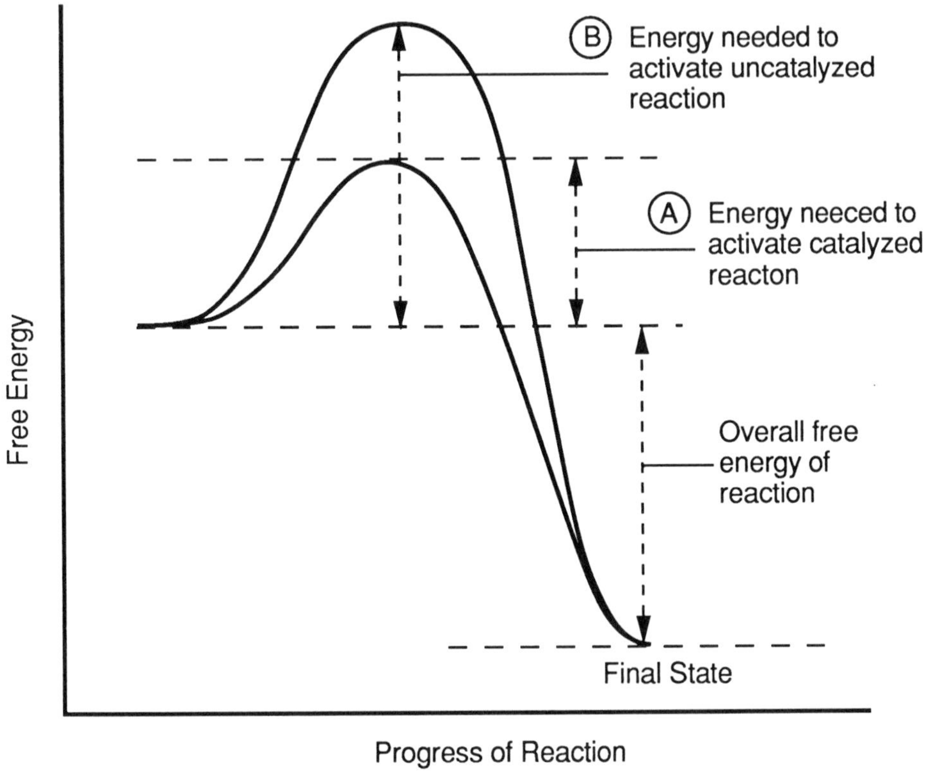

Fig. 3–7. Comparison of a catalyzed reaction *(A)* with a non-catalyzed reaction *(B)*. Enzyms accelerate reactions by reducing the energy required for the reaction to occur.

is phosphorylated, it is either used immediately for energy in the glycolytic pathway or stored in the cell as glycogen.

Glycogen is a large polymer of thousands of glucose units attached in chains (in 1 to 4 or 1 to 6 linkages), creating an almost pinwheel appearance. The fact that all the circulating glucose not used by the body is consolidated into large glycogen molecules is not by accident, but out of necessity. If glucose were stored as individual molecules instead of combined into glycogen, the osmotic gradient established would be so great that large amounts of water would be pulled into the cell, rupturing it. Sugars are therefore stored in cells as glycogen to keep the osmotic pressure inside the cell at normal levels. Even with this osmotic advantage, glycogen still carries with it four times its weight in water (Fig. 3–9).

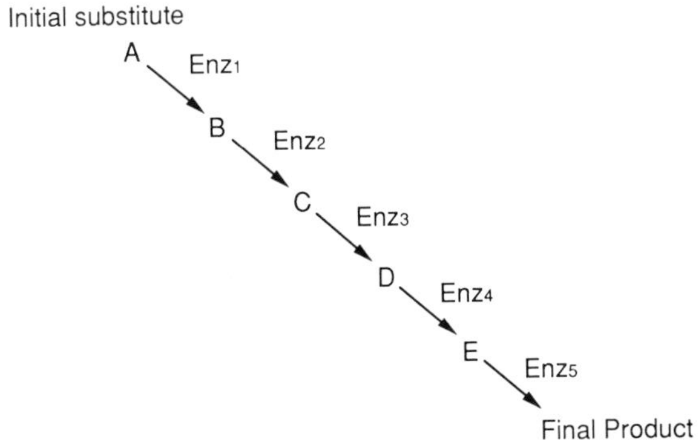

Fig. 3–8. A metabolic pathway, where the product of one enzyme becomes the substrate of the next in a multienzyme system.

Muscles normally contain about 1.5 g of glycogen per 100 g of wet muscle (1.5%) or 15 g per kg. This level can be raised dramatically by carbohydrate loading techniques (which will be discussed later) to 3.5–4.0 g per 100 g of muscle (3.5 to 4.0%). Since muscle makes up about 40% of the body weight of an average person, a 70 kg person would have about 28 kg of muscle (70 kg × 40% = 28 kg) and 420 g of total glycogen under normal circumstances (28 kg muscle × 1.5% = .420 kg or 420 g of glycogen). This level could be in-

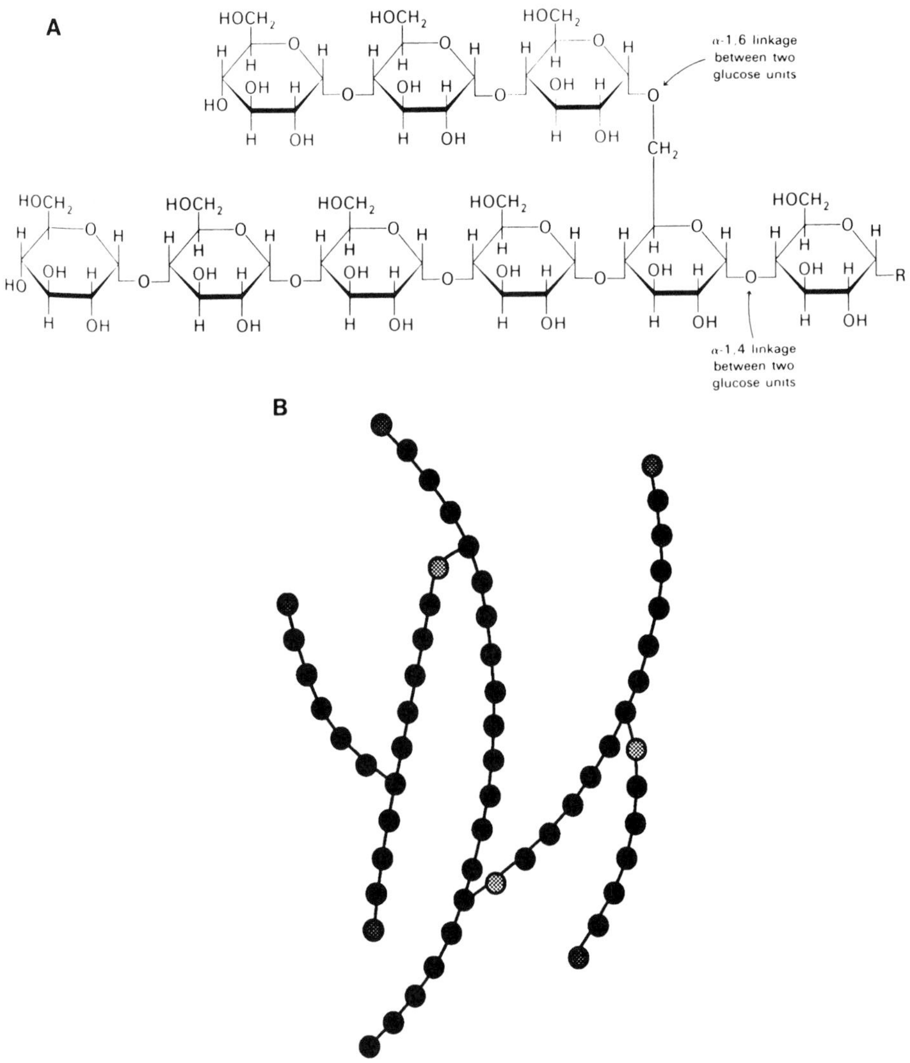

Fig. 3–9. *A.* Glycogen is a polysaccharide composed of glucose subunits joined together to form a large, highly branched molecule. *B.* Cross section of a glycogen molecule. (From Stryer, L. *Biochemistry.* Courtesy of W.H. Freeman, 1975.)

creased to over 1100 g of glycogen by glycogen loading (28 kg muscle × 4.0% = 1.2 kg or 1120 g).

GLYCOGENESIS AND GLYCOGENOLYSIS

If a cell is working and requires immediate energy, the glucose that enters the cell is phosphorylated and processed directly through the *glycolytic* pathway. If there is little need for immediate energy (the usual situation following a meal), glucose-6-phosphate (G-6-P) can be converted to glycogen for storage by a process called glycogenesis (glyco = sugar + genesis = to produce). In this process, G-6-P is converted to its isomer glucose-1-phosphate (G-1-P), to UDP glucose, and then to glycogen under the influence of an enzyme called *glycogen synthetase* (Fig. 3–10).

Glycogen represents a storage source of glucose, which can be liberated from the glycogen molecule through a process called *glycogenolysis* (glycogen + lysis = to break). When activated, the enzyme *phosphorylase* selectively releases a glucose molecule in the form of G-1-P. The G-1-P is then changed to G-6-P which in turn is broken down to glucose in the liver, and the glucose is subsequently

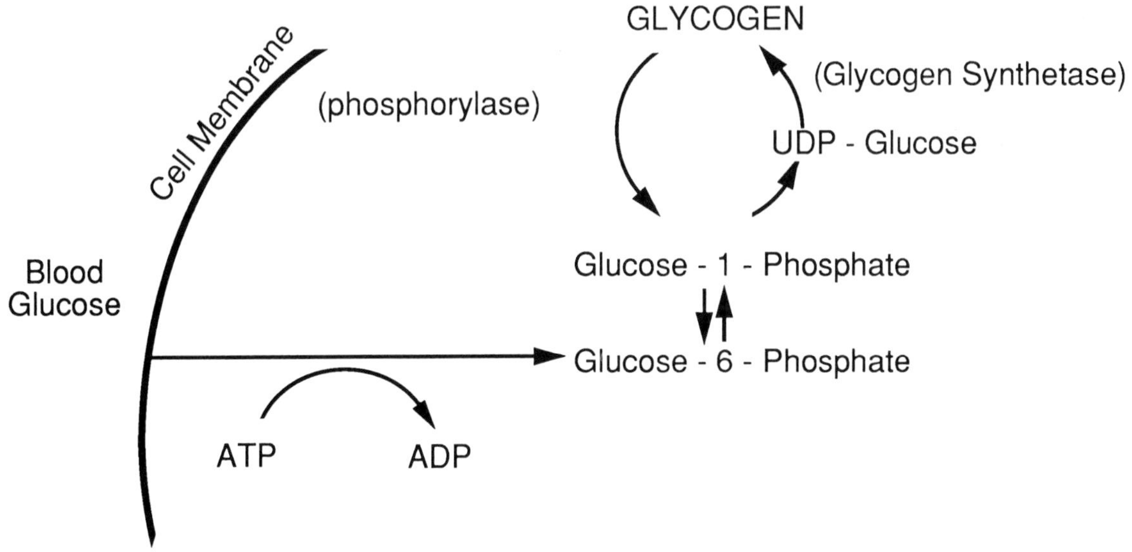

Fig. 3–10. Blood glucose that enters the tissue cells is rapidly converted to G-6-P. This intermediate can be converted to glycogen by glycogen synthetase. Glycogen represents a storage form of carbohydrates, which can be used as a source for new G-6-P through the activation of phosphorylase.

released into the blood to be transported to the tissues for use as energy. If in the muscle, the G-6-P is processed through the glycolytic pathway for ATP production.

In the muscle, phosphorylase is activated by two mechanisms: (1) By the hormone *epinephrine.* When exercise begins, epinephrine is released from the adrenal medulla, attaches to an epinephrine receptor on the cell, and stimulates a series of reactions mediated by cAMP that changes phosphorylase b (the inactive form) to phosphorylase a (the active form) (see Fig. 3–5). With rapid changes in activity, this mechanism is too slow to account for the glycogenolysis that has been observed, so the second mechanism is thought to be related to (2) the calcium released from the sarcoplasmic reticulum when muscles are stimulated to contract. According to this theory, the rate of glycogen degradation is related to the frequency of muscle contraction, with each stimulus resulting in activation of phosphorylase b kinase, which activates phosphorylase b to form phosphorylase a.

It should be pointed out that the hormonal signals that activate glycogenolysis also reciprocally inactivate glycogen synthetase to inhibit glycogenesis (glycogen synthesis). On the other hand, as glycogen synthesis is activated, phosphorylase activity is shut down, all by the presence or absence of cAMP.

GLYCOLYSIS (ANAEROBIC)

If the amount of creatine phosphate were the only means of regenerating ATP, man (and woman) would be severely limited in terms of the types of activities that could be carried out. Luckily, the body can overcome this limitation in the immediate availability of high energy intermediates by processing glycogen (or glucose) through the *glycolytic pathway,* forming lactic acid. Using anaerobic glycolysis, the work that can be done at high energy levels can be increased almost tenfold. In glycolysis, G-6-P coming directly into the cell, or more likely, G-6-P produced from glycogenolysis can be energized with another phosphate to form glucose 1,6 diphosphate, and then produce a total of 4 ATP's and 4 hydrogen atoms as it is processed to *pyruvate* and finally to *lactate.* In this process, the 6-carbon glucose is split in half to form two pyruvates and two lactates, both of which contain 3 carbons (Fig. 3–11).

Hydrogen production during metabolism is important because pairs of hydrogens are carried from all of the pathways by some hydrogen carrier (usually nicotinamide adenine

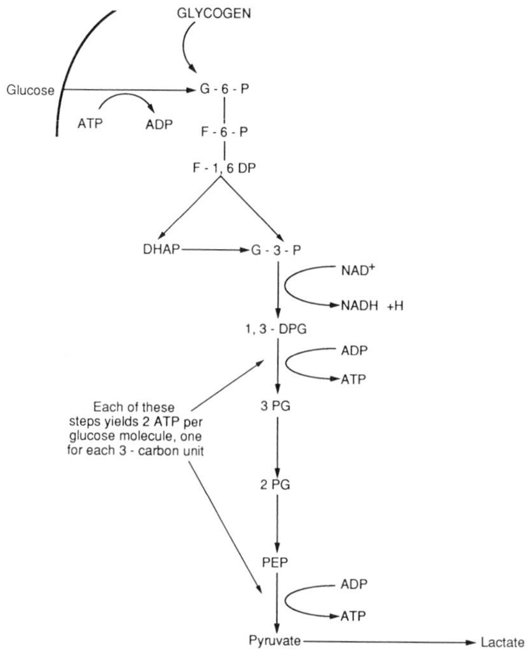

Fig. 3–11. A simplified drawing of glycolysis. Note that two pyruvate molecules are formed for each glucose processed.

dinucleotide (NAD) or flavoprotein adenine dinucleotide (FAD)) to the *electron transport system* (ETS) where they are used to produce large quantities of ATP oxidatively. These carriers (NAD and FAD) are not used up in the process, but must unload their hydrogens and return to pick up more or the metabolic process they are supporting would be unable to continue. During high intensity work, many type II (more glycolytic) fibers are recruited and the energy need of even ST fibers is greater than the amount of oxygen available. Under these conditions, many hydrogen carriers are unable to unload their hydrogens because of insufficient oxygen and must therefore find another place to unload or glycolysis must stop. Luckily, under the influence of an enzyme called lactate dehydrogenase (LDH), NADH$^+$H (the carrier and its hydrogens) can unload onto pyruvate forming *lactic acid* (Fig. 3–12). The only difference then between pyruvate and lactate is the two hydrogens unloaded by NAD.

The problem with producing lactic acid is twofold: first, lactic acid dissociates to form a hydrogen ion and lactate.

lactic acid -------------> H^+ + lactate$^-$

The H^+ or proton is positively charged and probably interferes with the contractile mechanism in the muscle when the proton level builds up. Second, when high levels of lactate build up, it begins to diffuse back into the cell as rapidly as it diffuses out and probably begins to inhibit glycolysis. In any event, a person cannot depend on energy from this source for too long (less than a minute at maximum levels of work), but it does make it possible to work at high rates for much longer than would be possible with only CP. The fate of the lactate produced from anaerobic glycolysis will be discussed later in this chapter.

THE BIOCHEMISTRY OF GLYCOLYSIS

Glycolysis (Embden-Meyerhoff pathway) is the sequence of reactions that converts glucose into pyruvate while producing ATP in the process. All reactions in glycolysis are reversible except for those indicated by only one arrow as shown in Figure 3–13.

Note that the lower portion of the cycle occurs twice because of the splitting of the glucose molecules to form two 3-carbon molecules of glyceraldehyde 3-phosphate.

As glucose enters the cells, it is immediately phosphorylated (phosphate added) by the enzyme *hexokinase* (No. 1) and is converted to G-6-P. This essentially traps the glucose in the cell. As the level of G-6-P increases, the activity of hexokinase decreases. On the other hand, as the demand for glu-

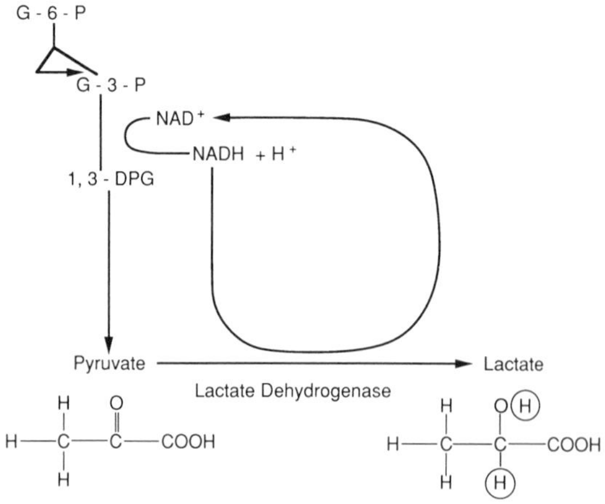

Fig. 3–12. Hydrogens from anaerobic glycolysis are unloaded onto pyruvate (see Ⓗ in lactate structure) instead of being carried to mitochondria for aerobic processing.

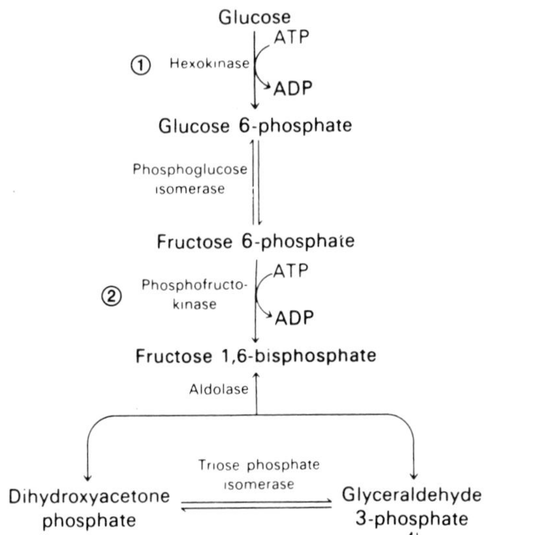

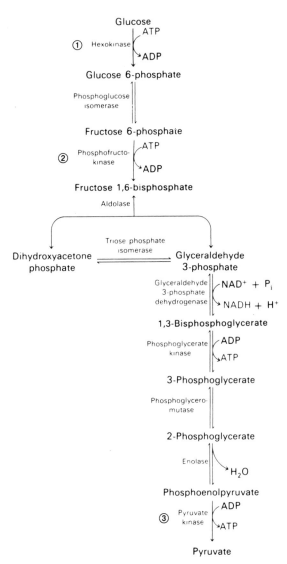

Fig. 3–13. The glycolytic pathway. (Modified from Stryer, L. *Biochemistry.* Courtesy of W.H. Freeman, 1975.)

cose increases, the inhibition of hexokinase is decreased, allowing additional glucose to enter the cell.

Phosphofructokinase (PFK) (No. 2) is the predominant regulating enzyme and is rate limiting (that is, it controls a series of reactions). During exercise, when glycolysis is rapid, PFK is totally activated; however, during rest, the levels of ATP, CP, and citrate (all products of aerobic metabolism) alter the conformation of PFK thus inhibiting its activity. Conversely, during exercise, where ATP, CP, and citrate levels fall, the presence of ADP, P_i, AMP, and decreased pH all serve to enhance the activity of PFK.

The third and final regulating step in glycolysis, *pyruvate kinase* (No. 3) is also controlled by the level of ATP and CP. Although not a major limiting enzyme, a pyruvate kinase deficiency results in abnormally high concentrations of glycolytic intermediates, since the terminal step in glycolysis is blocked.

GLYCOLYSIS (AEROBIC)

During rest or steady state work, most of the hydrogens produced in the glycolytic pathway are carried via a shuttle system to the ETS in the mitochondria instead of forming lactic acid. In highly aerobic muscle, the shuttle system is called the *malate-aspartate* system and the $NADH^-$ and H^+ from glycolysis unloads its hydrogens onto another NAD carrier molecule. In other muscles, the $NADH^-$ and H^+ utilizes the *glycerol phosphate* shuttle system which carries the hydrogens from glycolysis via FAD (Fig. 3–14). This makes the two pyruvic acid molecules produced from each glucose entering glycolysis available for further degradation and entry into the Krebs cycle (sometimes called the citric acid cycle).

Getting pyruvate ready for Krebs cycle processing is a major step, since glycolysis occurs in the cytoplasm and aerobic metabolism occurs in the mitochondria. Pyruvate (a 3-carbon piece of the original 6-carbon sugar) must lose a carbon (as carbon dioxide) and 2 hydrogen molecules that are carried by NAD to the ETS. The 2-carbon remains of pyruvate (called acetic acid) are then attached to a carrier molecule called coenzyme A forming a structure called acetyl CoA. Acetyl CoA is then carried into the mitochondria so it can be utilized.

It is important to realize that mitochondria are the site of *oxidative metabolism* in the cell and that most of the oxygen that is used is used by the processes that take place in this important structure. Because of their role in oxidative metabolism, these large double membraned, sac-like organelles are sometimes called the "powerhouses of the cell." There are more mitochondria in type I (slow-oxidative) than in type IIa (fast oxidative glycolytic) fibers, and the type IIa fibers have

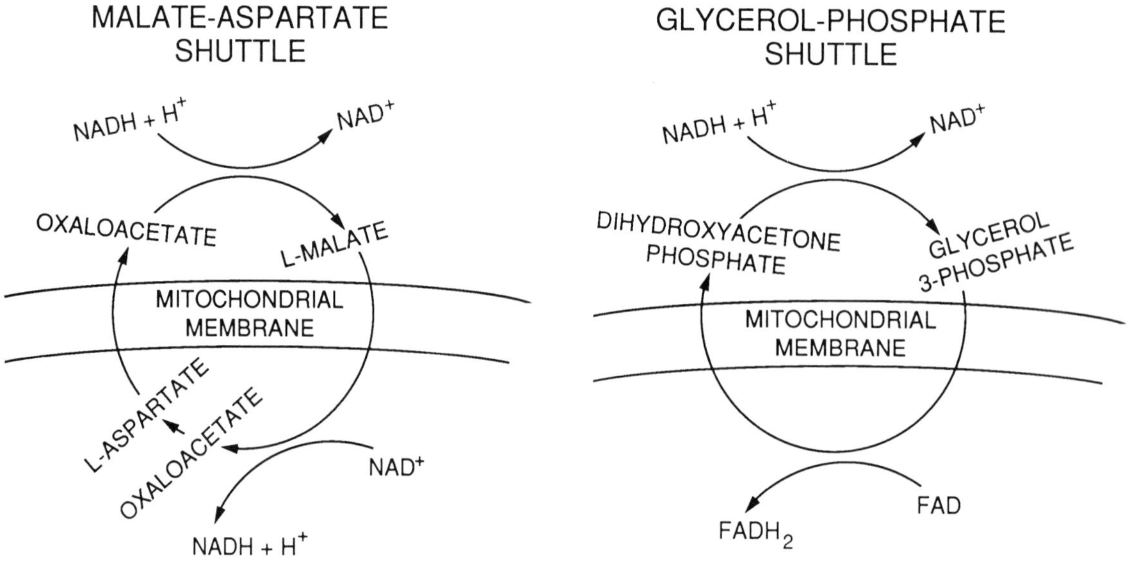

Fig. 3–14. *A and B.* Hydrogens are shuttled into the mitochondria by two different systems.

more mitochondria than in the type IIb (glycolytic) fibers. It is clear that the ability to do long-term activity is related to mitochondrial content of the muscles. Part of the red color of oxidative muscles comes from the mitochondrial content of these fibers.

Some mitochondria are located just beneath the sarcolemma and are used primarily to maintain the membrane integrity. Others are found deep in the muscle and these are used to provide energy to the contractile processes. Some evidence exists that mitochondria are connected in a complex branching network rather than being individual structures. The metabolic pathways and enzymes of metabolism are arranged in the various inner structures of the mitochondria, and the carbon structures from the food we eat are passed from one to another as the metabolic processes proceed. The *Krebs cycle* enzymes are located in the matrix within the cristae and the hydrogens released from the various pathways are processed by the *electron transfer system (ETS)* located on small "stalks" or "knobs" on the inner membrane structure (Fig. 3–15).

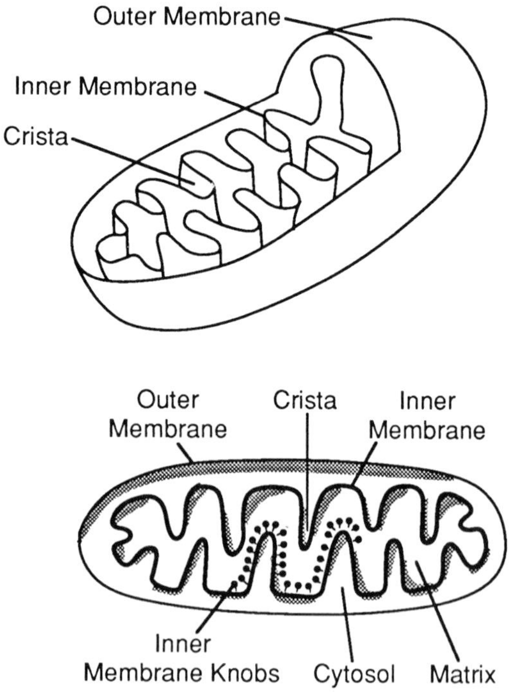

Fig. 3–15. *A.* Membranes' partition form the cristae within the organelles. *B.* A schematic diagram of a mitochondrion showing the inner membrane knobs. (From Armstrong, F.B. *Biochemistry.* Courtesy of Oxford Univ. Press, 1989.)

KREBS CYCLE

It is clear that the major purpose of the Krebs cycle is to generate hydrogen molecules to be processed for energy in the electron transfer system (ETS). The process starts when the 2-carbon acetate molecule (the remnant of the pyruvate) is delivered by CoA, which will return for the other half of the original glucose molecule that started through glycolysis. The 2-carbon unit joins with a 4-carbon oxaloacetate to form a 6-carbon citric acid. This product is then processed through a series of enzymes located on the cristae of the mitochondria. These enzymes are arranged in sequential order so the products of the reactions can be relayed from enzyme to enzyme as the chemical reactions occur.

The overall results of one revolution of the Krebs cycle can be summed up as follows: (1) two carbons released as two carbon dioxide molecules, (2) the production of GTP (guanosine triphosphate) which is converted to ATP, (3) three pairs of hydrogen atoms carried to the ETS bound to reduced NAD^+, and (4) one pair of hydrogen atoms carried to ETS by FAD^+ (Fig. 3–16). Remember that for each glucose molecule at the beginning of glycolysis, two acetate molecules enter the Krebs (this is because there were two pyruvates produced from each glucose). The total of two cranks of the Krebs results in the production of two ATP's, four CO_2 molecules, and 16 hydrogen. The four hydrogen atoms from glycolysis, the four from pyruvic acid breakdown, and the 16 from the Krebs cycle yield a total of 24 hydrogen atoms (Fig. 3–16).

Although the Krebs cycle is considered part of the aerobic metabolism, very little ATP is produced during this stage, and the NADH and $FADH_2$ cannot be used directly by any of the Krebs enzymes to produce energy. The primary role of energy production is reserved for the final series of catabolic reactions that remove the hydrogen ions from the NAD and FAD (from glycolysis and the Krebs) and combine them with oxygen. The energy released is harnessed to resynthesize ATP from ADP and P_i. These activities occur in the *electron transport system (ETS)* located on "stalks" of the inner membrane of the mitochondria. Since the process of forming ATP involves the binding of free inorganic phosphate (P_i) to ADP and oxygen to the hydrogen ions, the overall process is referred to as *oxidative phosphorylation.*

BIOCHEMISTRY OF THE KREBS CYCLE

The Krebs cycle begins with the coming of the 2-C acetyl group (from Acetyl CoA) with the 4-C oxaloacetate to yield citrate and CoA. Citrate is then changed to isocitrate under the influence of the enzyme aconitase in a series of steps to allow for a decarboxylation (loss of a carbon as CO_2) to occur. The first oxidative decarboxylation is catalyzed by isocitrate dehydrogenase which yields the 5-carbon alphaketoglutarate and a pair of hydrogens carried from the cycle by NAD. The second oxidative decarboxylation yields the 4-carbon succinyl CoA (with the release of more CO_2) and another pair of hydrogens carried by NAD. This reaction is catalyzed by the alpha-ketoglutarate dehydrogenase enzyme complex. Following this step is the only direct energy production of the Krebs cycle. The generation of a guanosine triphosphate (GTP) molecule from GDP is an example of a substrate-level phosphorylation, a reaction catalyzed by the enzyme succinyl CoA synthetase. The phosphoryl group of GTP can be easily transferred to ADP to form ATP so it can be counted the same as other ATP production.

The four carbon succinate is converted to oxaloacetate in three steps: an oxidation (loss of hydrogen), a hydration (adding water), and a second oxidation reaction. Oxaloacetate is thereby regenerated for another round of the cycle. The oxidation to fumarate is different in that the two hydrogens are carried by FAD under the influence of succinate dehydrogenase. FAD is used because there is insufficient energy in this step to reduce (add hydrogens to) NAD. The next step requires water to be added (with the enzyme, fumarase) to form malate, and then malate is oxidized (catalyzed to malate dehydrogenase) and the hydrogen pair is carried away by NAD (Fig. 3–17).

ELECTRON TRANSPORT SYSTEM (ETS)

The hydrogen atoms released from the glycolytic pathway and the Krebs cycle (and the pathways that process fat) represent a large

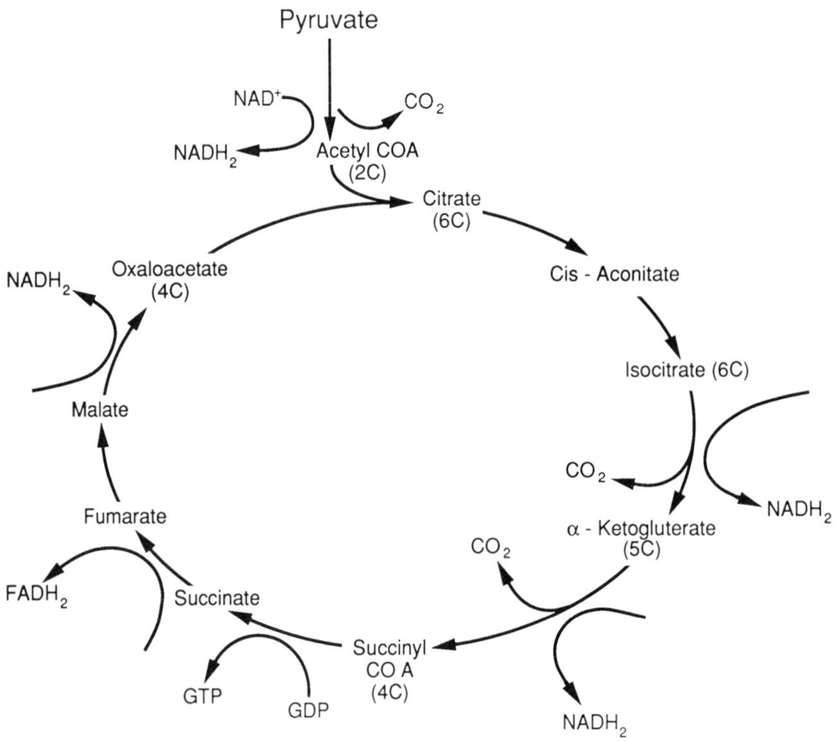

Fig. 3–16. A schematic representation of the Krebs cycle. Note that 1) two carbons are lost via CO_2, 2) three pairs of H are carried away by NAD, 3) one pair of H is carried by FAD, and 4) one molecule of ATP is produced for every acetyl COA entering the mitochondrion.

source of unharnessed energy that must be oxidized to realize the full potential of the metabolic system. In fact, over 90 percent of the total ATP produced in the metabolic pathways comes from the processing of these hydrogens through the ETS. These hydrogens are carried to the ETS by the carrier molecules and NAD and FAD, but the pair of hydrogens carried by NAD yield more energy than the pair carried by FAD because they enter the ETS at a higher level. Figure 3–18 is a schematic representation of the energy output from the ETS. Note that three ATP are released for every pair of hydrogens carried by NAD, but that only two ATP are produced for the hydrogen pairs carried by FAD.

Producing energy through the ETS is called *oxidative phosphorylation,* a two step process where the hydrogen atoms lose their electrons (oxidation) and the energy released is used to phosphorylate ADP to form ATP. Phosphorylation takes place as hydrogen atoms carried by NAD or FAD enter the ETS, their electrons are stripped from them, and the electrons are transferred down a series of electron carriers (called the respiratory assembly) to atomic oxygen (which is provided by the oxygen we breathe). The protons (the basic hydrogen molecule without its electron) are pumped outside the mitochondria, producing a chemical and osmotic difference between the inside and outside of the membrane. These protons then enter the mitochondria at a "stalk" (on the inner membrane) to combine with oxygen and the energy released from this movement is used to couple a phosphate ion to ADP, thus forming ATP. Of course, this coupling occurs at three different places in ETS for hydrogens carried by NAD and at only two places for those carried by FAD. The entire process occurs because oxygen is available as the final electron acceptor, and the hydrogen ion and its electron move from an area of electronegativity (NADH and $FADH_2$) to an area of electropositivity (atomic oxygen). Without oxygen, there would be no reason for hydrogen ions nor electrons to move through the ETS and

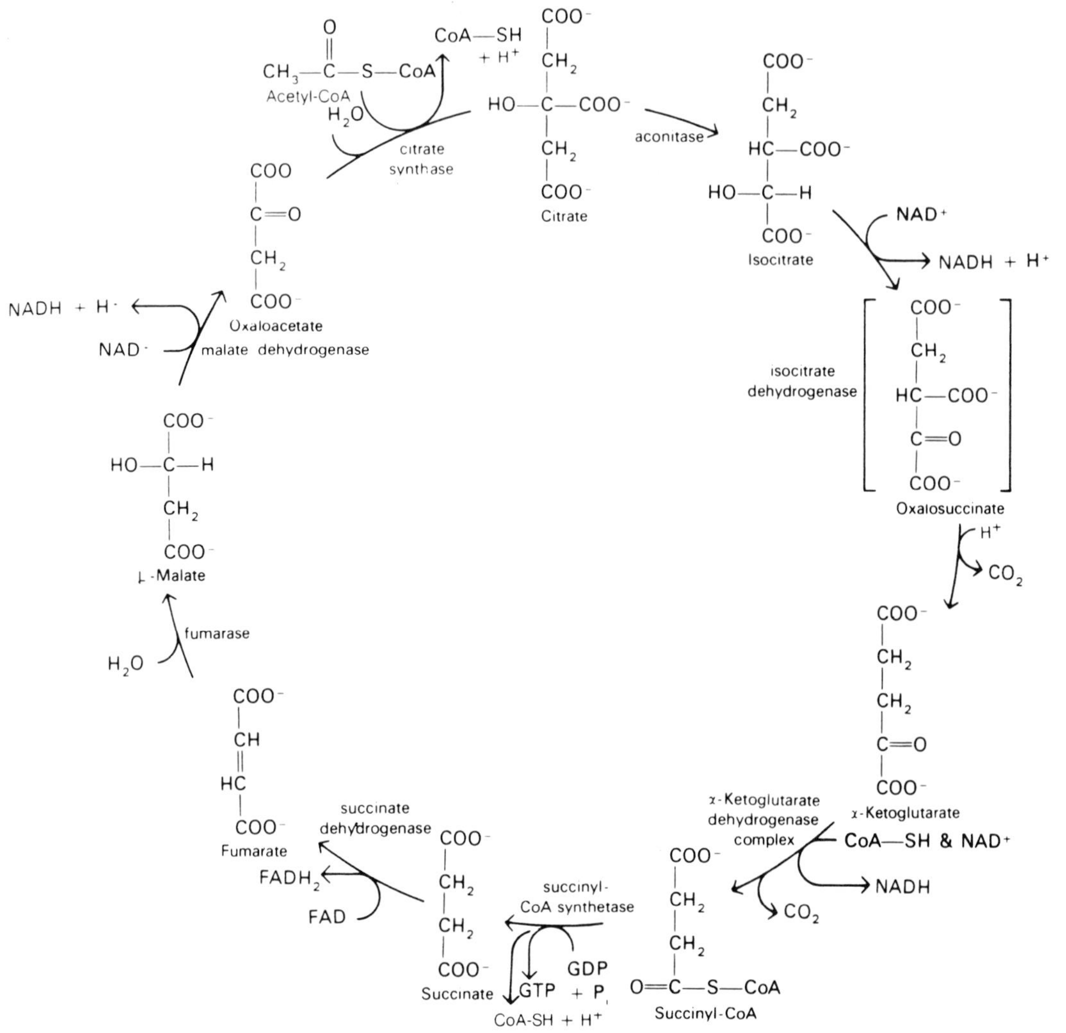

Fig. 3–17. Chemical structure, enzymes, and reactions of the Krebs cycle. (From Armstrong, F.B. *Biochemistry.* Courtesy of Oxford Univ. Press, 1989.)

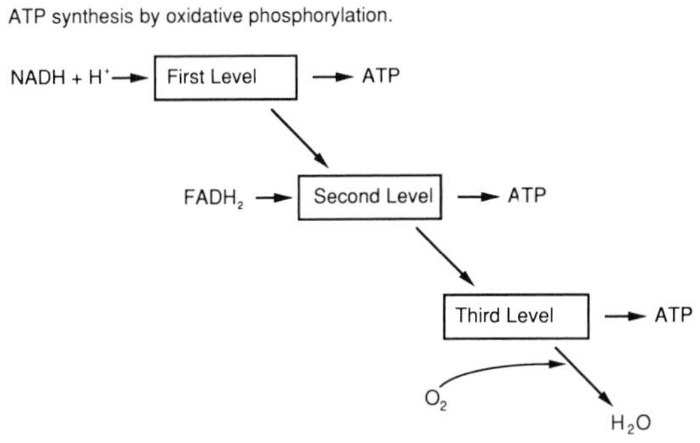

Fig. 3–18. ATP synthesis by oxidative phosphorylation.

energy production would not be possible (Fig. 3–19).

ENERGY PRODUCTION FROM AEROBIC GLYCOLYSIS

Now the total energy production from aerobic glycolysis can be calculated by looking at each stage of metabolism from glucose to the final degradation product, water:

1. Anaerobic glycolysis.
   a. A pair of hydrogens are carried by NAD to mitochondria by one of the shuttle systems for each 3 carbon G-3-P that travels down to pyruvate.

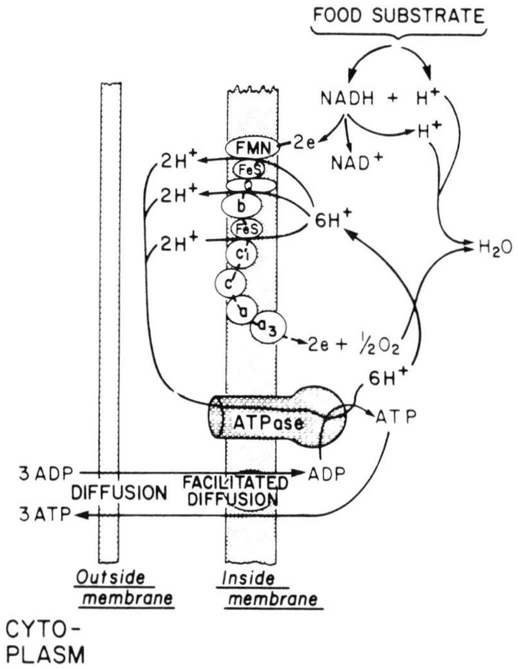

Fig. 3–19. The chemiosmotic theory of oxidative phosphorylation for forming great quantities of ATP. Electrons are carried down a series of electron carriers to atomic oxygen. (From Guyton, A.C. *Human Physiology and Mechanism of Disease*, 4th Ed. Courtesy of W.B. Saunders Co., 1987.)

There are two 3 carbon pieces for each glucose molecule that starts, so

if carried by the glycerol phosphate system they enter ETS with FAD as the carrier

$$2\ FADH_2 = 4\ ATP$$

if carried by the malate aspartate system they enter ETS with NAD as the carrier

$$2NADH + H = 6\ ATP$$

b. 2 ATP's are produced directly for each 3-carbon piece that is processed. There are two three carbon pieces so the total =

$$4\ ATP$$

2. Intermediate step (between glycolytic pathway and Krebs).
   a. A pair of hydrogens are carried to ETS by NAD for each pyruvate processed. For two pyruvates per glucose there are 2 pairs.

$$2\ NADH + H = 6\ ATP$$

   A CO_2 is also lost at this point, but no energy is directly produced.
3. Krebs cycle.
   a. 3 pairs of hydrogen are carried by NAD for each cycle and the cycle occurs twice for each glucose

$$6\ NADH + H = 18\ ATP$$

   b. 1 pair of hydrogen are carried by FAD for each cycle

$$2\ FADH_2 = 4\ ATP$$

   c. 1 GTP (ATP) is produced each cycle and the cycle goes twice

$$2\ cycles = 2\ ATP$$

Total ATP

1. Anaerobic glycolysis	
From hydrogens carried to ETS	4 ATP
or	(6 ATP)
Direct energy	4 ATP
2. Intermediate step	
From hydrogens carried to ETS	6 ATP
3. Krebs cycle	
From hydrogens carried by NAD	18 ATP
From hydrogens carried by FAD	4 ATP
Produced directly	2 ATP
Total	38 (or 40)
(depending on shuttle)	
Subtract 2 ATP to start glycolysis	−2 ATP
	36 (or 38)

A summary of the yield described above can be seen in Table 3–1.

FAT METABOLISM

About 40% of the calories ingested in the normal diet are from fat. In addition, some of the carbohydrates eaten are converted to fat and used later for energy. For this reason, fat metabolism is an important factor in en-

Table 3–1. Summary of Yield

Phase of Respiration	*High Energy Products*	*ATP from Oxidative Phosphorylation*	*ATP Subtotal*
Glycolysis (glucose to	4 ATP	—	4
pyruvic acid)	2 NAD_{red} or 2 FAD	6–4	10–8
Pyruvic acid to acetyl CoA	1 NAD_{red} (×2)	6	16–14
Krebs Cycle	1 ATP (×2)	—	18–16
	3 NAD_{red} (×2)	18	36–34
	1 FAD_{red} (×2)	4	40–38
	Total (aerobic) 2 ATP		36–38 ATP

ergy production. Triglycerides make up the majority of fats consumed in the diet. Dietary triglycerides, as well as cholesterol and some phospholipids, undergo little digestion in the mouth or stomach. However, in the small intestine, bile from the liver emulsifies fat molecules so that enzymes can act on their surfaces. Pancreatic lipases complete the process by breaking the emulsified fats into free fatty acids (FAA), glycerol, and monoglycerides. These particles are then processed by the epithelium of the small intestine and encased into globules with a protein coat. These globules are called *chylomicrons,* and are carried through the lymph system to the great veins of the neck where they enter the blood stream.

Dietary fats in the blood are cleared within a few hours of eating by either the liver or other body tissues. The liver is an important organ in the processing of fats. It not only uses fat as a fuel, but converts lipids from chylomicrons into other blood lipid products such as *lipoproteins.* Remember, fats are hydrophobic and must be tied to proteins in some manner in order to be transported in the blood. Lipoproteins are mixtures of triglycerides, phospholipids, cholesterol, and proteins and are classified according to their density as *low* or *very low density* (LDL or VLDL), which function to carry triglycerides from the liver to adipose tissue, or as *high density lipoprotein* (HDL).

Tissues (especially adipose tissue, the heart, and skeletal muscle) have the enzyme lipoprotein lipase (LPL) in the cell walls of capillaries flowing through them. This enzyme is responsible for clearing fats from the blood. LPL in adipose tissue is activated at meal time by increases in blood glucose and insulin. Muscle and heart LPL is activated during exercise, when insulin falls and glucagon rises.

During exercise, fats are released from adipose tissue by the action of *hormone-sensitive lipase.* The process is called *lipolysis* (lipo = fat). Lipolysis results in the release of *free fatty acids* (FFA) from triglyceride breakdown in the fat cell. FFA's are carried primarily by the blood protein *albumin.* Although the quantity of FFA's in the blood is not extremely high, the turnover is rapid and they are a major supply of energy during work. The rate of lipolysis has a major effect on the uptake of FFA's in muscle since about half of the circulatory FFA's are extracted from blood flowing through the muscles. These fat molecules are then transported to the mitochondria of the cell and degraded for energy.

The most common form of fat, the *triglyceride,* consists of a glycerol portion and three fatty acids (Fig. 3–20). Note that fatty acids (FA) are long, even numbered carbon compounds with hydrogen atoms on most or all of the carbons and a carboxyl group on the end. Free fatty acids (FFA) are FA that are released in the blood and carried by the plasma proteins for muscle fuel. Formation of fat *(lipogenesis)* occurs in a number of tissues, primarily the liver and adipose tissue, in response to elevated blood glucose levels. Fat represents the largest supply of stored energy. In a non-obese man of 160 pounds, it is estimated that 80 to 85% of his body's energy (approximately 140,000 calories) is stored as fat, compared to less than 2,000 calories attributed to glycogen storage.

USING FATS FOR ENERGY

Making fats available for energy involves four major steps or processes: (1) release of

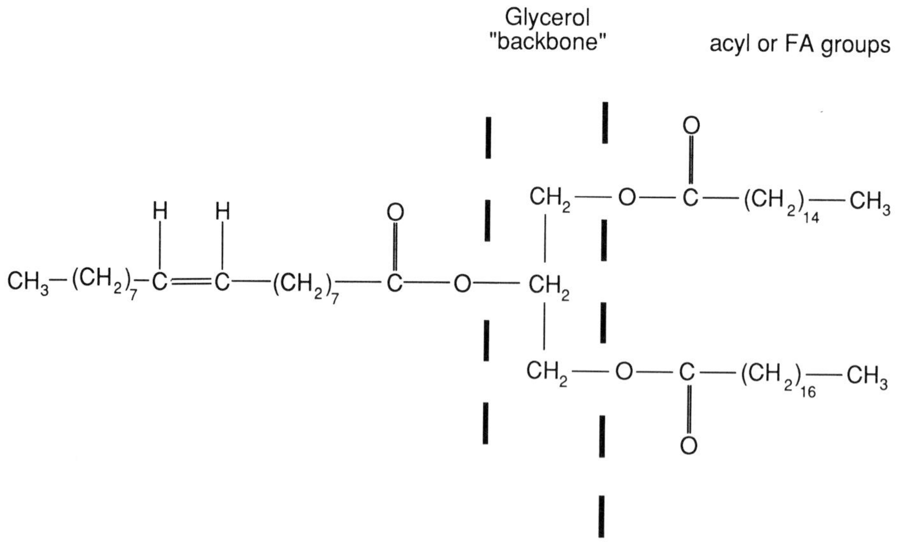

Fig. 3–20. A triglyceride (Triacylglycerol). Note the long chain fatty acid (FA) on each of the three carbon glycerol molecules. The FA on the center carbon is unsaturated because it contains fewer hydrogens than it can hold.

adipose FFA's into the blood, (2) movement of FFA's into the muscle from the blood, (3) processing of the FFA to prepare it for metabolism, and (4) metabolizing fats for energy.

Release of FFA from Fat Cells

The entry of FFA's into the fat cell is facilitated by adipose tissue lipoprotein lipase (AT-LPL). After entry, the FFA's are *esterified* (made into triglycerides) for storage. The opposite process or breakdown of triglycerides for release from the fat cell is called *lipolysis.* This process is stimulated by a hormone-sensitive lipase, which is turned on by both epinephrine and norepinephrine during exercise as well as by growth hormone (GH). Epinephrine and norepinephrine initiate lipolysis, whereas GH helps maintain it during prolonged exercise. Mobilized FFA's are carried by the protein albumin to the active muscle beds.

Movement of FFA's into the Cell

The uptake of FFA's from the blood occurs at a specific receptor site on the muscle cell membrane. There are many receptor sites on the cell membrane and FFA's are extremely soluble because of the membrane's basic structure, so that the entry of the FFA's into the membrane is rapid if FFA's are available in the blood. In fact, nearly half of all FFA's are removed in the muscle capillary beds during each circulation of blood through the muscle, regardless of the FFA level or blood flow.

Processing FFA

Once the fatty acids enter the cytoplasm of the cell they are activated by ATP and carried by coenzyme A to the mitochondrial membrane. Since the site of fatty acid oxidation is the mitochondria, a carrier molecule *carnitine* and the enzyme *carnitine translocase* are responsible for the transport of the FFA into the mitochondria. The CoA is stripped off and the FFA combines with *carnitine* to form *fatty acyl-carnitine,* which moves across the membrane where carnitine is released and the fatty acid is carried into the matrix by CoA (Fig. 3–21).

Metabolizing Fats for Energy (Beta Oxidation)

Once fatty acids have been carried into the mitochondria, they can be metabolized for energy using a process called *beta oxidation.* In this process, the long, even-numbered fatty acids are broken apart two carbons at a time, forming a structure (acetate) that is the same as the two carbon piece produced when pyruvate loses a carbon as it is carried to the Krebs cycle. In fact, the two carbon piece broken off from a fatty acid is also carried to the

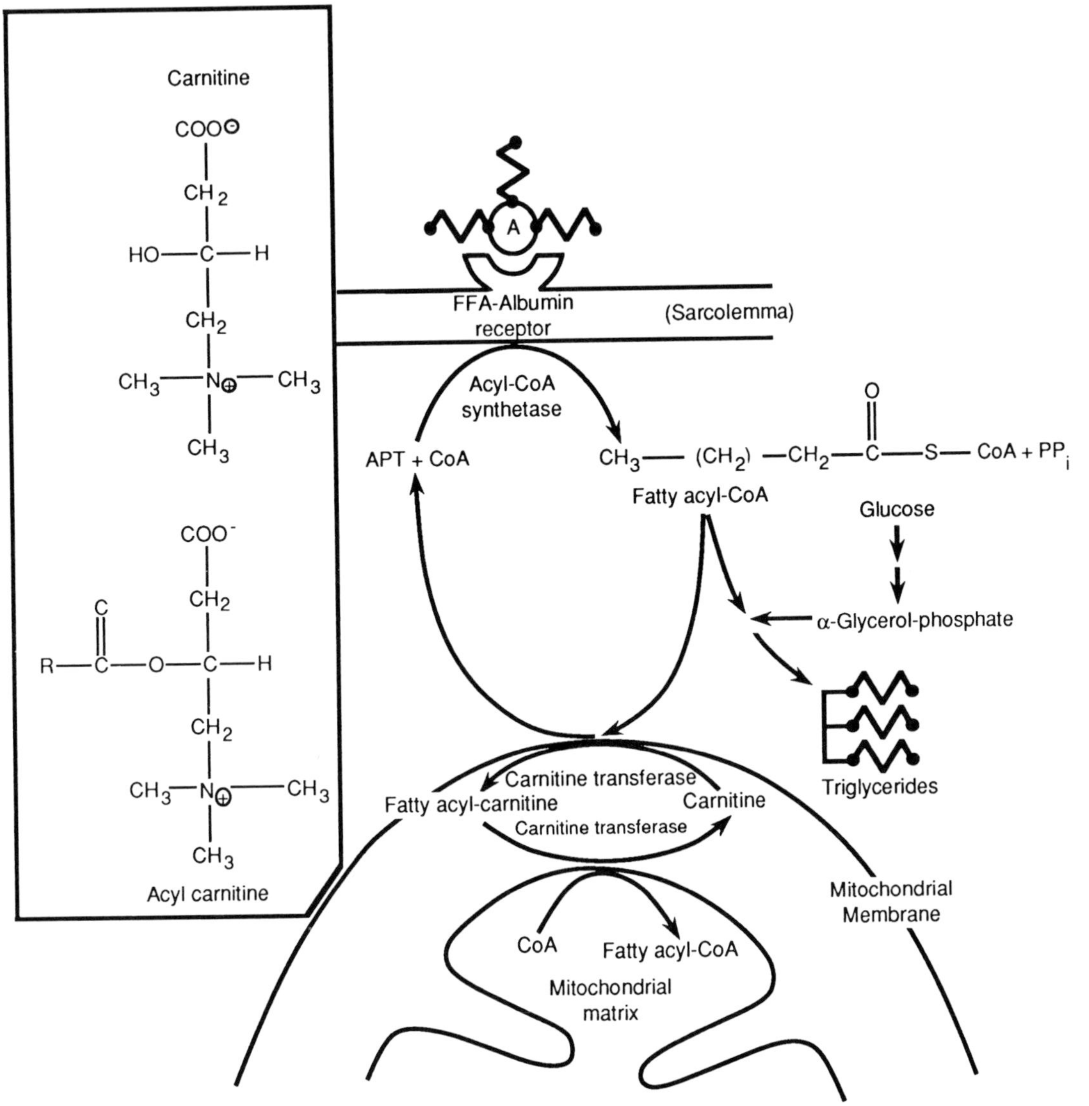

Fig. 3–21. Free fatty acid (FFA) activation and carnitine translocase. Prior to either oxidation or storage as triglycerides in muscle, fatty acids delivered by the circulation must be activated; this involves ATP and coenzyme A (CoA). To gain entry into the mitochondrial matrix for oxidation, the activated fatty acid must combine with a carrier substance, carnitine, which exists in the mitochondrial membrane. An enzyme, carnitine transferase, facilitates the formation of the fatty acyl carnitine complex, as well as the dissociation of the complex and release of the activated fatty acid into the matrix. The translocation of activated fatty acids from the cytosol into mitochondria is a rate-limiting step in lipid metabolism. (From Brooks, G.A., and Fahey, T.D. *Exercise Physiology.* Courtesy of John Wiley and Sons, 1984.)

Krebs cycle by coenzyme A as Acetyl CoA. The Krebs cycle cannot tell the difference between the acetyl CoA formed from fat degradation and that formed from sugars. Four hydrogen atoms are also released each time a two carbon segment is broken off from a FFA. Two of these are carried to ETS by NAD, and two by FAD. If a fatty acid had 18 carbons (stearic acid), there would be nine pair of carbons but only eight breaks as shown in Figure 3–22.

It is easy to calculate the energy available from any fatty acid. Since two of the four hydrogens available from the break are carried by NAD, there are three ATP's produced in ETS from those two. The other two are carried by FAD so only two ATP's are produced from them. The gross yield from each

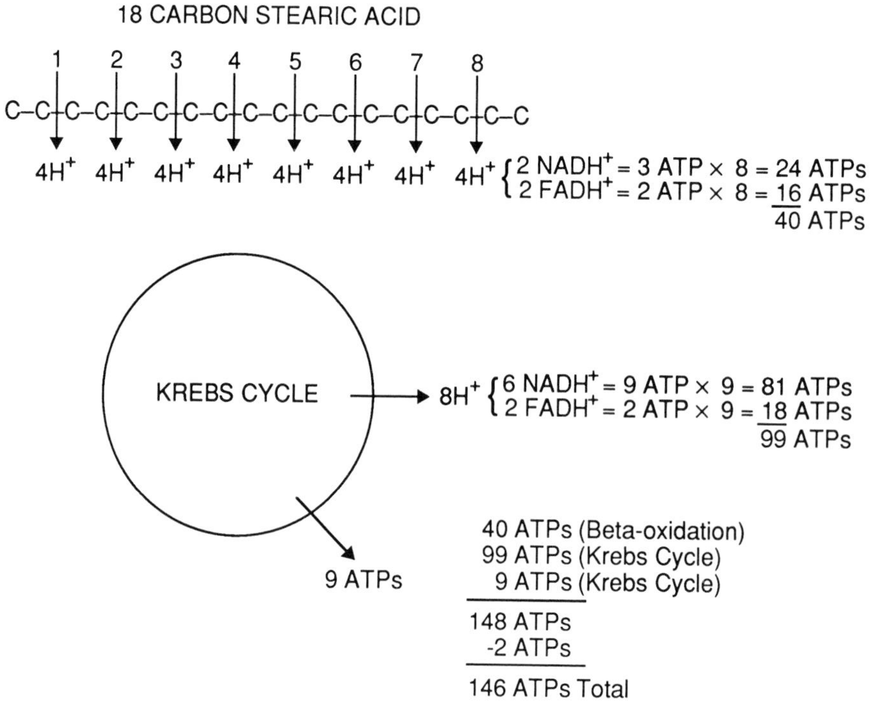

Summary of the energy output from our 18 carbon fatty acid.

Fig. 3–22. Summary of energy output from an 18 carbon fatty acid. Note that stearic acid has nine pairs of carbons but only eight breaks.

break is therefore five ATP's. The two carbon pieces are metabolized through Krebs just like the two-carbon pieces from glucose and produce six hydrogens carried by NAD for nine ATP, two hydrogens with FAD for two ATP, and one GTP that counts as an ATP. This totals 12 ATP for each two carbon carried away. For the 18 carbon fatty acid above, there would be eight breaks at five ATP per break = 40 ATP, plus nine pair of carbons through Krebs at 12 ATP per pair = 108 ATP. The grand total would be 149 ATP per 18 carbon fatty acid. However, two ATP are needed for the process to begin so the *net* gain is 146 (Fig. 3–22).

It is interesting to note that the rate of free fatty acid turnover in the blood is extremely rapid. One-half of the circulating fatty acids are replaced every two to three minutes. Normal fatty acid levels are about 150 mg/liter.

If liver cells contain sufficient ATP so that further ATP production through the Krebs cycle is not needed, some of the fatty acids are channeled into an alternate pathway. This pathway converts two 2-carbon segments into *acetoacetic acid* or *beta-hydroxybutyric acid.* These products are known as *ketone bodies.* If the production of ketone bodies exceeds the rate they can be decomposed in the Krebs cycle, the body eliminates them through the kidneys or lungs in the form of acetone. Ketosis occurs in people who have been dieting or fasting, where fatty acid metabolism is forced into action. Acetone breath or ketones in the urine are two excellent indicators of ketosis. A high level of circulating acidic ketones causes acidosis in the blood.

BETA-OXIDATION

Beta-oxidation is a cyclic series of reactions that (1) degrades fatty acyl CoA separating acetyl CoA molecules by cleaving two carbon atoms off the long hydrocarbon chain of fatty acyl CoA for use in the Krebs cycle, and (2) produces NADH and FADH for oxidation in the electron transport system.

Starting from the carboxyl end of the fatty

acid, the saturated acyl CoA is degraded first, by the oxidation of *acyl CoA by Acyl CoA dehydrogenase* to enoyl CoA, with the release of a pair of hydrogen atoms to FAD. The second reaction involves the hydration of the double bond between the second and third carbons by the enzyme *enoyl CoA hydrase to form betahydroxyacyl CoA*. The third reaction involves an oxidation reaction, which converts the hydroxyl group of the third carbon atom into a keto group catalyzed by *3-hydroxyacyl CoA dehydrogenase* and generates NADH in the process. The fourth and final step is the cleavage of ketoacyl CoA by *beta-ketothiolase* with the addition of a CoA molecule which yields acetyl CoA and an acyl CoA shortened by two carbon atoms.

The shortened acyl CoA then undergoes another cycle of oxidation, each time shortened by 2 carbon strands (acetyl CoA) and generating NADH and FADH in the process, and continues through the cycle until the fatty acid chain is completely chopped up (Fig. 3–23).

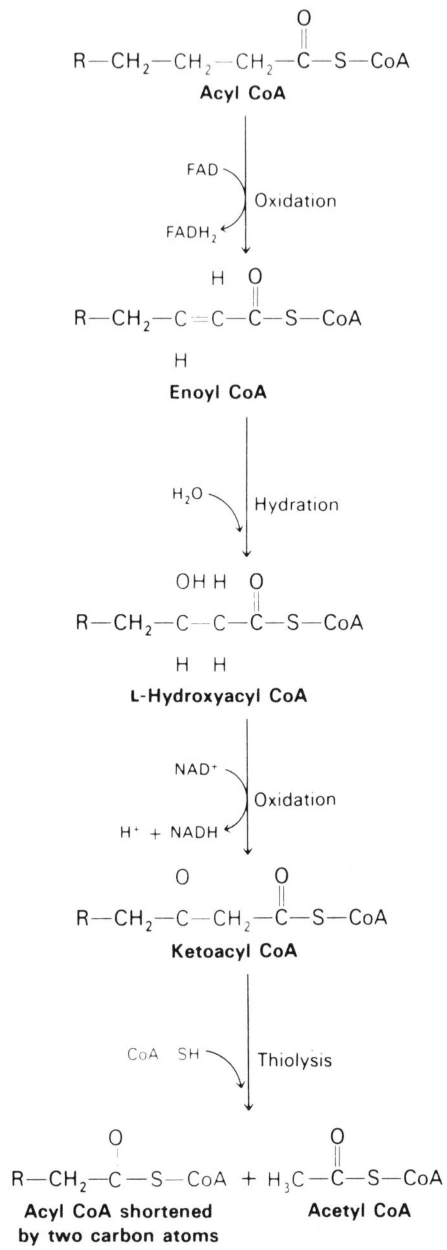

Fig. 3–23. In the beta-oxidation cycle, saturated fatty acid chains that have been transported into the mitochondrial matrix are processed to form three products (acetyl CoA, NADH, and FADH) with each crank of the cycle. These products will eventually be used for further ATP production. Note that with each crank of the beta-oxidation mechanism, the long-chain fatty acid is reduced in two-carbon segments that will eventually enter the Krebs cycle. (Modified from Stryer, L. *Biochemistry.* Courtesy of W.H. Freeman, 1975.)

PROTEIN METABOLISM

Proteins have many important roles to perform in the body. They form the building blocks for tissues and steroid hormones, are found in plasma membranes, are used for enzymes, bind substances, and act as a buffer in the blood. They can also be used for energy. Experiments have shown that a 160-pound man uses 400 g of protein each day. Of this total, 330 g of protein are reincorporated and reused while the remaining 70 g are converted to glucose and oxidized to produce energy. Approximately 70 to 100 g of proteins must be replenished daily. On the average it is recommended that a normal adult consume 0.8 g of protein per kg of body weight each day.

Proteins are large molecules made from smaller carbon subunits called *amino acids* (Fig. 3–24). Note that amino acids contain carbon and hydrogen just like fatty acids, but also contain nitrogen.

Each of the 20 naturally occurring amino acids can be catabolized and converted to energy through different pathways in the Krebs cycle. The first step in this process is *deami-*

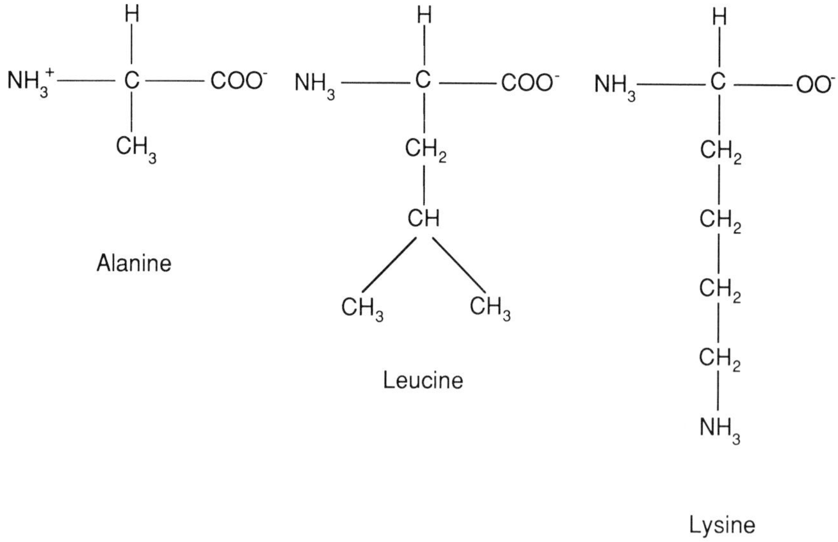

Fig. 3–24. Examples of common amino acids. Note that each contains a nitrogen group (NH_3^+).

nation, where the nitrogen ($-NH_2$) portion is removed from the amino acid, leaving a deaminated AA and the $-NH_2$, which is converted to urea and excreted in the urine. Depending on the carbon structure, this deaminated amino acid can enter the Krebs cycle at different levels of acetyl-CoA, pyruvate, oxaloacetate, alpha-ketoglycerate, succinyl CoA, or fumarate (Fig. 3–25).

When amino acids are used for energy, the nitrogen unit must be removed and excreted. If enough protein is eaten to match the amount of protein used, *nitrogen balance* is said to exist. The body is in *positive* nitrogen balance when intake exceeds excretion. This is very common in growing children, where large amounts of nitrogen are utilized for the building of muscle and bones. A *negative* nitrogen balance occurs when the output of nitrogen is greater than that consumed. The body catabolizes muscle and connective tissue to provide the necessary amino acids. Even if adequate amounts of protein are consumed every day, muscle tissue will be catabolized to act as the primary fuel if carbohydrate and fat intake is insufficient.

GLUCONEOGENESIS

Cardiac muscle is endowed with the ability to utilize many different types of substrates produced by the body, such as lactate, glucose, and fatty acids. However, the other tissues of the body, especially the brain, are dependent upon the constant supply of glucose as their primary fuel. The normal daily requirement of glucose for an adult is about 160 grams, of which the brain uses 120 grams. The normal stores of glucose consist of 5–6 grams circulating in the blood, and an additional 400 grams of glycogen in the muscles. Under normal conditions, this amount of glucose is enough to meet the body's needs. However, if the glucose stores are depleted by long exercise bouts or by periods of starvation, the body must be able to produce additional glucose from noncarbohydrate sources to survive. The process of producing new carbohydrates from these sources is called *gluconeogenesis.*

The major site of gluconeogenesis is the liver. Some occurs in the cortex of the kidney, but because of the kidney's smaller gluconeogenic mass, only about 10 percent of all new sugar is produced there. The main starting point of the gluconeogenic pathway is pyruvate whether the new sugar is to be made from lactate or some amino acid. Since the end point of the glycolytic pathway is pyruvate, it is easy to visualize gluconeogenesis as a simple reversal of glycolysis forming a new sugar molecule at the top. However, there are several irreversible steps in the glycolytic pathway and glycolysis is a reaction that goes

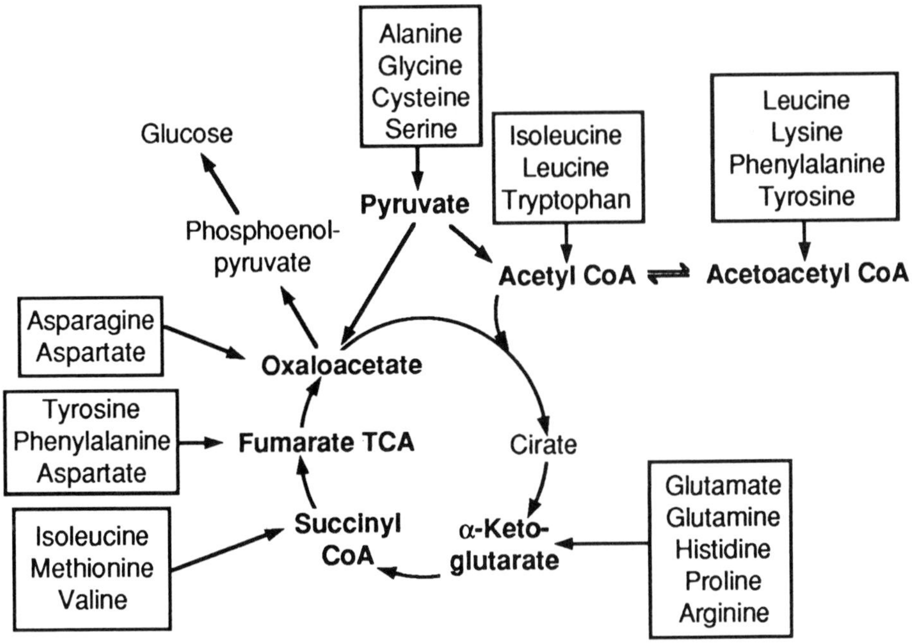

Fig. 3–25. Various points at which the carbon skeletons of the 20 amino acids enter the Krebs cycle for oxidation. (From Stryer, L. *Biochemistry.* Courtesy of W.H. Freeman, 1975.)

"downhill" from high to lower energy levels. Because of this, pyruvate must bypass the irreversible steps of glycolysis and have a significant amount of energy added to it to return to the higher energy molecule, G-6-P. In fact, the conversion of pyruvate to glucose requires six high-energy phosphate bonds.

FATE OF LACTATE

As discussed before, the major by-product of anaerobic glycolysis is lactic acid. In fact, the accumulation of lactate in muscle tissue and blood during heavy exercise is suspected of being one of the primary causes of fatigue. Obviously, lactate is not a molecule the body needs or wants to store for any purpose. Research in 1980 by Brooks and Gaesser using radioactive carbon isotopes traced the destination of lactate in rats as it was removed from the blood and muscle after intense exercise (Fig. 3–26). A summary of their findings follows:

1. By far the greatest amount of lactate produced from exercise was metabolized in aerobic respiration by skeletal muscle, heart muscle, the kidneys, and the liver. Lactate is, in fact, converted to pyruvate and eventually to CO_2 and H_2O in the Krebs cycle, and the radioactive carbon was expelled as CO_2 in the expired air. Seventy-two percent of the lactate was converted to pyruvate and channeled through the aerobic oxidative pathways.

2. Lactate was also resynthesized, to glucose and glycogen (gluconeogenesis). However, resynthesis of glycogen from lactate is a slow process, and therefore acounts for only about 18% of the total lactic acid removal. This conversion occurs mainly in the liver and muscle and is sometimes referred to as the Cori cycle.

3. Some lactate is converted in the liver to pyruvate by LDH, and then transaminated to the amino acid *alanine*. As exercise intensity increases, the production of alanine in the muscle also increases. Alanine released from the muscle is transported by the blood to the liver, where it is deaminated to pyruvate, and converted back into glucose (gluconeogenesis). This glucose is, in turn, released into the blood to help maintain blood glucose levels and is also used as a fuel by the active muscles. It has been proposed that alanine indirectly supplies as much as 10 to 15% of the total energy supply during exercise. Although only about 8% of the lactate is removed by this pathway, it is unique because it has long been

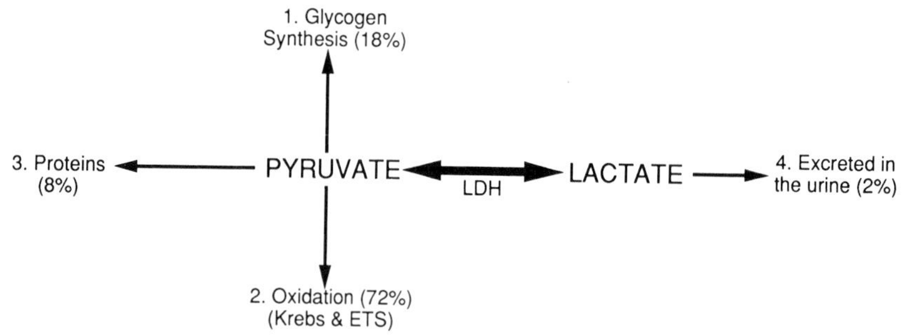

The fate of lactic acid. The lactic acid removal from blood and muscle during recovery can be converted to glucose, protein, or CO_2 and H_2O (oxidized).

Fig. 3–26. The fate of lactic acid. The lactic acid removed from blood and muscle during recovery can be converted to glycose, protein, or CO_2 and H_2O (oxidized).

felt that muscle was incapable of producing substrates for metabolism.

4. Finally, lactate can be excreted directly into the urine or sweat. However, this only accounts for about 2% of the lactic acid removed.

CONTROL OF METABOLISM

Metabolism is primarily regulated by four hormones: *insulin, glucagon, epinephrine,* and *norepinephrine.*

Insulin

Insulin, a hormone secreted by the beta cells of the pancreas, is the most important regulator of metabolism. After a meal, the amount of glucose entering the bloodstream increases (high blood glucose level), and in response the pancreas secretes insulin, which promotes entry of glucose into the cell. This rise in insulin is a signal that the body is fed, stimulating the storage of fats in the liver and the increased synthesis of proteins. The enzyme *glycogen synthetase* is stimulated in both muscle and liver, increasing glycogen synthesis and conversely suppressing gluconeogenesis.

Glucagon

Insulin is secreted by the beta cells of the pancreas in response to elevated blood glucose. Glucagon is secreted from the alpha cells of that same gland in response to low blood glucose levels. Glucagon acts on the liver by stimulating the breakdown of glycogen and inhibiting glycogen synthesis by the feedback of cAMP, which switches off glycogen synthetase and switches on phosphorylase. Obviously, if the body is low in energy as reflected by blood glucose level, fatty acid metabolism is diminished, while gluconeogenesis is enhanced by the hormone glucagon. In summary, glucagon increases the release of glucose by the liver, while increasing the level of cAMP in adipose tissue (promotes the breakdown of the triglycerides), and in the cell (promotes glycogen breakdown). The major role of glucagon, however, is gluconeogenesis.

Epinephrine and Norepinephrine

The two catecholamines, epinephrine and norepinephrine, are important regulators of metabolism. Norepinephrine is released from the terminal ends of the sympathetic nerve endings, while epinephrine is released from the adrenal medulla in response to low blood glucose level or exercise. These catecholamines increase the amount of glucose released into the blood by stimulating the mobilization of glycogen. This is accomplished by triggering cAMP, thus stimulating glycogenolysis (breakdown of glycogen to glucose). Although these catecholamines have very similar actions to those of glucagon, they differ in that the breakdown of glycogen is greater in muscle than in the liver (Table 3–2).

HEAT FROM METABOLIC PROCESSES

Metabolism can be defined as the sum total of all the chemcal reactions of the body. Met-

Table 3–2. Summary of Hormonal Regulation of the Metabolism of Carbohydrates, Fats, and Proteins

Hormone	*Actions*
Insulin	Stimulates glucose uptake by the cells, especially muscle
	Stimulates conversion of glucose into glycogen (glycogenesis)
	Stimulates fat synthesis and inhibits fat breakdown
	Stimulates active transport of amino acids into cells, especially muscle
	Stimulates protein synthesis
Glucagon	Stimulates conversion of glycogen into glucose (glycogenolysis)
	Stimulates conversion of noncarbohydrates into glucose (gluconeogenesis)
	Stimulates breakdown of fats (fat mobilization)
Epinephrine	Stimulates conversion of glycogen into glucose (glycogenolysis)
	Stimulates breakdown of fats (fat mobilization)
	Stimulates conversion of noncarbohydrates into glucose (gluconeogenesis)

abolic rate is expressed in units of heat (calories). A calorie (cal) is the amount of heat required to raise 1 g of water 1°C. The kilocalorie, or large Calorie (with a capital "C"), is equal to 1000 calories, and is commonly used to express energy expenditure of the body.

Direct Calorimetry

Since the amount of heat released from the body is indicative of the metabolic rate, any means used to measure this output is an excellent measurement of metabolism. To measure the amount of heat released from the body *directly*, a subject is placed in a large insulated chamber where the heat from the body warms the air of the chamber. The air in the chamber is kept at a constant temperature, however, and the warm air from the body is forced through pipes in a cool water bath. The rate of heat gain by the water bath is equal to the total heat output of the body.

This method has several disadvantages: (1) the equipment is expensive and difficult to use; (2) the equipment is inflexible and cannot be used except under ideal laboratory conditions; and (3) the test cannot be used as a maximal work test without great difficulty.

Luckily, metabolic heat production can also be measured *indirectly* using the amount of oxygen used by the metabolic processes and the amount of carbon dioxide produced. The amount of oxygen used by the body each minute is called "oxygen consumption" and is often expressed as "$\dot{V}O_2$" (volume of oxygen used per minute). The number of kilocalories (a measure of heat usually abbreviated kcals or simply Cals) released per liter of oxygen varies with the type of food burned, but on average, is about 5 kcals of heat per liter of oxygen. At rest, oxygen cost is about .25 liters per minute. Using the conversion above, the resting caloric cost would be about 1.25 kcals per minute. Walking uses about a liter of oxygen a minute, so about 5 kcals of heat are released during this activity. This concept will be more fully discussed in Chapter 6.

SELECTED READINGS

Brooks, G.A., Brauner, K.E., and Cassens, R.G.: Glycogen synthesis and metabolism of lactic acid after exercise. Am. J. Physiol. *224*:1162–1166, 1973.

Brooks, G.A., and G.A. Gaesser: End Point of Lactate and Glucose Metabolism after Exhaustive Exercise. J. Appl. Physiol. *49*:1057–1069, 1980.

Conlee, R.K. et al.: Reversal of phosphorylase activation in muscle despite contained contractile activity. Am. J. Physiol. *237*:5, R291–R296, 1979.

Cori, C.F.: Mammalian carbohydrate metabolism. Physiol. Rev. *11*:143–275, 1931.

Dickerson, R.E.: Cytochrome C and the evolution of energy metabolism. Sci. Amer. *242*(34):136, 1980.

Esmann, V. (ed.): *Regulatory Mechanisms of Carbohydrate Metabolism.* New York: Pergamon Press, 1978.

Favier, R.J. et al.: Endurance training reduces lactate productin. J. Appl. Physiol. *61*(3):885–889, 1986.

Fox, S.I.: *Human Physiology.* Dubuque: William C. Brown, Co., 1981.

Gollnick, P.D., and D.W. King: Energy release in the muscle cell. Med. Sci. Sports Exer. *1*:23–31, 1969.

Guyton, A.C.: *Textbook of Medical Physiology.* 6th ed. Philadelphia: W.B. Saunders Co., 1981.

Ganong, W.F.: *Review of Medical Physiology.* 10th ed. Los Altos, CA: Lange Medical Publications, 1981.

Goldsby, R.A.: *Cell and Energy.* 3rd ed. New York: Macmillan, 1977.

Hermansen, L.: Anaerobic energy released. Med. Sci. Sports *1*:32–38, 1969.

Hill, A.V.: The oxidative removal of lactic acid. J. Physiol., *48*:x–xi, 1914.

Homsher, E., and Kean, C.J.: Skeletal muscle energetics and metabolism. Annu. Rev. Physiol. *40*:93, 1978.

Hultman, E., et al.: Energy metabolism in muscle. Prog. Clin. Res. *136*:257–272, 1983.

Klachko, D.M. et al. (eds.): *Hormone and Energy Metabolism.* New York: Plenum Press, 1978.

Lithell, H., Helking, K., Lundquist, G., et al.: Lipoprotein-lipase activity of human skeletal muscle and adipose tissue after intensive physical exercise. Acta Physiol. Scan. *105*:312–315, 1979.

Lund-Anderson, H.: Transport of glucose from blood to brain. Physiol. Rev. *59*:305, 1979.

Munon, Z.A.: *The Structure of Mitochondria.* London: Academic Press, Inc., 1974.

McCarty, R.E.: How cells make ATP. Sci. Amer. *238*(3):104, 1978.

Newsholme, E.A.: The regulation of glycolysis in muscle during sprinting and marathon running. (abstract) Int. J. Sports Med. *1*:212, 1980.

Salans, L.B.: Obesity and the adipose cell. In: Bondy, P.K., and Rosenberg, L.F. (eds.): *Metabolic Control and Disease.* 8th ed. Philadelphia: W.B. Saunders Co., 1980, p. 495.

Stryer, L.: *Biochemistry.* 2nd ed. San Francisco: W.H. Freeman, 1981.

Wynn, C.H.: *The Structure and Function of Enzymes,* 2nd Ed. Baltimore: University Park Press, 1974.

4

Cardiovascular System

In the previous sections, you have seen that movement occurs only as the result of skeletal muscle contraction. Further, most contractions can occur only when motor neurons stimulate the muscles and the muscles have energy available in the form of ATP. The ultimate source of ATP was shown to be from the oxidative metabolism in the mitochondria, where food molecules (from digestion) were processed. In a complex system like the human body, the transportation of both food molecules and oxygen to the cells requires a circulatory system, powered by a pump (the heart) and regulated by circuits (the blood vessels) that can adjust to meet the needs of different muscles at various work loads. The circulatory system also helps maintain the internal homeostasis of the body by removing waste products; helps maintain temperature; and transports hormones and other chemicals throughout the system. The purpose of this section on the heart and circulatory system and the chapter to follow on respiration is to discuss how oxygen gets from the air around us to the mitochondria of the cell so that energy can be produced and muscle contraction can occur—thus allowing movement to take place.

THE HEART

The heart is a four-chambered muscular organ located in the thoracic cavity retrosternally, designed specifically to circulate blood throughout the body. It is roughly the size of a clenched fist and pumps over 700,000 gallons of blood each year.

Blood from the superior and inferior venae cavae and from the coronary sinus drains into the right atrium, then into the right ventricle. From there, it is pumped to the lungs through the pulmonary arteries. Oxygenated blood returns to the heart through the left atrium into the left ventricle. The left ventricle is responsible for pumping blood into the aorta, which carries it throughout the body (Fig. 4–1).

Structurally, the atria (top chambers) and ventricles (lower chambers) are joined by four rings of connective tissue called the *AV ring*, which forms the fibrous "skeleton" of the heart. Electrically, the atria and ventricles are connected by a specialized cardiac conduction system called the *bundle of His*. The atria serve as reservoirs for blood returning to the heart and contract to help fill the ventricles. The left ventricle has a larger muscle mass because it must circulate blood throughout the entire body. The right ventricle is slightly "moon-shaped" and smaller because less pressure is needed to pump blood through the lungs (Fig. 4–2).

Separating each of the four chambers of the heart are valves which prevent the backflow of blood. Between the atria and ventricles are two *atrioventricular* valves: the *tricuspid valve* is located between the right atrium and right ventricle: the *bicuspid* or *mitral valve* lies between the left atrium and left ventricle. Each of these valves is secured in place by strong tendon cords called the *chordae tendineae*. These tendons are attached to the ventricular wall by cone-shaped muscles called *papillary muscles*. The papillary muscle's contraction (during systole) applies tension to the chordae tendineae to prevent the valves from buckling into the atria. Blood is therefore

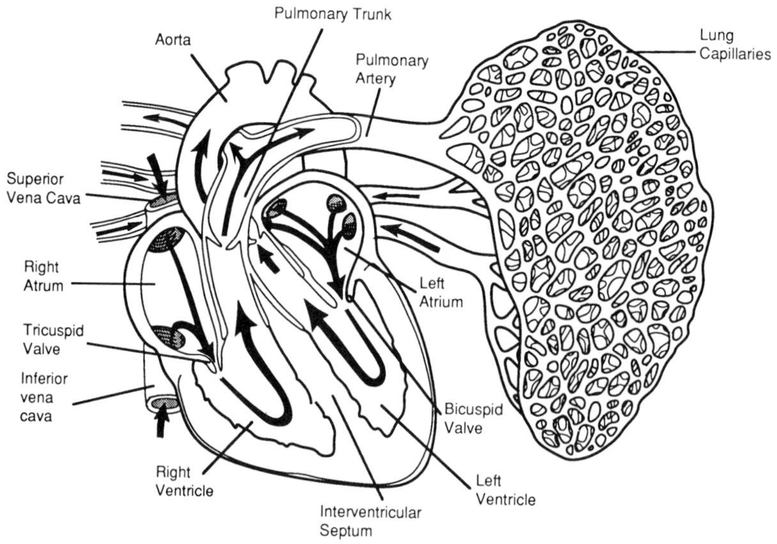

Fig. 4–1. Schematic diagram of blood flow in the heart. Blood enters the heart, is pumped to the lungs through the pulmonary arteries, reenters the heart, and is eventually pumped out through the aorta. (From Spence, A.P., and Mason, E.B. *Human Anatomy and Physiology.* Courtesy of Benjamin-Cummings, 1979.)

forced into the aorta and pulmonary artery. Each of these vessels has a valve which opens to allow blood to flow out of the heart, but closes (as the heart relaxes) to keep blood from flowing back into the ventricles. The valve between the right ventricle and the pulmonary arteries is the *pulmonary semilunar* (half-mooned shaped) *valve*. The valve which lies between the aorta and the left ventricle is referred to as the *aortic semilunar valve* (Fig. 4–3).

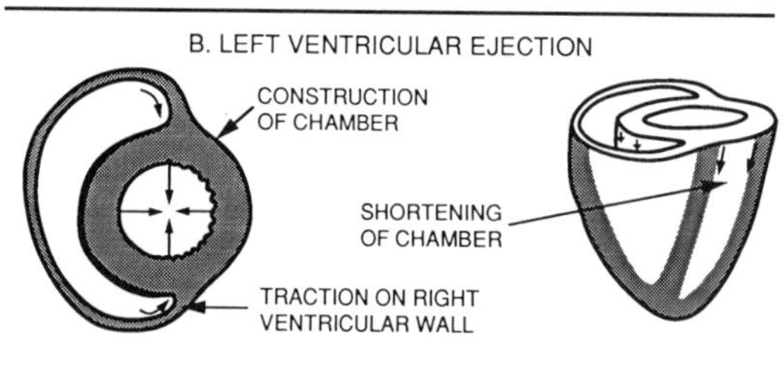

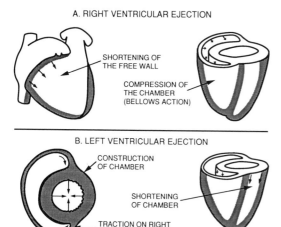

Fig. 4–2. *A and B.* Right and left ventricular ejection. (From Rushmer, R.F. *Structure and Function of the Cardiovascular System,* 2nd Ed. Courtesy of W.B. Saunders Co., 1976.)

The wall of the heart is composed of three layers of tissue: the *epicardium,* the *myocardium,* and the *endocardium.* The epicardium is the outer layer of the heart wall. The thick middle layer is called the myocardium, and is composed exclusively of cardiac muscle arranged in a spiraled pattern around the ventricles in such a way that a wringing action is produced during contraction, squeezing blood out of the heart. The greatest amount of cardiac muscle is found surrounding the left ventricle, creating the great force of contraction needed to eject blood from the chamber. The innermost layer of the heart wall is the endocardium. It consists of epithelial tissue that lubricates the lining of the heart. The entire heart is encased in a sac called the *pericardium,* which holds the heart much like a turnip in a plastic bag. The pericardium normally secretes a small amount of fluid to lubricate the heart within the sac.

Coronary Arteries

Despite the large quantity of oxygenated blood being pumped through the chambers of the heart, the myocardium depends entirely on its own circulatory system for oxygen to support the contractile process. Two major arteries (the left and right coronary arteries) arise from the anterior cusps of the aortic semilunar valve (Fig. 4–4). The left coronary

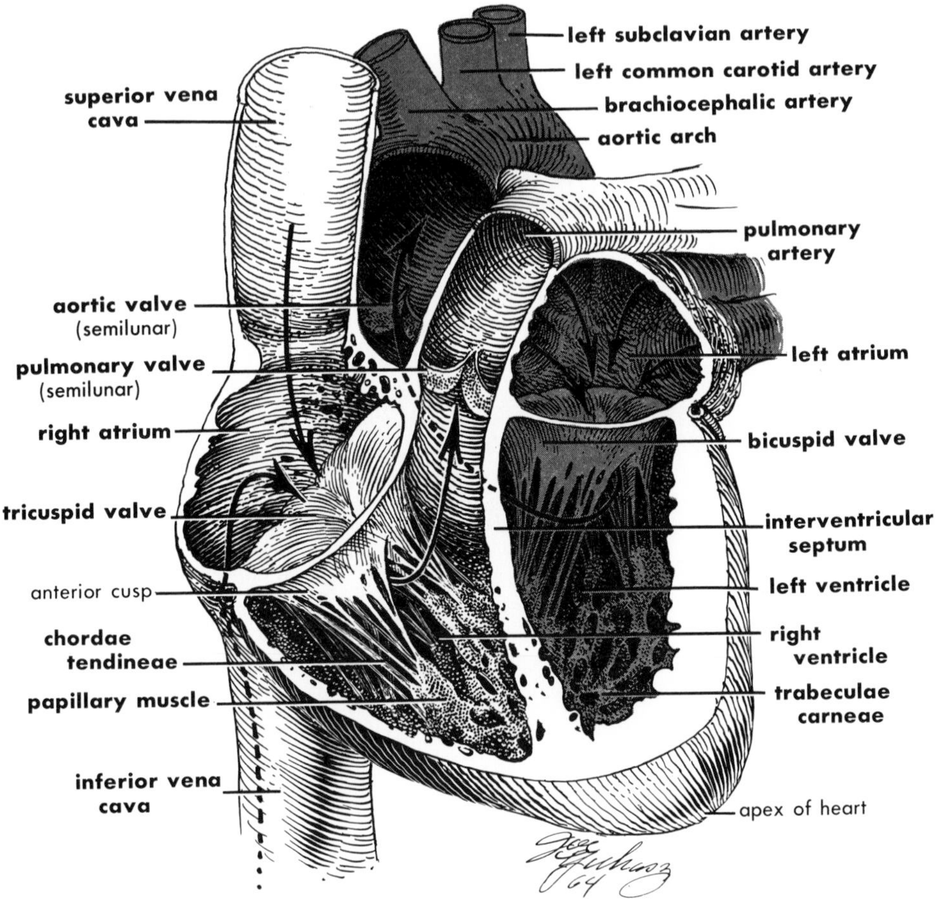

Fig. 4–3. Anterior view of opened heart showing chambers and valves. (From Crouch, J.E. *Functional Human Anatomy*, 4th Ed. Courtesy of Lea & Febiger, 1985.)

proceeds under the pulmonary artery where it divides to form the *circumflex* (which encircles the heart to the left in the atrial-ventricular groove) and the *left anterior descending* (sometimes called the anterior interventricular artery because it descends in the groove between the left and right ventricles over the interventricular septum). The *right coronary artery* proceeds around the heart to the right with a branch to the SA node, and in about 95% of all people, descends on the back side of the heart as the *posterior interventricular artery*. The point where the right and left arteries meet on the posterior side of the heart is referred to as the *crux*. Much of the blood supply to the AV node and the posterior intraventricular septum is supplied by the right coronary artery (Figs. 4–4 and 4–5).

During systole, as the cardiac muscle contracts, the blood vessels in the heart become partially occluded. Therefore, most of the flow through the coronary arteries occurs during diastole while the heart is relaxed. As blood exits the heart, it fills and stretches the aorta (the windkessel effect) but is prevented from flowing backward into the left ventricle during relaxation, by the closure of the aortic valve. This backward pressure on the valve and the relaxed state of the myocardium encourages effective blood flow through the coronary arteries. The arteries branch and get smaller in size, carrying the blood past each myocardial cell in a rich network of capillaries. From the capillaries in the myocardium, blood drains into three principal veins: the *great cardiac vein*, the *middle cardiac vein*, and the *coronary sinus*, where most is dumped into the right atrium and back into the circulation.

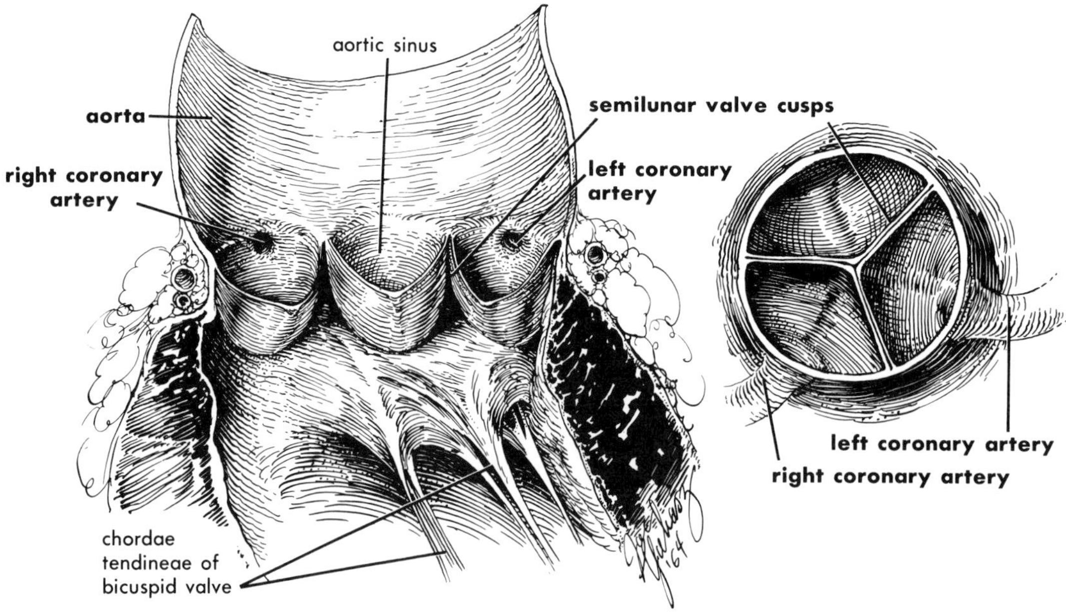

Fig. 4–4. *A and B.* The coronary arteries arise from the semilunar aortic valves. (From Crouch, J.E. *Functional Human Anatomy*, 4th Ed. Courtesy of Lea & Febiger, 1985.)

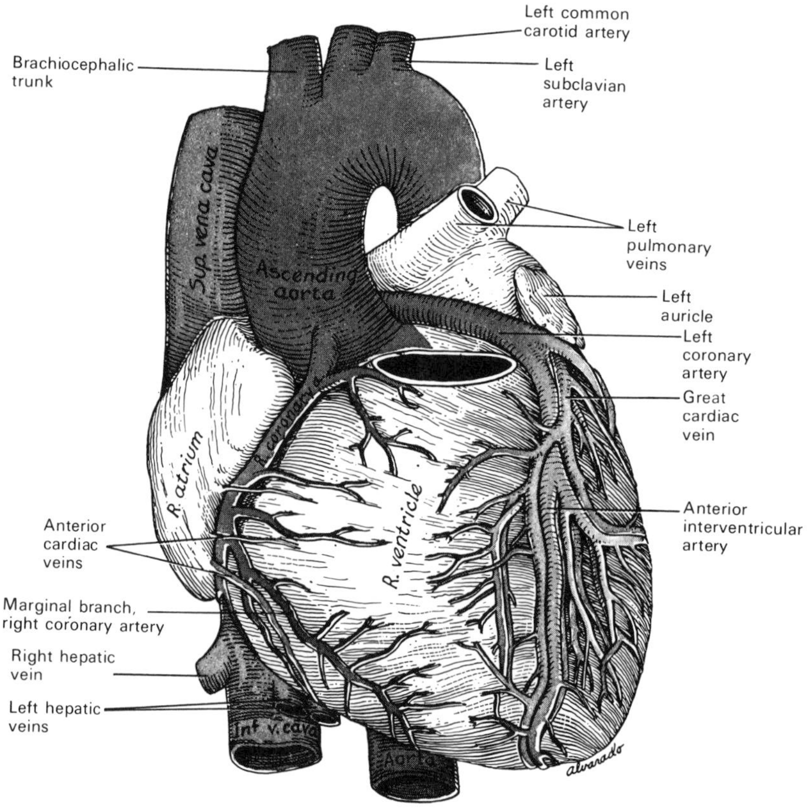

Fig. 4–5. The coronary vessels. (From Clemente, C.D. *Gray's Anatomy of the Human Body*, 30th Ed. Courtesy of Lea & Febiger, 1985.)

Coronary Artery Disease

Coronary artery disease (CAD) is the most common cause of death in America, and is caused by the blockage or occlusion of any one or all of the coronary arteries. Such a blockage results in a regional trauma to the myocardium. If prolonged, the lack of oxygen will result in permanent damage to the portion of the heart fed by the blocked vessel. The most common cause of coronary artery blockage is atherosclerosis, where fatty deposits form under the tunica media of the vessel, causing it to bridge into the lumen and decreasing the blood flow to the myocardium.

The most common treatment for blocked coronary arteries is coronary bypass surgery. In this procedure, a vein or artery from the leg is grafted above and below the blockage to allow restoration of blood flow to occur (Fig. 4–6).

Several alternate methods of treatment are now available:

1. *Angioplasty.* A balloon catheter is inserted through the arterial system into the blocked area and inflated to force the occluded vessel into opening.

2. *Steptokinase.* Steptokinase can be released directly onto the clot by placing a catheter in the plugged vessel or by simply injecting it into the circulatory system within a few hours of the heart attack. Both procedures have been shown to help if done soon enough after the blockage.

3. *Tissue Plasminogen Activator (TPA).* TPA is a new drug that is twice as effective as steptokinase. It dissolves clots circulating in the bloodstream, without altering the normal clotting response of the body.

The best way of reducing the risk of a heart attack is to exercise regularly, lose weight, stop smoking, and eat properly.

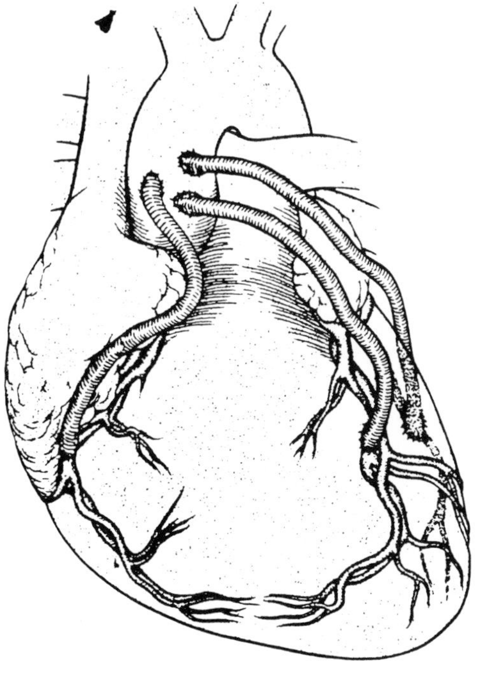

Fig. 4–6. Diagram of a coronary artery bypass. (Courtesy of the American Heart Association.)

Conduction System of the Heart

The muscle tissue in the conduction system of the heart is autorhythmic and requires no external stimuli to depolarize or fire. In addition, when any cell in either the upper or lower part of the heart depolarizes, the other cells in that part of the heart also depolarize, because each cell is connected to the next by a specialized part of the cell membrane called the *intercalated disc.* Depolarization in the atria can spread to the ventricles or vice versa via a connecting bridge called the *bundle of His.* The major components of this conduction system are the *sinoatrial node (SA Node),* the *atrioventricular node (AV Node),* and *bundle of His,* and the *right* and *left bundle branches* (Fig. 4–7).

The SA node, commonly called the *pacemaker* of the heart, is composed of a small mass of specialized myocardial tissue embedded in the posterior wall of the right atrium. The spontaneous depolarization wave which originates in the SA node spreads throughout the right and left atria at about 1 meter/second. The SA node is the pacemaker of the heart simply because it has the most rapid inherent rhythm (about 70 to 80 beats per minute) and thus it is the frst tissue in the heart to depolarize. The spontaneous signal produced from the SA node spreads over the atria, causing contraction of the atria (which pushes blood into the ventricles), then passes through the AV node located in the inferior portion of the interatrial septum. The AV node functions to delay the electrical impulse for 0.08 to 0.12 seconds allowing enough time for the ventricles to fill with blood. The impulse then branches and passes into the right and left bundle branches of the ventricles. These branches are composed of specialized muscle (not nervous) tissue called *Purkinje fibers* which

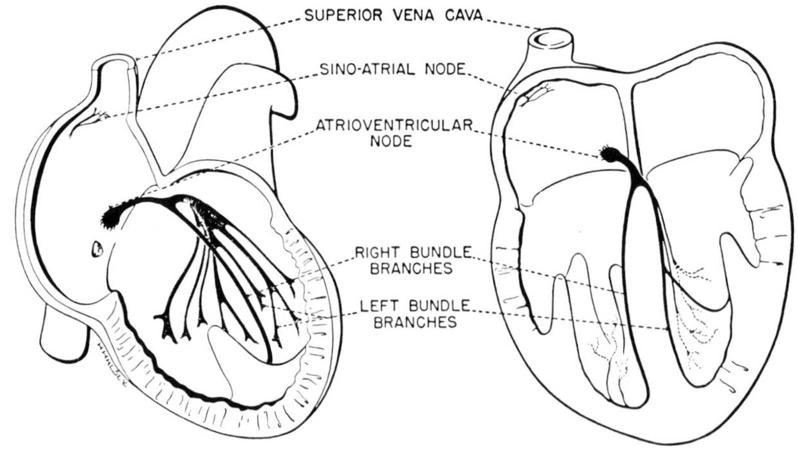

Fig. 4–7. Conduction system of the heart. (From Rushmer, R.F. *Structure and Function of the Cardiovascular System*, 2nd Ed. Courtesy of W.B. Saunders Co., 1976.)

carry the depolarizing wave (down right and left bundle branches) to all areas of the ventricles at about 4 to 5 meters/second. This high speed of conduction yields an almost simultaneous contraction of the ventricles.

Cardiac Tissue

Because of the difference in function, tissues from different areas of the heart have different electrical characteristics. For instance, the "working" muscle cells in the atrium and ventricles and the ventricular Purkinje fibers that transmit the signal into the ventricles are classified as "fast" response tissue (Fig. 4–8); the SA and AV nodes are classified as "slow" response tissue (Fig. 4–9). The resting membrane potential of the fast response cardiac tissue is about 90 mV, compared to a −60 mV for the slow. The threshold for the slow cardiac muscles is also lower, −40 mV compared to −65 mV for the fast. The amplitude of the depolarization wave is also much smaller for the slow tissue reaching only 0 mV compared to +35 or +40 mV for the fast (Fig. 4–9). Of course, the low amplitude waves have a much slower conduction speed, which explains why the conduction through the A-V node region is so much slower than the conduction down the Purkinje system.

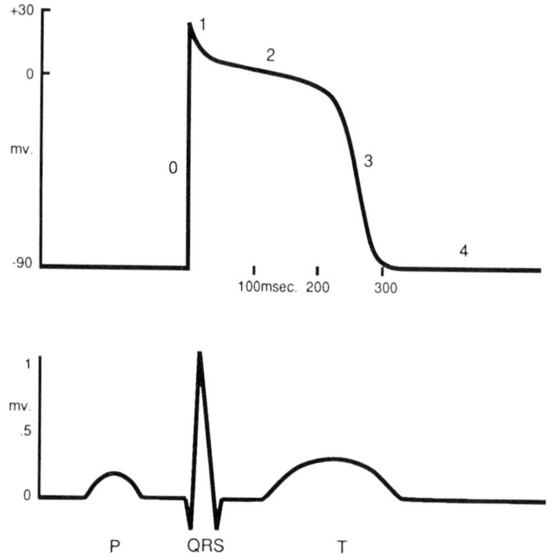

Fig. 4–8. Action potentials of fast response cardiac muscle as related to ECG. (From Rushmer, R.F. *Structure and Function of the Cardiovascular System*, 2nd Ed. Courtesy of W.B. Saunders Co., 1976.)

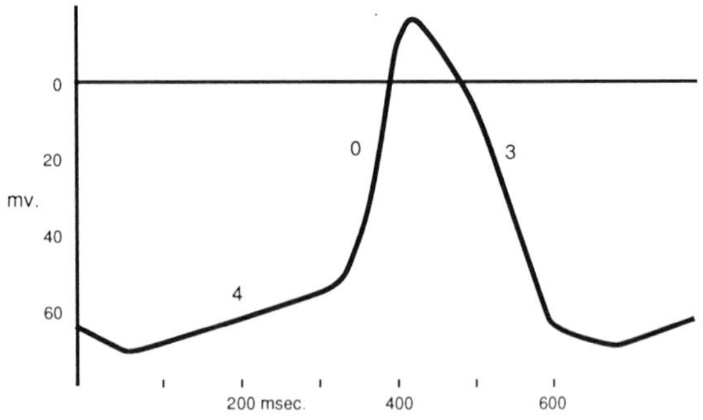

Fig. 4–9. Action potentials of slow response cardiac muscle. (From Rushmer, R.F. *Structure and Function of the Cardiovascular System*, 2nd Ed. Courtesy of W.B. Saunders Co., 1976.)

"Slow" cardiac muscle cells are autorhythmic because the membrane "leaks" sodium until threshold is reached and no outside stimulus is necessary.

Ionic Basis for the Difference in Action Potentials

Because of the differences between cardiac and skeletal muscle, there are some major differences in the ionic components of each action potential. Since skeletal muscle needs to fire rapidly and actually gains force as a result of tetany, the repolarization process is rapid and due mostly to the exit of potassium (K^+) following the influx of Na^+. On the other hand, cardiac muscle is an effective pump only when the muscle contractions are synchronized and working together and when it beats slowly enough to be filled with blood. Obviously, tetany would be detrimental to this process. Therefore, there is a long "refractory period" in which tetany cannot occur.

Each phase of the action potential is labeled by number for easier discussion. Since all cells in the heart are electrically connected, the stimulus that triggers contraction is usually the ionic flow from a neighboring cell.

As in skeletal muscle, the spike potential in *fast response tissue* (labeled #0 in Figs. 4–8 and 4–9) is caused by an increased membrane permeability to sodium. When threshold is reached, Na^+ flows rapidly into the cell, causing the interior of the cell to become more positive. This spike is called the *fast inward sodium current.*

The rapid repolarization phase (labeled #1) is believed to be related to increased membrane permeability to the chloride (Cl^-) ion, which causes the membrane to return to a more normal "negative" level. The plateau (labeled #2) is characterized by a slow inward calcium flow that not only helps provide calcium for cardiac contraction, but also maintains an "effective refractory period" so that the cell cannot be repolarized too quickly. The last stage (labeled #3) is related to the outward movement of potassium, much like skeletal muscle repolarization, that takes the membrane back to normal resting potential (#4).

The "slow" cardiac muscle cells (SA node, AV node, and Purkinje fibers) have a "slow" response time and are "autorhythmic;" that is, they require no outside stimulus in order to depolarize. These cells have slightly different ionic actions from the fast action potentials just discussed.

Both cells depolarize because of an increased permeability to Na^+ (labeled #0). However, slow cells repolarize using the slow inward calcium current and outward potassium current (labeled #2 and #3) and in the final phase (labeled #4), *decreased* permeability to K^+, which moves the resting potential back to threshold without outside stimuli.

Contractile Differences

There are major differences between cardiac muscle and skeletal muscle in their contractile characteristics. Skeletal muscle fibers are separate from each other and each requires a stimulus from a neuron for contraction to occur. Increased contractile force by any skeletal muscle group requires an increased frequency of stimulation from the motor neurons (which leads to tetany), and/or an increase in the number of motor units recruited. Since every cardiac muscle cell contracts each time the heart beats, and since tetany in cardiac tissue would make it impossible to pump blood, the mechanism for increased force of contraction in the heart must necessarily be different from those of skeletal muscle.

In cardiac tissue, the mechanism for increased force of contraction relates to the amount of calcium available to the cross-bridges. In skeletal muscle, most of the calcium available to trigger the contractile process, is stored in the lateral sacs and external calcium stores have little to do with contractile force. In cardiac muscle, external calcium plays a major role. During rest, only small amounts of external calcium are made available to the cross-bridge so fewer cross-bridges form and contractile force is moderate. During exercise or "fight or flight" situations, calcium "channels" are opened in the membrane and the increased calcium flux allows more cross-bridges to form, increasing the force of cardiac contraction. Both norepinephrine and epinephrine as well as various cardiac drugs (glycosides) open calcium channels and increase the force of contraction. Increased contractile forces yield increased ejection of blood from the heart which produces an increased pumping capacity.

BASIC ELECTROCARDIOGRAPHY

The electrical activity of the heart is recorded as an *electrocardiogram (ECG)*. The waves of depolarization and repolarization that pass through cardiac muscle fibers are recorded by sensitive electrodes on the skin and are manifest as deflections on the recording paper. The deflections (P, Q, R, S and T waves) on the ECG represent five distinct electrical activities of the heart (Fig. 4–10).

The *P-wave* is a small upward deflection that measures the depolarization wave traveling through the atria. Contraction of the atria follows immediately behind the wave of depolarization. The *QRS complex* begins as a short downward deflection (Q wave), immediately fires upward (R wave), and is then followed by a quick negative deflection (S wave). The QRS complex represents the depolarization of the ventricles. The *T-wave* is a positive deflection at the end of the recording produced by a repolarization of the ventricles. The ECG can be valuable during an exercise test because of the information it may contain.

ECG During an Exercise Test

ECG information is used by the cardiologist to evaluate the clinical status of cardiac patients both at rest and during graded exercise testing (GXT). However, there is much useful

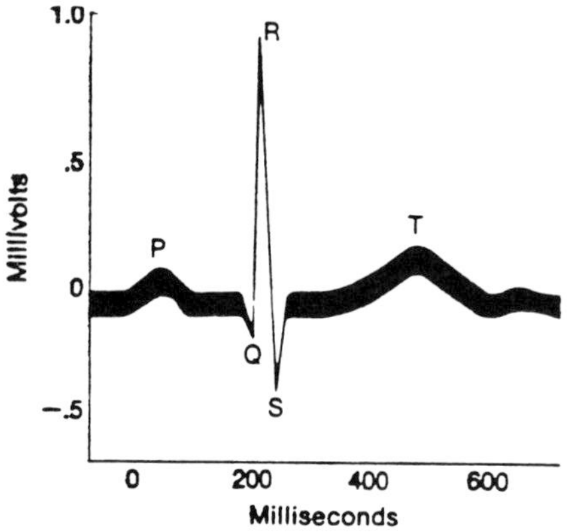

Fig. 4–10. Recording of a normal electrocardiogram (ECG). (From Fardy et al. *Cardiac Rehab., Adult Fitness, and Ex. Testing,* 2nd Ed. Courtesy of Lea & Febiger, 1988.)

information available from ECGs for the exercise physiologist who tests primarily healthy subjects.

Heart Rate. ECG is the best method for obtaining heart rate information during work and can be obtained from a basic three lead or five lead hookup.

Because the ECG recorder travels 1,500 mm/minute, rate can be calculated by dividing 1,500 by the number of mm between R waves (Fig. 4–11A). Many exercise physiologists memorize the heart rate related to each 5 mm box and can therefore estimate heart rate by rapid inspection during the graded exercise test. The number of 5 mm boxes from the 1st R wave to the 2nd tells the heart rate (e.g. 3 boxes = 100 bpm) (Fig. 4–11B).

Arrhythmias. The exercise physiologist usually runs the ECG continuously through a persistent oscilloscope (one that keeps the image visible for a short time) so that arrhythmias may be visualized. The most common arrhythmia is the premature ventricular contraction (PVC). A large number of PVC's (more than 1/3 of the total beats) would be a good reason to stop a test. Runs of PVC's (Fig. 4–12) would indicate a potentially dangerous situation.

Ischemia (Lack of Oxygen). Probably the most important reason for watching an ECG during a stress test (especially if testing adults) is to detect signs that the myocardium is getting too little oxygen (ischemia). With normal beats, the S waves (J point) return quickly to baseline and there is a positive T wave (Fig. 4–13A). If the S wave begins to sag below the baseline, especially if the ST segment is level or downsloping, there is reason to stop the test (Fig. 4–13B). Another sign of ischemia is an inverted T wave in leads V_4 to V_6 (Fig. 4–13C).

THE CARDIAC CYCLE

The cardiac cycle includes a combination of mechanical, electrical and valvular events whose interrelationship is essential to an understanding of how the heart functions. At a rate of 60 beats per minute, the complete cycle would take about 1.0 second to complete; at 75 bpm, about 0.8 seconds. The vertical lines in Figure 4–14 help relate the electrical ac-

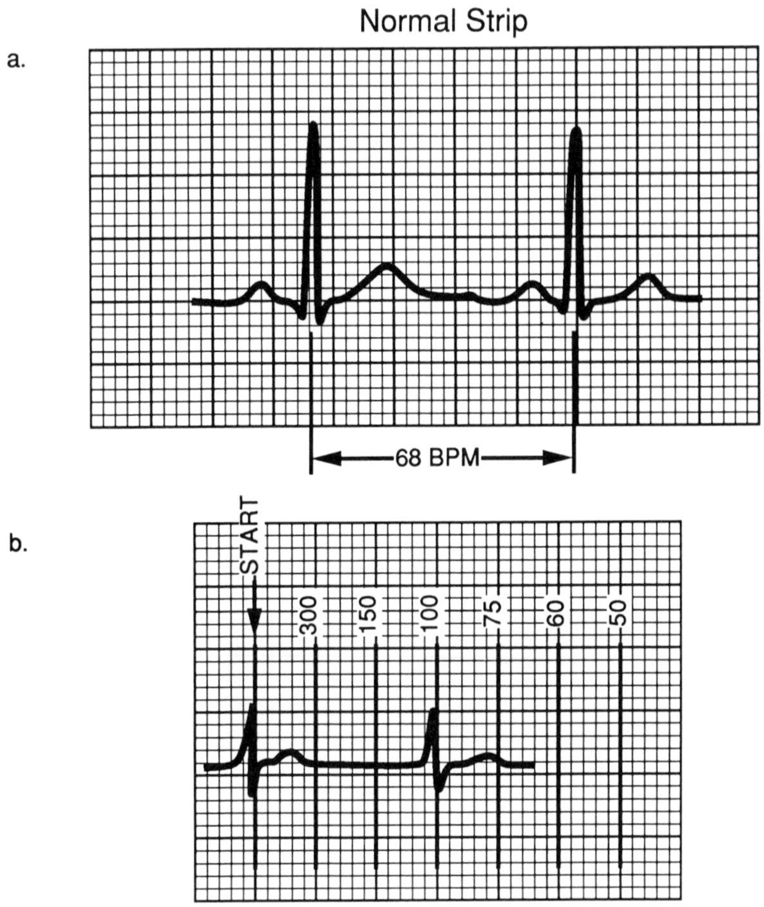

Fig. 4–11. *A.* EKG is the best method for obtaining heart rate information during work and can be performed with a basic three-lead or five-lead hookup. Because the EKG recorder travels 1500 mm/min, the rate can be calculated by dividing 1500 by the number of mm between R waves. *B.* The heart rate related to each 5 mm box can be memorized for rapid heart rate information.

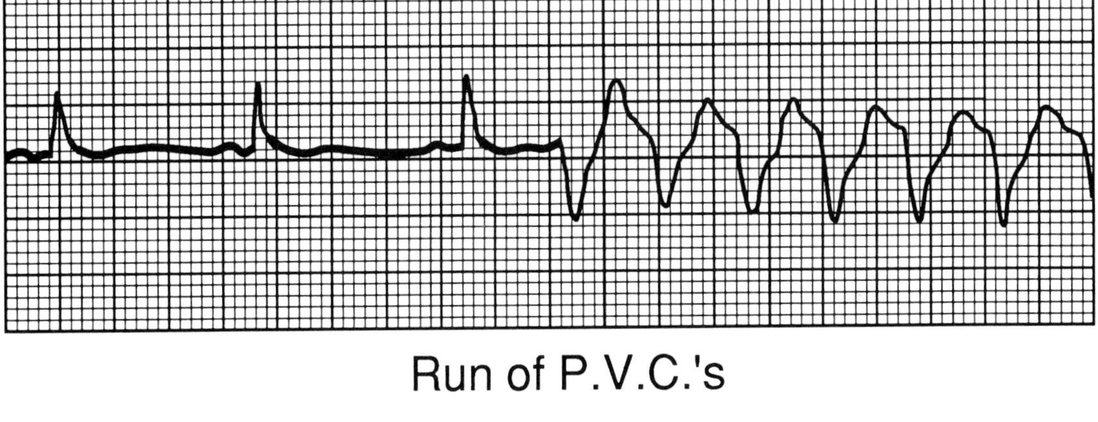

Fig. 4–12. Run of PVCs.

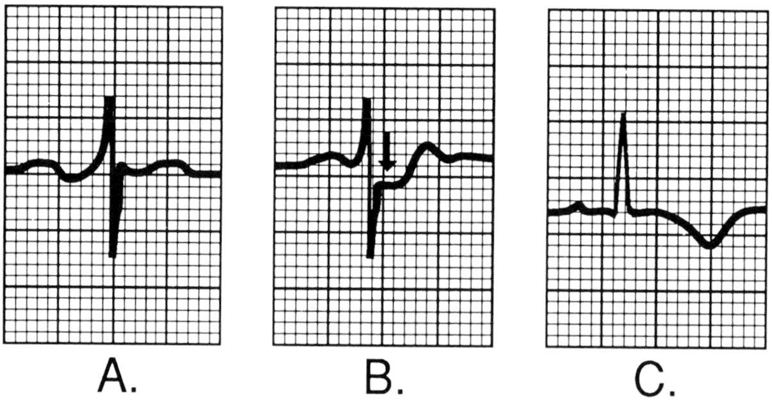

Fig. 4–13. *A.* Normal EKG. *B.* Depressed ST segment. *C.* Inverted T wave.

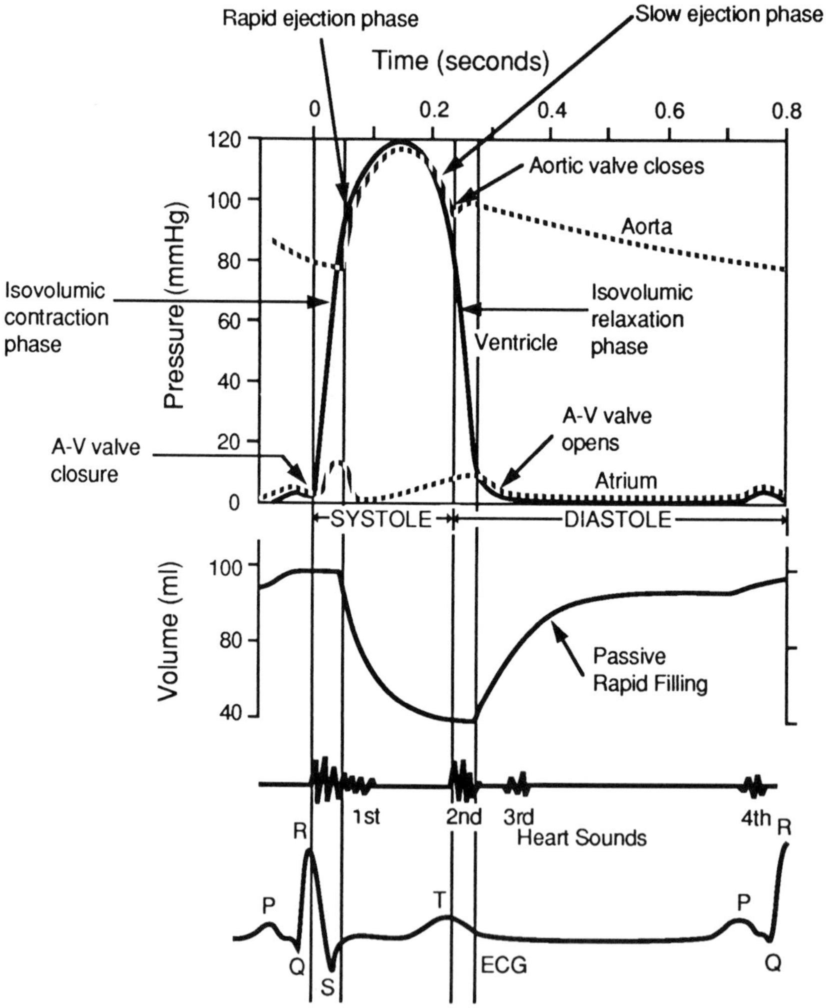

Fig. 4–14. Mechanical and electrical events of the cardiac cycle showing also the ventricular volume curve and the heart sounds. Note the isovolumic contraction period (ICP) and the relaxation period (IRP), during which no change in ventricular volume occurs because all valves are closed. The ventricle decreases in volume as it ejects its contents into the aorta. During the first third of systolic ejection—the rapid ejection period—the curve of emptying is steep. (Modified from Smith, J.J., and Kampine, J.P. *Circulatory Physiology,* 2nd Ed. Courtesy of Williams & Wilkins, 1984.)

tivity, the pressure and volume changes, and the sounds of the heart as it cycles first through *systole* (the contraction phase), and then *diastole* (the relaxation phase). At typical resting heart rates, systole will take only about one-third of the total cycle and diastole takes the remaining two-thirds. This allows ample time for ventricular filling and rest between beats. At higher heart rates (as during exercise), the length of the total cycle is reduced to about one-third of a second (at 180 bpm), and much of the reduction comes from diastole. At these higher heart rates, atrial contraction is critical and may provide as much as 25 to 30% of the total ventricular filling.

In order for contraction to occur, there must be a preceding action potential to trigger the event. The ECG is the recording from the body's surface of the electrical activity of the heart. As discussed in the previous section, the P-wave represents atrial depolarization and is followed immediately by atrial contraction. Ventricular depolarization is represented by the QRS complex which triggers the contraction of the ventricles. Both the atria and ventricles have repolarization waves, but the atrial wave is hidden in the QRS. Ventricular repolarization is represented by the T-wave.

As the ventricles begin to contract, the pressure change closes the A-V valves and the pressure in the ventricles begins to rise. Since the pressure changes are so much greater in the left half of the system, this will be the system discussed from this point on. The closure of the A-V valves causes heart sound one. With the A-V valves closed, the pressure increases until the pressure in the left ventricle reaches aortic (diastolic) pressure. Since pressure increases, but no blood leaves the heart, this phase is called the *isovolumic contraction phase.*

Once the pressure inside the ventricle is greater than the pressure in the aorta, the aortic valve opens and blood flows rapidly out of the heart. The initial period of flow (from aortic valve opening until the highest aortic pressure) is called the *rapid ejection phase* and about two-thirds of the ventricular volume is ejected. Toward the end of the ejection period, the ventricles begin to relax a little and flow decreases (the *slow ejection phase*). At some point during relaxation, the aortic pressure exceeds the left ventricular pressure and the aortic valve closes abruptly. The closing of the aortic valve causes heart sound two. Because the valves and aorta are distended, they recoil when the aortic valve closes, producing a secondary pressure wave which forms a notch on the pressure curve. This notch is called the *dicrotic notch.*

The period between aortic valve closure and the opening of the A-V valves is characterized by a rapid fall in pressure and is called the *isovolumic relaxation phase.* When ventricular pressure falls below atrial pressure, the A-V valves again open and the period of ventricular filling begins. The filling is rapid during the initial one-third of diastole and approximately two-thirds of all the returning blood enters the ventricles at this time. This rapid filling phase is called the *passive rapid-filling phase* and is associated with the third heart sound. (For unknown reasons, a physiologic third heart sound may be present in younger individuals; however, if it occurs after the age of 40 years, it is generally considered abnormal). Later in diastole the atria contract and help finish the filling process. This phase is called the *active rapid-filling phase.* The period between these phases is called *diastasis* (a slower filling phase).

CONTROL OF THE HEART

Although the heart has a basic autorhythmicity and will beat regularly with no outside influences, it must be carefully regulated to meet the changing demands of the body for oxygen and nutrients. There are two sets of controls that regulate the amount of blood that is pumped from the heart: those possessed by the heart itself, often called *intrinsic* controls and those from other areas of the body called *extrinsic* controls.

Intrinsic Control

During the first half of this century, two physiologists, Frank and Starling, found that a normal heart could increase the amount of blood it pumps to match the amount of blood returning to it. This special characteristic of myocardium—also called "heterometric autoregulation"—is an inherent, intrinsic property of the muscle fiber that is evident in the heart even when isolated from all neural and humoral influences. Using anesthetized dogs whose hearts were removed from the thoracic cavity, Frank and Starling plotted curves showing that, within physiologic limits, the force or tension generated by the contracting myocardium was greater if the muscle was "stretched" by an increased venous return. The value of this characteristic is apparent; any increase in the amount of blood returned to the heart during exercise would immediately yield an increase in the amount of blood pumped out of the heart. Further, since the heart must ultimately pump the same amount of blood from both ventricles or get a fluid back up (edema) in either the pulmonary system or in the body, it is fortunate that the heart can intrinsically increase or decrease the output from either ventricle to match the other.

Starling misunderstood the way this adjustment occurred. He thought that the heart was small when the output was small and large when the output was large, and ejected blood much like a balloon filled to different sizes. It is now clear that the heart size changes less than visualized by Starling, who experimented with the heart outside the chest cavity of the dog. Instead, the variability in volume pumped out during exercise primarily relates to how much of the total blood in the heart is ejected (an extrinsic factor). At rest, only about 60 to 70% of the blood in the ventricle is ejected and during work, the amount ejected may increase to 90% or more. The percentage of blood in the ventricles that is ejected when the heart contracts is called the *ejection fraction.*

Of course, ventricular size does vary within certain limits, and the amount of blood that returns to the heart is critical to its function. However, ventricles probably never decrease in size as much as did the heart that Starling used with anesthetized dogs. There is also an upper limit in size determined by the tough connective tissue coverings of the heart. Although this size can be increased slightly by training and to a greater extent by certain disease conditions, there is surely an upper size limit which cannot be exceeded acutely no matter how blood is returned. It is obvious that endurance athletes have greater upper size limits than normal people and therefore also have larger volumes of blood ejected each beat (stroke volumes).

Another heterometric mechanism is the *atrial stretch reflex.* An increased volume of blood returning to the right atrium can increase heart rate by 10 to 20 beats (sometimes called the Bainbridge reflex). This reflex also plays a role in the regulation of blood pressure by increasing urinary excretion when blood volumes are high.

Extrinsic Control

There are several important extrinsic control factors that help the heart either increase its force of contraction or how fast it beats. These factors include the autonomic nervous system, certain hormones, and various receptors.

The Autonomic Nervous System. As discussed in Chapter 2, the autonomic nervous system is composed of the sympathetic and parasympathetic divisions. Sympathetic postganglionic fibers from the cervical and upper four thoracic sympathetic ganglia supply the SA and AV nodes and much of the ventricular myocardium. Stimulation of these fibers activate adrenergic receptors (called beta receptors) and cause an increase in both the rate and conduction velocity in the heart as well as an increase in myocardial contractility. Parasympathetic influence comes from the vagus (tenth) cranial nerve. These fibers are distributed mainly to the SA and AV nodes and to the junctional fibers. Vagal stimulation activates cholinergic receptors in the heart which exert strong inhibitory effects by slowing heart rate and conduction velocity and by decreasing cardiac contractility, primarily of the atria.

The main nervous control of the circulation resides in several functionally diverse areas in the dorsal reticular matter of the medulla, known as cardiovascular centers. These centers have a close neural connection with the respiratory center and they are all essential for survival. As might be expected, the areas that control the heart functionally and anatomically overlap the areas that control peripheral blood vessels. They also function in a coordinated fashion to control arterial blood pressure. For instance, stimulation of certain areas (called pressor areas) will induce both an increase in cardiac rate and contractility and a generalized increase in peripheral resistance while depressor area stimulation usually elicits the reverse. A summary of the effects of the sympathetic and parasympathetic nervous system on cardiovascular function is shown in Table 4–1.

Note that the changes associated with the sympathetic nervous system (cardio-accelerating) are all associated with increasing the heart's effectiveness as a pump and shunting blood to active tissue.

Hormonal Control. Both exercise and the anticipation of exercise stimulates the sympathetic nervous system which in turn stimulates the adrenal medulla which releases epinephrine and some norepinephrine. As opposed to the direct effects of the nervous system on specific organs and systems, the circulating catecholamines have a rather general effect on the circulation, depending on the specific "receptors" in the target tissue. For instance, beta receptors are most prevalent in the heart and in blood vessels of skeletal muscle, and are activated by epinephrine. Therefore, epinephrine released from the adrenal medulla initiates an increased heart rate and contractile strength of the myocardium and a "pure" vasodilation of skeletal muscle blood vessels (more will be said about the receptors in the section on blood vessel control). Both thyroid hormone and glucagon increase heart rate and contractile strength directly, and other hormones (such as glucocorticoids, mineralocorticoids, ACTH, TSH, and GF) indirectly affect heart function.

Receptor Control. Of the other extrinsic controls, the most important is probably the *baroreceptors* (sometimes called stretch receptors, pressorreceptors or mechanoreceptors) of the aorta and carotid arteries. Afferent nerve fibers from these specialized pressure-sensitive receptors in the walls of the aortic arch and internal carotid arteries travel to cardiovascular centers of the medulla to help adjust the amount of blood ejected from the heart. These receptors respond to any change in pressure, but are especially sensitive to rapid changes. They also work most effectively in the range of pressure between about 80 and 150 mm Hg. Their major role is to help maintain adequate pressure (and therefore flow) to the brain and heart during ordinary circulatory stresses such as postural changes (dizziness upon standing) and elevated intrathoracic pressure (such as when lifting a heavy weight), which tend to decrease venous return and arterial pressure. However, they also work well to decrease heart rate and myocardial contractility with increased blood pressure. The responsiveness of these receptors may decrease with age, hypertension, and in coronary artery disease. These receptors are so sensitive that stimulating them by rubbing or even when taking pulse can slow or even stop the heart in extreme cases.

Although chemoreceptors may have some effect on circulation, their primary function relates to respiratory control. More will be said about them in the section on pulmonary function.

CARDIAC OUTPUT

Cardiac output is defined as the amount of blood ejected by one ventricle in 1 minute and is abbreviated as CO or $\dot{Q}$ (the dot over the "Q" is a shorthand way of indicating a *unit time* function). Normal cardiac output at rest is about 5 liters/min. (adults) and can increase to over 40 liters/min. in some world-class athletes during intense work. In fact, the amount of blood that can be expelled is probably the

Table 4–1. The Autonomic Nervous System and Cardiovascular Function

Sympathetic	*Parasympathetic*
Increased heart rate	Decrease heart rate
Increase strength of contraction	Decreased strength of atrial contraction
Vasodilation of coronary arteries	Vasoconstriction of coronary arteries
Mild vasoconstriction in abdomen (adrenergic), skin, and kidneys	Dilation of skin blood vessels
Vasodilation of muscle (cholinergic) of skin	

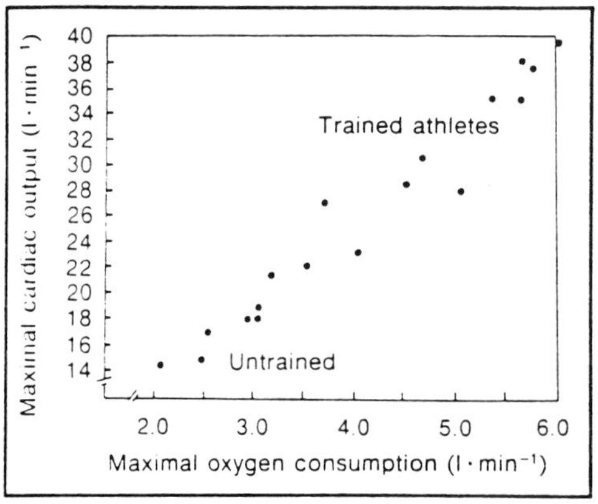

Fig. 4–15. Relationship between cardiac output and work in trained and untrained individuals. (From McArdle, W.D., Katch, F.I., and Katch, V.L. *Exercise Physiology,* 2nd Ed. Courtesy of Lea & Febiger, 1986.)

most important limiting factor during heavy exercise.

Cardiac output ($\dot{Q}$) is the result of two factors: heart rate (beats/min.) and stroke volume (the amount of blood ejected from the ventricle per beat). $\dot{Q}$ is calculated as the product of heart rate and stroke volume:

$$\dot{Q} = HR \times SV$$

The average heart rate in a resting adult is about 72 beats/min. and the average stroke volume averages about 75 ml/beat. The product of these two variables yields an average cardiac output of 5400 ml or 5.4 liters of blood per minute. Since the body contains only about 5 to 6 liters of blood, the total volume is, in effect, pumped each minute. Of course, as work increases (as during exercise), more blood is needed to supply oxygen to the working muscle cells. There is a definite relationship between the amount of work done and the cardiac output. The larger the cardiac output, the greater the total amount of work that can be accomplished (Fig. 4–15).

Both heart rate and stroke volume increase during exercise, but highly trained endurance athletes have a much higher maximal $\dot{Q}$ than the average person. Whereas the athlete may have a $\dot{Q}$ from 35 to 40 l/min during exercise, the average person will have from 20 to 30 l/min. Although ventricular size can probably be increased through training, the large volumes of the endurance athlete may never be reached without some genetic help. Since maximum heart rates are very similar among people of the same age, the difference in maximum $\dot{Q}$ is due mostly to differences in SV. Table 4–2 below will be helpful in seeing these differences.

Heart Rate

Heart rate is simply the number of times the heart contracts each minute. Resting heart rates vary from 35 to 45 in well-trained athletes to 70 to 90 in untrained adults. Maximum values relate to age and can be predicted using the formula 220 − age = maximum predicted heart rate. Thus a 30 year old would have a maximum predicted heart rate of 220 − 30 = 190 beats per minute.

Heart rate is linearly related to work and becomes the only factor in increasing cardiac output after stroke volume reaches its maximum level at about 40% (120 bpm) of maximum work (Fig. 4–16). Since heart rate can increase 300 to 400% (from 50 to 190 bpm) in young adults and since stroke volume increases only 50 to 75%, heart rate is the major factor in the increased cardiac output during work.

Stroke volume plays a major role in determining heart rate during submaximal work. For example, two joggers of similar size and metabolic efficiency will need similar cardiac outputs to maintain a given level of work. If one has a larger stroke volume, his heart rate will be lower (Table 4–3).

This explains why it is so difficult for runners of different fitness levels to jog together. One is working too hard (166 bpm) while the other is not really challenged (115 bpm).

Heart rate is affected by a wide variety of

Table 4–2. Comparison of Heart Rate, Stroke Volume, and Cardiac Output During Rest and Exercise in World-class Athletes and in an Average Athletic Person

	Rest			*Maximum Work*		
Subject	*HR*	*SV*	$\dot{Q}$	*HR*	*SV*	$\dot{Q}$
World-class athlete	50	100	5 l/min	200	200	40 l/min
Average athletic person	72	72	5 l/min	200	140	28 l/min

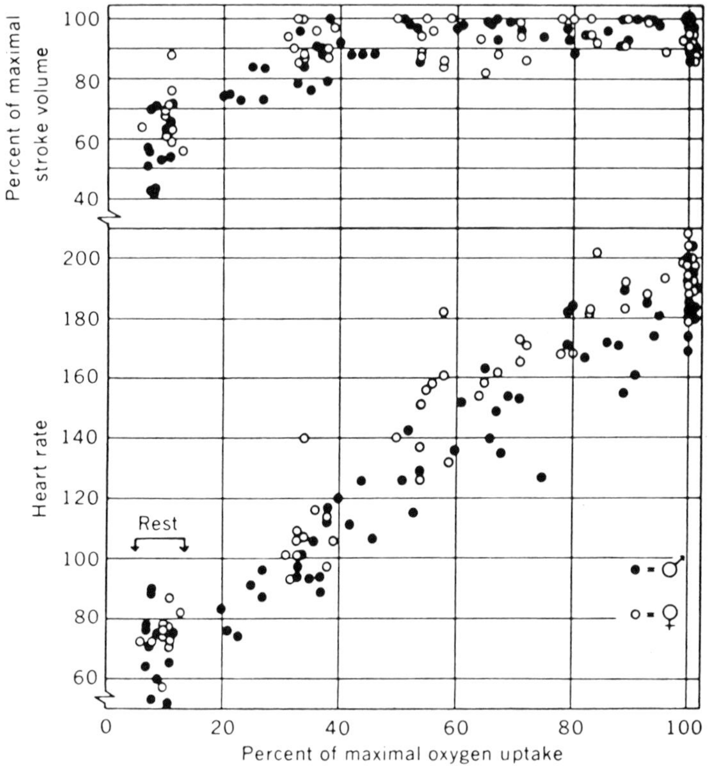

Fig. 4–16. Note that stroke volume levels off between 25 and 40% of max work whereas heart rate increases linearly with work. (From Astrand, P.O., and Rodahl, K. *Textbook of Work Physiology: Physiological Basis of Exercises*, 2nd Ed. Courtesy of McGraw Hill, 1986.)

factors such as anxiety, temperature, altitude, blood volumes (hydration), body position, etc., and responses will vary depending on the type of work being done. The use of smaller muscles such as the arm muscles during cranking or heavy lifting increases the heart rate out of proportion to the metabolic need.

There are several factors, called *pressors,* that increase heart rate: (1) Higher centers in the *CNS* can increase heart rate dramatically before any real need for oxygen is experienced. (2) Stimulation of the adrenal medulla releases epinephrine (and some norepinephrine) into the circulatory system. The effects of these hormones are similar to the direct effect of sympathetic stimulation except that they last longer because they are blood borne. (3) Movement of body parts may actually increase heart rate, perhaps by proprioceptor (muscle spindle) stimulation. (4) Stimulation of the aortic *chemoreceptors* can increase heart rate in an attempt to adjust for chemical byproducts of metabolism. (5) Stretching of the atria by increased venous return (Bainbridge reflex) can increase heart rate.

Other factors, called *depressors,* actually have a slowing effect on the heart. These are: (1) The parasympathetic nervous system, which exerts a depressing effect by releasing ACh onto the SA node. This mechanism may account for the low resting heart rate in well-trained athletes. (2) Baroreceptors located principally in the carotid arteries and aorta are stimulated by stretch and work by inhib-

Table 4–3. Comparison of Heart Rates and Stroke Volumes of Two Similar Joggers Who Need a $\dot{Q}$ of 15 l/min

	Heart Rate	*Stroke Volume*	$\dot{Q}$
Jogger 1	166 bpm	90 ml/beat	15 l/min
Jogger 2	115 bpm	130 ml/beat	15 l/min

iting the sympathetic cardioregulating center in the brain. This mechanism protects the system from a possible "blow-out" from pressures that are too great. Strong stimulation of the carotid receptors (as when taking a pulse in the neck) can result in a decreased heart rate and blood pressure response. Physicians sometimes use the carotid reflex to treat tachycardias. It should be noted that the heart's response to carotid sinus massage is often dramatic, and use of this maneuver is dangerous in the absence of an expert and a sufficient back-up support system.

Stroke Volume

The amount of blood forced out of the ventricles with each beat of the heart is the stroke volume. The stroke volume varies within certain limits and can change depending on body position and work load. The amount of blood forced out of the ventricles is limited by the initial size of the ventricles, which in normal subjects contain about 75 ml/square meter of body surface at the end of diastolic filling.

The role of stroke volume in the performance of endurance activities cannot be overstressed. There is a clear relationship between maximal aerobic work and cardiac output. What many people fail to realize is that, to a large extent, stroke volume determines the limits of cardiac output, because almost everyone has about the same heart rate parameters. Thus, stroke volume is the primary difference between a person with large cardiac output and one with only average output.

The resting stroke volume of untrained male subjects averages between 50 to 80 ml per beat depending on the size of the ventricle. In trained athletes, resting stroke volumes can average about 100 to 120 ml per beat. Prior to exercise, the stroke volumes of most subjects are between 50 to 75% of the maximum they can reach. As exercise begins, stroke volume increases and continues to increase with increasing work loads until the workload reaches from 25 to 40% of maximum. Stroke volume is maximal at this point, which corresponds to a heart rate of about 100 to 120 beats/min (Fig. 4–16). Even though diastolic filling time decreases significantly, there is little tendency for a decrease in stroke volume at maximal work.

The smallest stroke volume occurs in the erect standing position. This is also the position in which the heart functions at its smallest size. The heart probably functions at its greatest size during supine rest or heavy work. However, the greatest *stroke volume* occurs during work because of increased vigor and strength of the ventricular contraction, which yields a more complete emptying of the ventricle (larger ejection fraction).

Factors Affecting Stroke Volume. Stroke volume is defined as the amount of blood expelled from one ventricle each time it beats. The amount of blood moving out of the heart depends primarily on how much blood enters the ventricle during diastole *(end-diastolic volume)*, and how much blood is left within the chamber following its contraction *(end-systolic volume)*. The four basic factors that have the greatest effect on stroke volume are (1) an effective filling pressure (venous return), (2) distensibility of the ventricles (size), (3) contractility of the ventricles, and (4) systemic pressure.

1. *Effective Filling Pressure (Venous Return).* The volume of blood that enters a ventricle during the diastolic filling stage is controlled mainly by the condition in the peripheral vessels. Any factor that increases the venous pressure or slows the heart allows greater cardiac filling. The increased filling of the ventricles increases the *tension* exerted by the muscle, but the time to peak tension is constant. This means that the true *force* of contraction is *not* increased. There are several mechanisms that contribute to increased venous return during exercise: (1) the pumping force of the heart (by far the most important factor), (2) the rhythmic contraction of skeletal muscle during movement which pumps blood back to the heart as the muscles contract and relax and blood is pushed along through the one-way valves in the veins (the venous pump); (3) the act of breathing which helps pull the blood into the thoracic area: (4) an increase in venous tone mediated by the central nervous system which will help speed the blood back to the heart; and (5) an increase in blood volume which not only increases the cardiac output but also the oxygen carrying capacity of the body. Obviously, a large drop

in blood volume due to hemorrhage would greatly diminish cardiac output.

There is no doubt that cardiac muscle demonstrates a length-tension relationship which makes the heart more efficient when more blood is returned to it. Asmussen and Christensen elevated the legs of their subjects for about 10 minutes and then put pressure cuffs around the thighs to maintain a large venous return to the heart. Even though the heart rate was decreased, the cardiac output was about 30% higher because of the increased efficiency of the heart. The effects of a decreased volume of blood returned to the heart can be easily seen by performing a *valsalva* maneuver, such as lifting a heavy weight or straining. Because of the decreased volume of blood returning to the heart, the heart rate increases rapidly to maintain cardiac output. Conversely, recovery can be hastened after exercise by lying down or by moving around to aid the venous return of blood to the heart.

2. *Distensibility of the Ventricles.* Distensibility refers to the ability of the ventricles to be stretched. Normal ventricles will relax during diastole to accommodate the returning blood entering them. *Starling's Law of the Heart* states that all the blood that enters the heart will be pumped. With greater venous return, the ventricles will distend to accommodate the blood, and with the increased stretch, the muscle produces greater tension. It is impossible to expand the ventricles like a balloon, however, since the heart is contained in a relatively small cavity and is surrounded by tough connective tissue which prohibits any acute increases in size beyond its normal dimensions.

3. *Diastolic (systemic) Pressure.* The influence that diastolic pressure has on stroke volume is important. If this pressure were to increase to equal the contraction pressure, an isometric contraction would occur and no blood would flow from the heart. During heavy work, the diastolic pressure of endurance athletes often decreases. This decrease in pressure, along with the increase in contractile strength of the ventricle allows a greater percent of the blood in the ventricles to be expelled (increased ejection fraction).

4. *Contractility.* Contractility is the change in ventricular performance which causes the ventricle to produce more force per unit time (change in pressure/change in time, or $\Delta P/\Delta T$). Fortunately, increased force is a routine adjustment with increased heart rate as a response to exercise. In addition to causing the ventricles to empty more completely, this factor also yields greater time for diastolic filling because the systolic stroke is completed more quickly. Myocardial strength is enhanced in exercise by the action of the sympathetic hormones epinephrine and norepinephrine, which allow greater Ca^{++} flux.

CARDIAC FUNCTION CURVE

Sarnoff and Mitchell performed experiments that led to "cardiac function curves." These curves showed the "length-tension" or "pressure-volume" relationship of cardiac muscle under various conditions of filling and state of myocardial contraction. These relationships also have been studied by using samples of myocardium, particularly papillary muscles, in which the fibers are nearly parallel in orientation and are more easily studied. Although these curves may not completely represent the functional characteristics of myocardium, they are extremely helpful to an understanding of this function.

Figure 4–17 shows a simple cardiac function curve. Notice that muscle performance is altered (1) by change in initial muscle length and (2) by changes in the contractile state of the muscle. The initial length of the fibers is a product of increased or decreased venous return, which yields a larger or

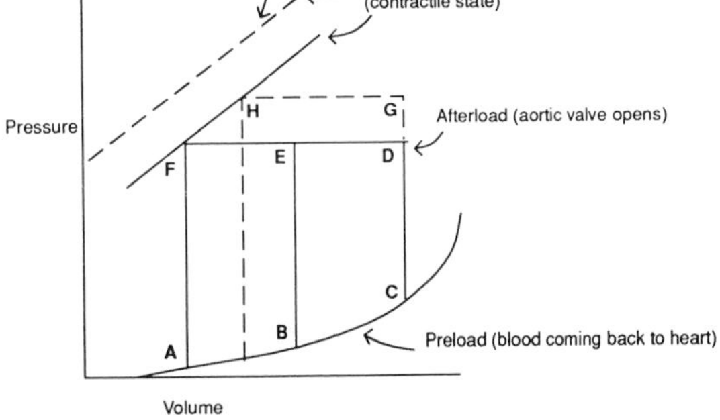

Fig. 4–17. Cardiac function curve. (From Jensen, C.R., and Fisher, A.G. *Scientific Basis of Athletic Conditioning*, 2nd Ed. Courtesy of Lea & Febiger, 1979.)

smaller volume as plotted on the passive pressure-volume line. The amount of blood returned is designated A (small return), B, and C (large venous return). Notice that the increased venous return causes the line to rise, indicating an increase in passive pressure with the increased filling. The isovolumic pressure line represents the force of myocardial contraction. It is plotted by filling the ventricle to some given volume, clamping the aorta, and plotting the pressure (isometric) exerted by the myocardium under that condition. Of course, with the aorta clamped, no flow occurs and the pressure rise is plotted for each increasing volume to form the isovolumic pressure line. If the muscle contracts with more force, a new isovolumic pressure line would result, which would be above the old line.

Cardiac performance can be plotted on the cardiac function curve using the following terms;

1. Preload—initial length of the fibers as a result of venous return.
2. Afterload—the load that the heart works against. This is the pressure in the aorta and is the point at which the aortic valve opens (diastolic pressure).
3. Contractile state—the vigor of the cardiac contraction, which depends on calcium flux within the individual cardiac fibers.

With a large venous return (preload) to point C, the heart contracts. The pressure in the heart rises until the aortic valve opens. At this point, the blood flows into the aorta and continues to flow until the isovolumic pressure line is reached (point F) and pressure returns to point A, where filling once again commences. If the subject were to stand, the venous return would be decreased (say, to point B). At the same aortic pressure, the pressure would rise to point E, and a decreased volume (point E to point F) would result. An increase in aortic pressure (point G) would also decrease the amount of blood pushed out, since the volume would flow only to point H.

This curve explains why stroke volume, or the amount of blood pumped each beat, decreases with standing and increases with exercise. With exercise, the isovolumic pressure line rises because of the increased force of contraction caused by sympathetic activity. At any given venous return, the stroke volume increases because the emptying continues until the new isovolumic pressure line is reached.

CIRCULATION

One of the most important factors in the ability to do intense work is the amount of blood circulated past the cells. Once the blood leaves the heart, there are many factors which affect its flow. The purpose of this section is to discuss these "peripheral" factors.

Vascular System

Blood leaving the heart passes through vessels of progressively smaller diameters referred to as *arteries, arterioles,* and *capillaries.* Blood returning to the heart from the large capillary beds passes through vessels of progressively larger diameters called *venules,* and *veins.*

Most of the vessels have an internal endothelial layer and are reinforced by a network of elastic fibers, smooth muscle, fibroblasts, or collagenous fibers, depending on the size and function of the vessel. The true capillaries are thin-walled endothelial tubes with no muscle or fibrous tissue.

The major *arteries* are large, thick-walled vessels that carry blood away from the heart and act as pressure tanks (windkessel vessels) during the systolic ejection phase. These arteries are large in diameter and have a low resistance to blood flow, with the ability to absorb great increases in pressure near the heart, and convert those pressures to continuous flow through the system.

Arterioles are small vessels located between the arteries and capillaries whose major role is to control the flow of blood to the various capillary beds by vasoconstriction and vasodilation. A layer of smooth muscle (tunica media) surrounding arterioles can be stimulated by the sympathetic nervous system to contract or a lack of stimulation can allow them to relax. A decrease in vessel diameter is called *vasoconstriction* and an increase *vasodilation.* It is important that vasoconstriction of one set of arterioles is balanced by the vasodilation of another.

Capillaries are the basic functional unit of the circulatory system. True capillaries are about 1 mm in length and just large enough to allow red blood cells to pass. The capillary wall is composed of a single layer of endothelial cells with no muscle or elastic fibers. This wall must be thin to allow the proper transport of materials into and out of the cell. Although capillaries are small, there are so many of them that the total cross-sectional area is estimated to be 600 times that of the aorta.

The distribution of blood through capillaries is regulated primarily by concentric bands of smooth muscle referred to as *precapillary sphincters* (Fig. 4–18). The precapillary sphincters are located at the entrance of the capillaries or capillary beds and constrict or dilate according to the metabolic needs of the tissue they feed and not by the nervous stimulation. Some capillary beds are bypassed by arteriovenous shunts.

Venules carry "used" blood and waste materials away from the capillaries and connect to larger vessels called *veins.* Veins gradually increase in caliber and in the thickness of their walls as they get nearer to the heart. The thinner walls of veins and venules allow greater distention than in the arteries. For this reason, more than 60% of the total blood supply is found in the venous system at any one time.

The pressure of the blood as it leaves the capillaries is only about 10 mm Hg, which is not enough pressure to return blood to the heart effectively by itself. To enhance greater venous return, the skeletal muscles squeeze blood toward the heart as they contract. This is possible because the venous system also contains valves to prevent backflow and pooling of blood in the lower extremities (Fig. 4–19). The smooth muscle that surrounds veins and venules is also important in terms of returning blood to the heart. Constricting these veins makes them less compliant, which in turn elevates venous pressure and enhances venous return during exercise.

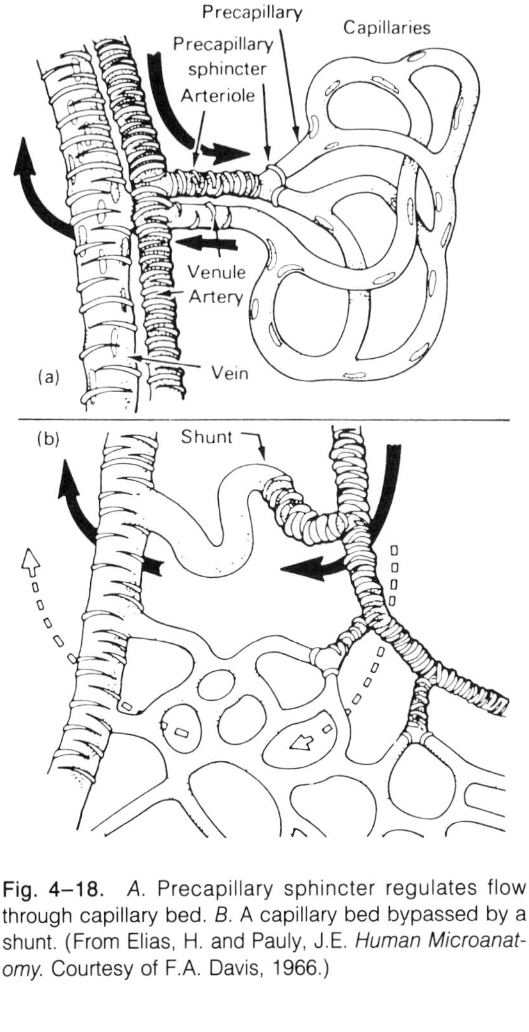

Fig. 4–18. *A.* Precapillary sphincter regulates flow through capillary bed. *B.* A capillary bed bypassed by a shunt. (From Elias, H. and Pauly, J.E. *Human Microanatomy.* Courtesy of F.A. Davis, 1966.)

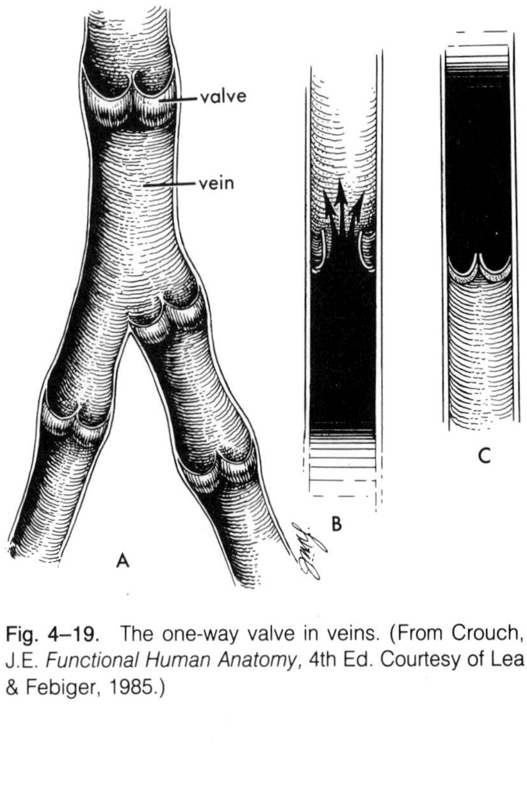

Fig. 4–19. The one-way valve in veins. (From Crouch, J.E. *Functional Human Anatomy,* 4th Ed. Courtesy of Lea & Febiger, 1985.)

Microanatomy of Vessels

Arteries and veins have many structural similarities. They both have three distinct layers or *tunicas* (tunica = coat), which collectively form the hollow center or *lumen* of the arteries and veins. The layers of the arterial and venous walls from the innermost layer outside are the *tunica intima, tunica media,* and *tunica externa* (Fig. 4–20). Note that the tunica of the arteries are much thicker than those of the veins. The thicker walls allow the arteries to handle greater pressure without rupturing.

The innermost layer (tunica intima) is called the endothelium and serves to protect the red blood cell from damage. In the development of the artificial heart and artificial arteries, the researcher's greatest challenge was to develop a synthetic lining smooth enough to protect the fragile membrane of the red blood cells as they pass through the heart.

The walls of the arteries and veins are too thick to be nourished by diffusion from the blood within the vessel itself. Instead, they are supplied by blood vessels called *vaso vasorium* which arise from the tunica externa of the vessel itself or from some neighboring blood vessel.

Body Fluids and Blood

The body contains a great deal of water; in fact, the average man is 63% water by weight (40 liters) while a female averages 52%. The purpose of water in the body is to provide a fluid medium for the processes that must be carried on to maintain life.

The body's water is stored in two major compartments: (1) the *intracellular fluid compartment,* which includes all fluid within the cells, and (2) the *extracellular fluid compartment,* which includes all fluid outside of the cell. The extracellular fluid compartment can be further divided into *intravascular* (the fluid in the circulatory system) and *interstitial* (the fluid around the cells).

Blood functions as a vehicle to carry oxygen and nutrients to the cell and carry carbon dioxide away from the cells. There is approximately 5 to 6 liters of blood in the average size person. Blood consists of a liquid *plasma* component and *formed elements* such as red blood cells (erythrocytes), platelets (thrombocytes), and white blood cells (leukocytes). A

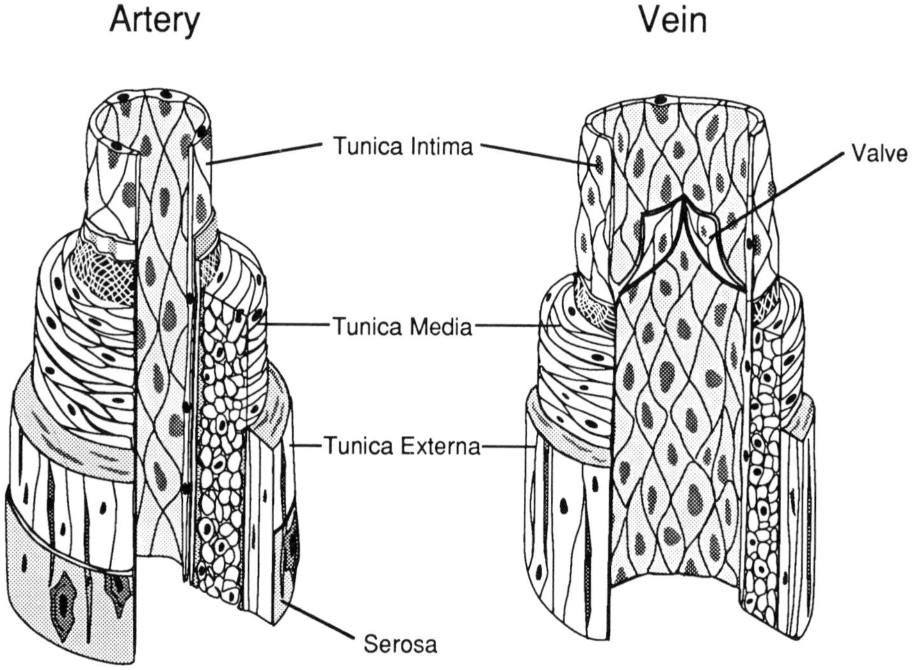

Fig. 4–20. Structure of an artery and a vein, showing the relative thickness and composition of each of the three tunicas. (From Van De Graaff, K.M. *Human Anatomy.* Courtesy of William C. Brown, 1984.)

typical blood sample is about 55% plasma and 45% formed elements.

When a test tube filled with blood is centrifuged, the heavy formed elements such as erythrocytes and leukocytes will settle to the bottom of the tube, and the liquid plasma fraction will rise to the top (Fig. 4–21). The percentage of formed elements to the total amount of blood is known as the *hematocrit.* Men generally have hematocrit levels between 44 and 48, where women have significantly lower levels of 36 to 45.

A low hematocrit would decrease the work capacity of a person while an infusion of extra red blood cells (a process known as "blood doping") has been shown to increase the oxygen carrying capacity of the individual and thus increase his performance. A detailed discussion of blood doping is covered later in the book.

During exercise, the hematocrit will tend to increase 5 to 10% as fluid shifts from the blood stream into the active muscles. A reduction in plasma volume is referred to as *hemoconcentration.*

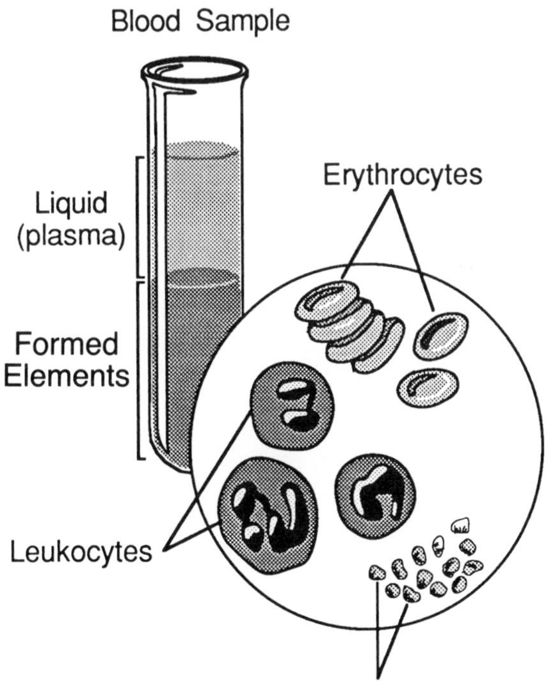

Fig. 4–21. Formed elements in the blood. Note separation of these elements in the test tube. (From Van De Graaff, K.M. *Human Anatomy.* Courtesy of William C. Brown, 1984.)

Athletes have a higher blood volume, plasma volume, total hemoglobin and erythrocyte volume.

Red blood cells (RBC's) serve as the transport mechanism for oxygen and carbon dioxide. The red blood cell is a small (7.5 μ) non-nucleated biconcave (concave on each side) disc. The unusual shape aids in the transport of oxygen. It is estimated that one cubic millimeter of blood contains 5.1 to 5.7 million red blood cells in men and 4.3 and 5.2 million red blood cells in women. The distinctive red color of the erythrocyte is produced by a molecule which makes up ⅓ of the red blood cell called *hemoglobin.* Red blood cells are produced in the bone marrow. In the early stages of development, erythrocytes are nucleated, but lose their nucleus as they reach maturity. Even with the loss of the nucleus, the erythrocyte continues to live for only a limited time; after 90 to 120 days, the cell becomes less active, eventually dies and is degraded by the liver. The body therefore replaces its entire blood supply every four months.

Plasma is the liquid portion of the blood that suspends and carries the red blood cells, white blood cells, and platelets. Plasma is almost entirely water (90%) with the remaining 10% consisting of large proteins, salts, carbohydrates, lipids, gases, amino acids, vitamins, and hormones. The plasma transports small amounts of gases, nutrients, and acts as a buffering system in maintaining the body's pH.

The main difference between plasma and other fluids of the body are the large blood-borne proteins. These proteins constitute 7 to 9% of the plasma and are grouped into three separate types: *albumin, globulins,* and *fibrinogens.* The albumin is the smallest of the proteins but by far the most numerous of the three, making up 60% of the plasma proteins and functioning to maintain the osmotic pressure of the blood. The globulins which make up 36% of the total plasma proteins are separated into three distinct categories called: (1) *alpha globulin,* (2) *beta globulin,* and (3) *gamma globulin.* Alpha and beta globulins have a number of different functions, one of which is the transporting of lipids and fat-soluble vitamins. The gamma globulins are used in the production of antibodies. The remaining 4% of the plasma proteins consist of fibrinogens, whose primary role is involved with the clotting mechanism of the blood. Collectively, these large proteins increase the osmotic pressure of blood as it passes through the capillaries (Table 4–4).

Plasma and tissue fluids are continuously interchanged in the capillaries through the action of filtration and colloid osmotic pressure. In the capillaries, the hydrostatic pressure from within the capillary wall is about 30 to 40 mm Hg at the arteriole end. As a result, some of the larger molecules (such as glucose, inorganic salts, and certain ions) and water are forced out of the capillary into the interstitial space. Fluid loss within the capillaries causes a significant drop in hydrostatic pressure at the venule end to about 10 to 15 mm Hg. The osmotic pressure of the plasma proteins in the capillary (referred to as *colloid osmotic* or *oncotic pressure*) is about 28 mm Hg throughout the entire capillary. As hydrostatic pressure drops below osmotic pressure, fluid containing waste products is pulled back into the capillaries. Fluid not recovered by this process (edema) is removed by the *lymphatic system* (Fig. 4–22).

It is easy to understand tissue edema caused by heart failure in terms of this concept. For instance, if the left ventricle of the heart is unable to maintain its pump responsibilities, the pressure at the distal end of the pulmonary capillaries rises, which causes a net outflow of fluid. The build-up of tissue fluid results in pulmonary edema, which can literally drown a person in his own fluids. Right heart failure can cause similar problems in the extremities as fluid builds up in these tissues.

Physics of Blood Flow

Poiseuille's Formula. In 1846, a French physician named Poiseuille described the factors that govern the flow of a homogeneous fluid through a rigid tube. He stated first that flow, $\dot{Q}$ was directly proportional to the driving pressure gradient, or ΔP. If two garden hoses are hooked together and attached to separate taps, no flow would occur. Only when there is a pressure difference is there a flow of fluid. In the circulatory system, the point of highest pressure occurs where blood is pumped out of the heart. At rest, this pressure varies between 120 and 80 mm Hg, with a mean of about 96 mm Hg because there is more time in diastole. The lowest pressure is at the vena cava as blood returns to the right heart (usually about 0 to 5 mm Hg at rest). The difference in pressure or pressure gradient (ΔP) is about 90 to 100 mm Hg (see Fig. 4–23, pressure gradient in the body). During work, ΔP increases as the heart contracts with more force and total blood flow increases as well.

Pressure gradient was not the only factor affecting flow—Poiseuille saw that flow was directly related to vessel size (radius) to the fourth power and inversely proportional to the length of the tube and the viscosity or thickness of the fluid. The formula describing this relationship is shown below (the terms π and "8" are proportionality constants):

$$Q = \frac{\pi \, Pr^4}{nL8}$$

Although blood is a non-homogeneous fluid, and it flows through distensible tubes, this formula has proven helpful in understanding circulation. As the heart beats with more force, the ΔP rises to increase the flow of blood. At the same time, the body squeezes some blood vessels and relaxes others to be sure that blood flows to the area of greatest need. Because the resistance in the vessels changes with the fourth power of the radius, only small changes in vessel size yield a large change in flow. For example, a vessel squeezed

Table 4–4. Protein Components and Their Functions in Blood

Protein	*Percentage*	*Origin*	*Function*
Albumin	60%	Liver	Maintenance of blood osmotic pressure and transport of FFA
Globulins	36%	Liver	Transport of lipids, and fat-soluble vitamins, and antibody production
Fibrinogen	4%	Liver	Blood clot formation

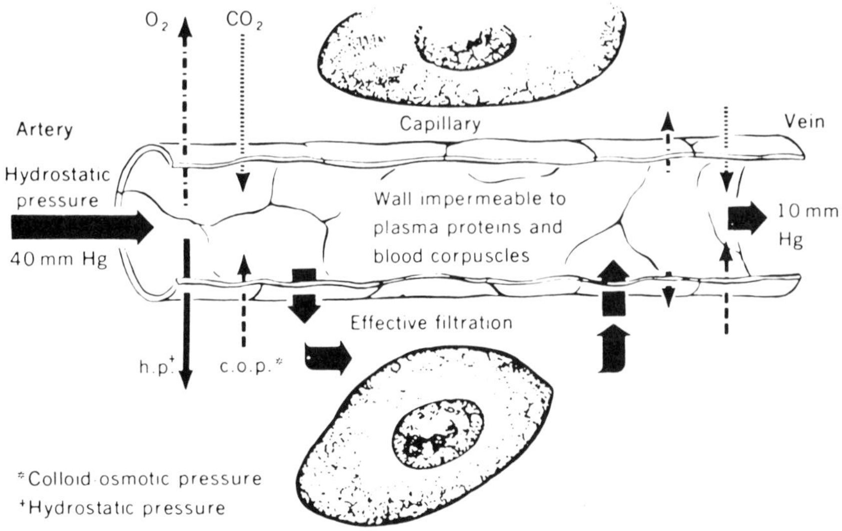

Fig. 4–22. Movement of fluid out of the capillary, due to hydrostatic pressure as balanced by the movement of fluid in the opposite direction, due to colloid-osmotic pressure. (From Astrand, P.O., and Rodahl, K. *Textbook of Work Physiology: Physiological Basis of Exercises*, 2nd Ed. Courtesy of McGraw Hill, 1986.)

to half its normal size would have a flow 16 times less than normal.

Luckily, a large majority of the circulatory system is designed in parallel circuits (as opposed to a series arrangement). This allows flow through one circuit to be increased or decreased with little affect on total arterial pressure or flow in other systems.

Resistance. The ΔP in the Poiseuille formula can be considered a "pushing" factor and the rest of the factors are actually factors that resist flow. If these other factors are collected together, inverted, and called resistance (R), the formula can be simplified to:

$$\dot{Q} = \frac{\Delta P}{R} \qquad \text{where } R = nLr^4$$

In any given vascular bed, neither the length of the circuit nor blood viscosity would ordinarily change dramatically so the most important factor is r^4. Although blood is quite viscous (about 3.6 times as viscous as water under normal conditions), its viscosity increases exponentially as the number of red blood cells go up and can become viscous enough to reduce work capacity and increase blood pressure, with certain diseases, dehydration or blood doping.

This simplified Poiseuille formula can be mathematically rearranged to solve for resistance:

$$R = \frac{\Delta P}{\dot{Q}}$$

Using this arrangement, total body resistance sometimes called PRU (pressure-resistance units) can be solved. For example, at rest the average driving pressure (ΔP) is about 100 mm Hg (the average of the systolic and diastolic pressure). The cardiac output is about 5 l/min. Therefore, the PRU = 20 (100/5). During exercise, the ΔP goes up to 140 (driving pressure = 200/80) or so and the $\dot{Q}$ may increase to 30 l/min. PRU in this case has decreased to about 5 (140/30 = 4.6).

Blood Pressure

Arterial blood pressure, because of its role in blood flow, is probably the most important controlled variable in the circulatory system. Rearranging the simplified Poiseuille formula ($\dot{Q}$ = P/R), reveals that blood pressure is, in effect, the mathematical product of cardiac output and peripheral resistance or P = $\dot{Q}$ × R. The body, through the cardiovascular control centers, must control blood pressure through adjustments of these two important variables. However, these centers are themselves governed by reflex responses to pressure changes and by impulses from higher neural centers. Thus, the arterial pressure, acting through classical feedback mechanisms, is both the controlled and the controlling variable.

As was mentioned in a previous section (extrinsic controls of the heart), the control of circulation resides in several areas or centers in the dorsal reticular matter of the medulla, which are collectively known as cardiovascular (CV) centers. These centers function in a coordinated manner to maintain arterial pressure within normal limits. Most of the intrinsic and extrinsic reflexes discussed earlier affect not only the heart, but the circulatory system as well. For instance, the pressure within the aortic arch and carotid sinuses often falls upon standing as blood pools into the lower extremity. This decreases the stretch of the baroreceptors and causes an increase in heart rate and strength of contraction as well as a vasoconstriction of blood vessels in the lower extremities via the sympathetic nervous system to prevent fainting. If for some reason the vasoreceptors are unable to maintain blood flow to the brain after standing, a person can feel dizzy or even faint because of inadequate perfusion of blood to the brain. The lack of sensitivity of the baroreceptors is called *orthostatic hypotension.* Conversely, chronic hypertension (high blood pressure) may be due to baroreceptor insensitivity.

Measuring Blood Pressure. As blood is ejected from the left ventricle (systole) the pressure produced in the artery is about 120 mm Hg. During diastole, blood pressure drops to about 80 mm Hg. The blood pressure in the arteries and arterioles is collectively referred to as *systemic pressure,* and is normally expressed as systolic pressure over diastolic pressure as 120/80 mm Hg.

Blood pressure can be most accurately measured by inserting a small cannula directly into the artery. Indirectly, blood pressure measurements are based on the correlation of blood pressure and arterial sounds. An inflatable cuff or *sphygmomanometer* is wrapped around the upper arm, at the same level of the heart, with a stethoscope placed over the brachial artery.

The cuff is then inflated (usually at 180 mm Hg) to be sure that the flow of blood through the artery is stopped. The air in the cuff is then slowly released until the pumping pressure of the heart equals the constrictive pressure of the cuff. Flow through the artery is usually silent, but when the artery is pinched, the blood flow becomes turbulent. As blood first begins to flow through the tightly constricted vessel, the vibrations can be heard with a stethoscope. The first vibrations or Korotkoff sounds represent the *systolic pressure* (about 120 mm Hg). As the pressure on the cuff is further decreased, the sound of the blood flow changes to a low quiet thump, and finally disappears. Remember that blood flowing through a vessel cannot be heard unless the vessel wall is pinched dispersing the smooth laminar flow. The last vibrations or sounds occur when the cuff pressure is equal to the *diastolic pressure* (80 mm Hg) (Fig. 4–24).

There are basically five stages of the Korotkoff sounds, identified as the following:

Stage 1. Systolic—the point at which blood can be heard as it begins to rush through the vessels once the cuff pressure is released.

Stage 2. Loud Tapping—the blood pulsing through the vessels is very distinct.

Stage 3. Muffled with Tapping—the loud tapping sound heard in stage 2 begins to become muffled.

Stage 4. Quicker—the sounds become quicker at this point. This stage is usually defined as the pediatric blood pressure and is also recorded as the exercise diastolic pressure.

Stage 5. Diastolic—the point at which the pulsative Korotkoff sounds totally disappear.

Blood Pressure During Work. Blood pressure increases with work to increase the amount of blood pumped. Normally only systolic pressure increases because an increase in diastolic pressure (afterload) would decrease stroke volume (see the cardiac function curve if this idea is still not clear). Therefore, the "pulse pressure" or difference between diastolic and systolic pressure increases. An increase in diastolic pressure indicates a maladjustment to exercise and would cause an exercise test to be stopped if it increased to levels above 100 mm Hg (Fig. 4–25).

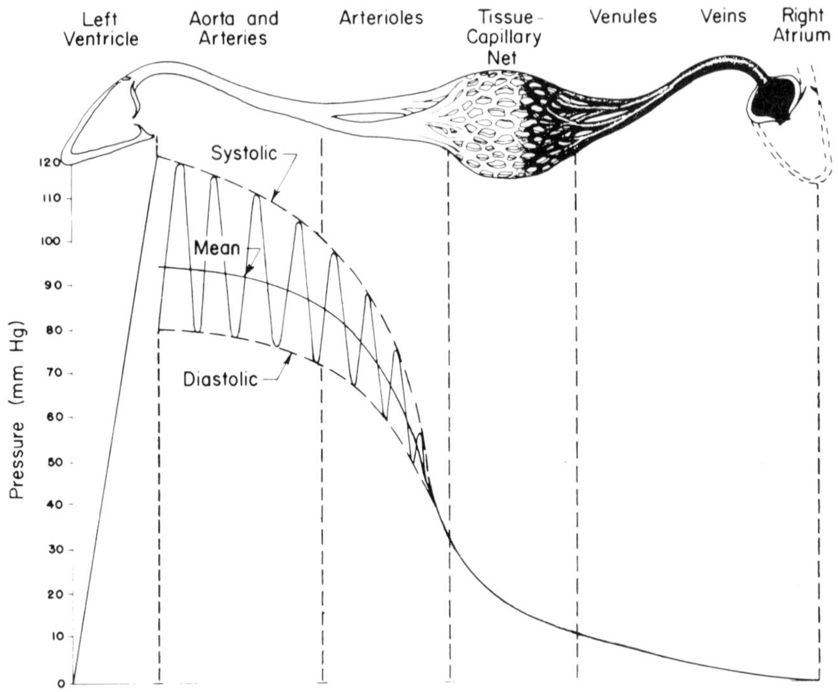

Fig. 4–23. Blood pressure differential along the systemic vascular tree. Blood always flows from an area of high pressure to one of low pressure. Note also that the pressure (and thus the flow of blood) fluctuates in the arteries and arterioles, but that it is steady in the capillaries. Systolic pressure is the highest pressure obtained, diastolic the lowest; the average of the two is the mean arterial pressure. (From Mathews, D.K. and Fox, E.L. *Physiological Basis of Physical Education and Athletics,* 2nd Ed. Courtesy of W.B. Saunders Co., 1976.)

Measuring blood pressure during work is difficult, especially in running subjects. However, exercise blood pressure can be measured in walking subjects after a little practice, and may be important when testing older or postcardiac subjects. Sometimes the diastolic sounds can be heard all the way to zero during exercise or recovery. This phenomenon is caused by the rebound action of the blood in the vessels and is not a cause for concern. This blood pressure is recorded as 180/90-0, which indicates that the systolic pressure is 180 mm Hg, a change in sound from bright to dull occurred at 90 mm Hg (stage 3), and that the dull sound could be heard all the way to 0 mm Hg.

Arterial blood pressure is significantly higher in arm exercise than in leg exercise because the cardiac output is forced into the smaller muscle bulk of the arms instead of those of the legs. This explains why it is dangerous for cardiac patients to shovel snow or do other heavy work involving the arms. There is also a powerful cardiovascular reflex associated with sustained static muscle contraction. The pressure response is largely independent on the muscle bulk involved, and is just as strong with arm-muscle work as with leg-muscle work, *if* the same percent of maximum force is used. This reflex is most often noticed in cardiac patients who carry a suitcase (sustained contraction of the forearm) and causes a significant increase in blood pressure and heart rate. It also increases the myocardial oxygen need, which may lead to angina (chest pain) or other cardiac aberrations.

Control of Circulation

Since there is potentially much more room in the circulatory system than there is blood and since the needs of the various tissues vary depending on their activity, the body must be able to control the flow of blood so that it goes where it should.

It is also important to maintain a fairly stable blood pressure throughout the system, so when the body opens one area to increased flow, it must close down some other area and/

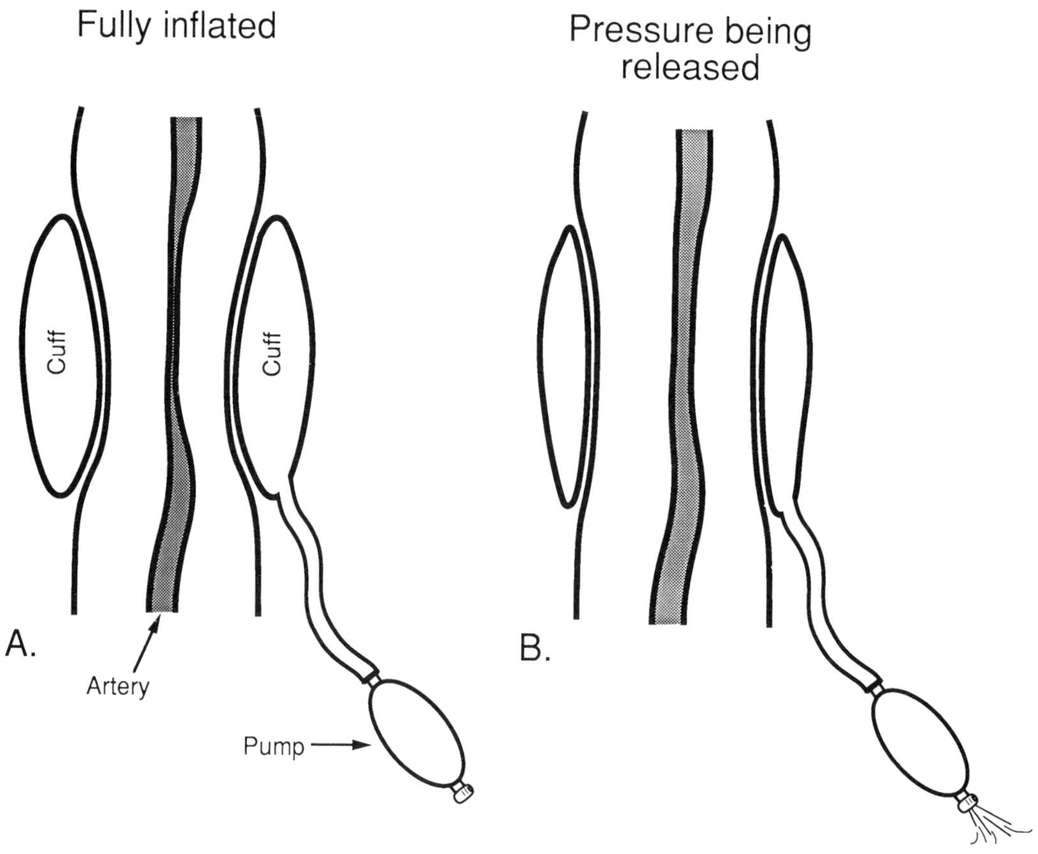

Fig. 4–24. *A.* The blood pressure cuff, fully inflated, cuts off blood flow. *B.* As pressure is released, the sound of blood jetting through the arteries (Korotkoff sound) is heard until the diastolic pressure equals the cuff pressure.

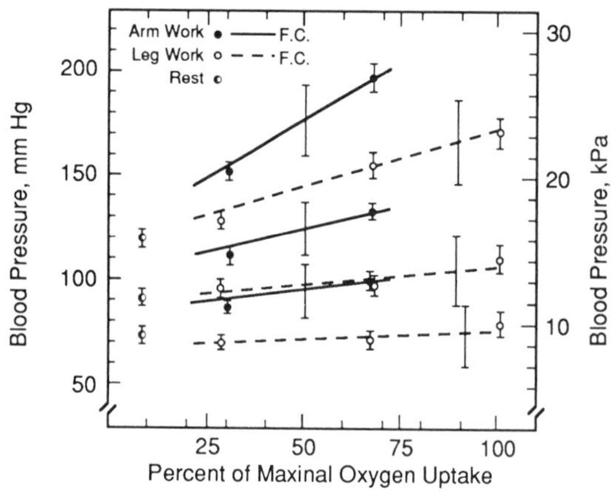

Fig. 4–25. Effect of exercise on blood pressure. Regression lines of arterial systolic, mean, and diastolic blood pressures, respectively, in relation to oxygen uptake during leg and arm exercise. (From Astrand, P.O., and Rodahl, K. *Textbook of Work Physiology: Physiological Basis of Exercises,* 2nd Ed. Courtesy of McGraw Hill, 1986.)

or increase the total output enough to maintain pressure.

At rest, the brain, liver, kidney and muscle receive the greatest amount of blood (14, 25, 20 and 21%, respectively). During severe exercises, cardiac output can increase 4 to 8 times the resting rate, and the skeletal muscles can receive up to 90% of the total flow. In the body, changes in flow to different tissues occurs because of changes in vessel size. These changes may occur passively with transmural pressure changes or through active contraction (vasoconstriction) or relaxation (vasodilation) of circular smooth muscle. A wide variation in flow occurs with only moderate changes in vessel diameter because of the fourth power effect of the radius on flow (Poiseuille's Law).

There are two main ways that control of circulation occurs. One, *central control* involves control by either the sympathetic nervous system or humoral agents which are released into the blood. Both of these are central because they originate from a source other than the tissue affected. The second control system is *local control,* which involves local hormones or ions derived from the individual tissues that act directly on the nearby capillary beds.

Central Control. The autonomic nervous system (ANS) is responsible for integrating and modulating the functions of all the autonomous organs of the body, including the cardiovascular system. This occurs as a result of nerve impulses that release specific neurotransmitter chemicals onto the tissues being controlled. There are basically three transmitter chemicals in the ANS: (a) acetylcholine (ACh), which is released at all ANS presynaptic endings, parasympathetic endings, and at myoneural junctions: (b) norepinephrine (NE) which is released at all adrenergic endings, and (c) epinephrine (E), released mostly by the adrenal medulla into the blood. Interestingly, when any one of these chemicals is released, there are different responses, depending upon which tissue is affected. This is because each tissue has its own "receptor system" that causes the effect of the chemical to be specific for that tissue's role in circulation.

The first type of receptors (called *alpha* receptors) are found in the vessels of skin, kidney, splanchnic area and skeletal muscle. Alpha receptors are strongly activated by NE (less strongly by E) and vasoconstrict virtually all blood vessels to help maintain peripheral resistance in the system. The second type, *beta* receptors, are related to factors that help the body increase metabolic rate (the "flight or fight" response). There are two specific beta receptors; beta 1 receptors work more specifically with the heart where they increase heart rate, stroke volume, and at the same time, increase lipolysis. Beta 2 receptors dilate bronchioles, increase glycogenolysis, and dilate certain skeletal muscle blood vessels to increase the flow to working muscles. Table 4–5 outlines the most common function of the various receptors discussed above.

With exercise, stimulation of the sympathetic NS activates beta adrenergic receptors causing an increase in the output of the heart (both stroke volume and heart rate) while other fibers activate alpha adrenergic receptors to produce a general vasoconstriction, especially in the veins, to help blood get back to the heart more effectively. This stimulation also activates peripheral beta receptors which tend to produce vasodilation, particularly to the skeletal muscle, and preganglionic fibers supplying the adrenal medulla to release epinephrine into the blood stream. However, the "humoral" chemicals (those released into the blood stream) have only minor cardiovascular effects compared to neurostimulation. Interestingly, epinephrine in low doses causes vasodilation through beta receptor effects, but in high doses, has alpha constrictor effects.

Table 4–5. Summary of Action of Alpha and Beta Receptors.

Receptor Type	*Action*
Alpha	General vasoconstriction
$Beta_1$ (found in heart tissue)	Increased heart rate Increased lipolysis Increased contractility
$Beta_2$	Vasodilation of skeletal muscle arterioles Bronchodilation Increased glycogenolysis

Local Control. When tissues increase their metabolic activity, they also cause a local vasodilation to allow blood to flow directly to the area of most need. The mechanism for this effect is not certain, but it is probably related to either the accumulation of metabolites produced because of the increased metabolic activity (CO_2, lactic acid, K^+, or H^+, etc.) or to increased heat production. If blood flow is cut off to a muscle bed for a short time, there will be an increased flow to the area after the blood flow is restored (called reactive hyperemia). Body builders use this technique to "pump" their muscles prior to competition.

In summary, the regulation of circulation during exercise is a complex series of events. The changes that must occur are initiated from the brain and affect many functions. The increase in sympathetic activity stimulates the heart and reciprocally decreases parasympathetic activity, allowing the heart (pump) to increase both rate and force. The skeletal muscles begin to receive a larger share of the circulation because of their innervation with sympathetic cholinergic vasodilator fibers, which opens the vessels near muscles that are metabolically active. The activity of these muscles in turn, causes local vasodilation, all of which allows an increased flow of blood past each cell. At the same time, the flow of blood to the gut and other organs is decreased by the action of the sympathetic adrenergic vasoconstrictor fibers. The veins are also constricted and increase their pumping action due to the contraction of the working muscles, which increases venous return. Later, as heat is produced, the vessels of the skin open and blood flow increases to that area to aid the cooling process. Through this series of actions, the cardiac output is increased and the circulation is adjusted to pump the blood where it is needed most.

SELECTED REFERENCES

Alpert, N.R., et al.: Heart muscle mechanics. In *Annual Review of Physiology,* vol. 41, edited by I.S. Edelman, et al., Palo Alto, Calif.: Annual Reviews, 1979, p. 521.

Baez, S.: Microcirculation. In *Annual Review of Physiology,* vol. 39, edited by Ernst Knobil, et al., Palo Alto, Calif.: Annual Reviews, 1977, p. 391.

Benditt, E.P.: The origin of atherosclerosis. Sci. Amer. 1977.

Bezucha, G.R., Lenser, M.C., Hanson, P.G., et al.: Comparison of hemodynamic responses to static and dynamic exercise. J. Appl. Physiol. *53*:1589–1593, 1982.

Bing, D.H. (ed).: *The Chemistry and Physiology of the Human Plasma Proteins.* New York: Pergamon Press, 1979.

Bishop, V.S., et al.: Factors influencing cardiac performance. Int. Rev. Physiol. *9*:239, 1976.

Brodal, P., Ingjer, F., and L. Hermansen: Capillary supply of skeletal muscle fibers in untrained and endurance trained men. Am. J. Physiol. *232*:H705–H712, 1977.

Cranefield, P.F.: *Conduction of the Cardiac Impulse.* Mount Kisco, N.Y.: Futura Publishing Co., 1975.

Dickhuth, H.H., et al.: Two Dimensional Electrocardiographic measurements of left ventricular volume and stroke volume of endurance trained athletes and untrained subjects. Int. J. Sports Med. *4*:21, 1983.

Donald, D.E., and J.T. Shepard: Autonomic regulation of the peripheral circulation. In *Annual Review of Physiology,* vol. 42, edited by I.S. Edelman, et al., Palo Alto, Calif.: Annual Reviews, 1980, p. 419.

Dubin, D.: *Rapid Interpretation of EKGs.* Tampa, Fla: Cover Publishing, p. 1–43, 1980.

Durrer, D., et al.: Human cardiac electrophysiology. In Dickinson, C.J., and J. Marks (eds): *Developments in Cardiovascular Medicine.* Lancaster, Eng.: MTP Press, 1978, p. 53.

Ferge, E.D.: "Coronary Physiology." Physiol Red., *63*:1, 1983.

Fozzard, H.A.: Heart: Excitation-contraction coupling. Annu. Rev. Physiol. *39*:201, 1977.

Gore, R.W., and P.F. McDonagh: Fluid exchange across single capillaries. In *Annual Review of Physiology,* vol. 42, edited by I.S. Edelman, et al., Palo Alto, Calif.: Annual Reviews, 1980, p. 337.

Guyton, A.C., et al.: Pressure-volume curves of the entire arterial and venous systems in the living animal. Am. J. Physiol. *184*:253, 1956.

Guyton, A.C.: *Textbook of Medical Physiology.* 6th Ed. Philadelphia: W.B. Saunders Co., 1981.

Guyton, A.C.: Arterial Pressure and Hypertension. Philadelphia: W.B. Saunders Co., 1980.

Hilton, S.M., and K.M. Spyer: Central nervous regulation of vascular resistance. In *Annual Review of Physiology,* vol. 42, edited by I.S. Edelman, et al., Palo Alto, Calif: Annual Reviews, 1980, p. 399.

Hurst, J.W. ed: *The Heart.* New York: McGraw-Hill, 1979.

Jarvik, R.K.: The total artificial heart. Sci. Amer. Jan. 1981.

Kanstronp, I.L. and B. Elkblom: Blood volume and hemoglobin concentration as determinants of maximum aerobic power. Med. Sci. Sports. Exerc., *16*:256, 1984.

Lowenthals, David T., et al.: Cardiovascular Drugs and Exercise. In Pandolf, K.B. (ed), ESSR, Vol. 15, 1987, p. 67.

Nilsson, H.: Adrenergic nervous control of resistance and comparative vessels. Acta Physiol. Scand. *124* (Suppl. 541), 1985.

Nobel, D.: *The Initiation of the Heartbeat.* New York, Oxford: University Press, 1979.

Roach, M.R.: Biophysical analysis of blood vessel walls and blood flow. Annual. Rev. Physiol. *39*:51, 1977.

Rushmer, R.F.: *Structure and Function of the Cardiovascular System.* 2nd ed. Philadelphia: W.B. Saunders Co., 1976.

Sagvig, M. et al.: Aging and the effect of increased afterload on left ventricular contractile state. Med. Sci. Sports Exer. *20*,(3):281–284, 1988.

Scheuer, J., and C.M. Tipton: Cardiovascular adaptation to physical training. In *Annual Review of Physiology,* vol. 39, edited by Ernst Knobil, et al., Palo Alto, Calif: Annual Reviews, 1977, p. 221.

Shepard, J.T., and P.M. Vanhoutte: *The Human Cardiovascular System: Facts and Concepts.* New York: Raven Press, 1979.

Smith, J.J. and J.P. Rampine: *Circulating Physiology—The Essentials.* Baltimore: Williams & Wilkins, 1980.

Spence, D.W., L.H. Peterson, and V.E. Friedewald: Relation of Blood Pressure During Exercise to Anaerobic Metabolism. Am. J. Cardio. *59*:1342–1344, 1987.

Sperelakis, N.: Propagation mechanisms in heart. Annual. Rev. Physiol. *41*:441, 1979.

Starling, E.H.: *The Linacre Lecture on the Law of the Heart.* London: Longmans, Green and Co., 1918.

Stehbens, W.E. (ed): *Hemodynamics and the Blood Vessel Wall.* Springfield: Charles C Thomas, 1978.

Strobeck, J.E. and E.J. Sonneyblick: Myocardial Contractile Properties and Ventricular Performance. In Fozzard, H.A., et al., (eds). *The Heart and Cardiovascular System,* Scientific Functioning, vol. 1, pp. 31–49, New York, Raven Press, 1986.

Westfall, V.A.: Electrical and mechanical events in the cardiac cycle. Am. J. Nursing, February, 1976.

5

Respiration

The circulatory system is assigned the task of providing oxygen and nutrients to the cell and carrying carbon dioxide and other products of metabolism away so that energy production for the support of muscular contraction can occur. Since oxygen is found naturally in the air around us, it makes sense to use air as the basic source of this important element and to provide a series of exchanges to get oxygen to the final end point, the cell. Total respiration involves three different exchanges of gases: (1) The exchange of air into and out of the lungs (ventilation), (2) the exchange of gases between the lungs and the blood, and (3) the exchange of gases between the blood and various tissues of the body.

In this system the lungs are designed to move the proper amount of air into close proximity to the blood supply in such a way to allow an exchange of O_2 and CO_2 to occur. This process not only supplies the O_2, but also removes the CO_2. The purpose of this section is to discuss how the lungs function to support the metabolic needs of the body through the circulatory system and to analyze the factors that affect the exchange of gases.

VENTILATION

Ventilation is the exchange of air into and out of the lungs. Air enters the mouth and nose and goes through the pharynx, larynx, and trachea into the bronchial tree. The bronchial tree bifurcates (branches) into bronchioles, terminal bronchioles, respiratory bronchioles, alveolar ducts, and alveolar sacs. The first 16 branches are primarily conducting pathways, covered by a tough continuous cartilaginous material (Fig. 5–1). The inner surface is lined by ciliated cells interspersed with mucous cells at regular intervals. As the bronchioles divide into ducts, they lose their cartilage and ciliated cells.

The blood vessels in the lungs generally follow the respiratory ducts and terminate at the alveoli in a dense network of capillaries. Diffusion of gases takes place through the thin membranes that separate the millions of alveolar sacs from the capillary beds. The area from the respiratory bronchioles to the alveoli is referred to as the transitory and respiratory zone, which is the site of all gas exchange, and constitutes 90% of the total lung volume (Fig. 5–2).

Since the alveolar tissues are so thin and delicate (so that gas exchange can occur through them) (Fig. 5–3), inspired air must be saturated with water, brought to body temperature, and cleaned regardless of how hot or cold, dry or humid or dirty it may be. Air is saturated by the moisture from mucous cells lining the respiratory ducts. It is warmed or cooled as it comes into contact with the mass of body tissue whose temperature is 37°C. It is cleaned as particles in the air are caught by the mucus and removed by the beat of the cilia that line the airways. Larger particles or particles that get deeper into the lung are attacked and destroyed by macrophages. As the air is expelled, the respiratory tract is able to recover some but not all of the heat and moisture. Excess moisture can be easily seen on a cold day as it condenses.

MECHANICS OF PULMONARY VENTILATION (BREATHING)

At rest, air is pulled into the lungs by the contraction of the diaphragm and the *external*

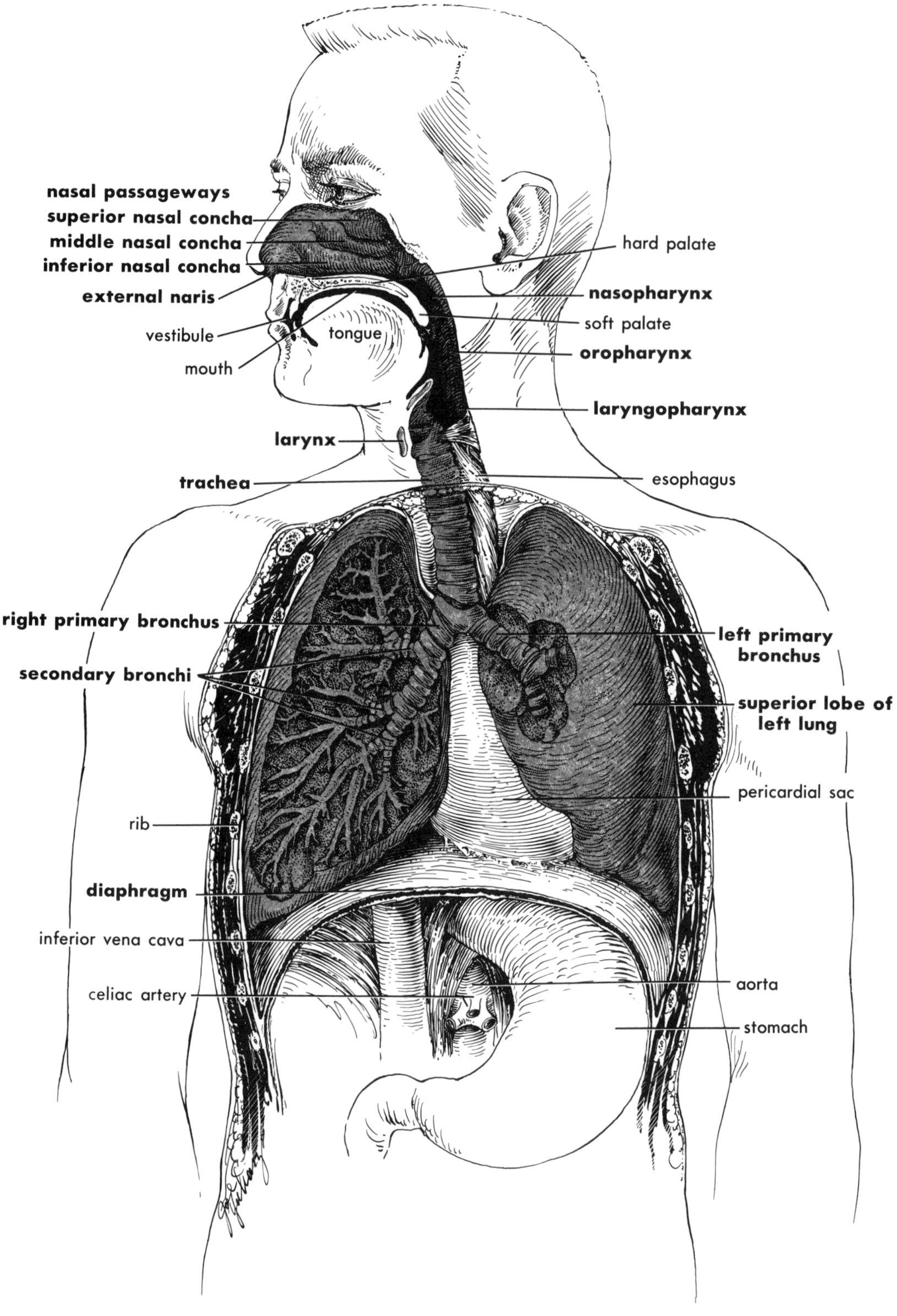

Fig. 5–1. Schematic diagram of respiratory system showing airways and lungs. (From Crouch, J.E. *Functional Human Anatomy,* 4th Ed. Courtesy of Lea & Febiger, 1985.)

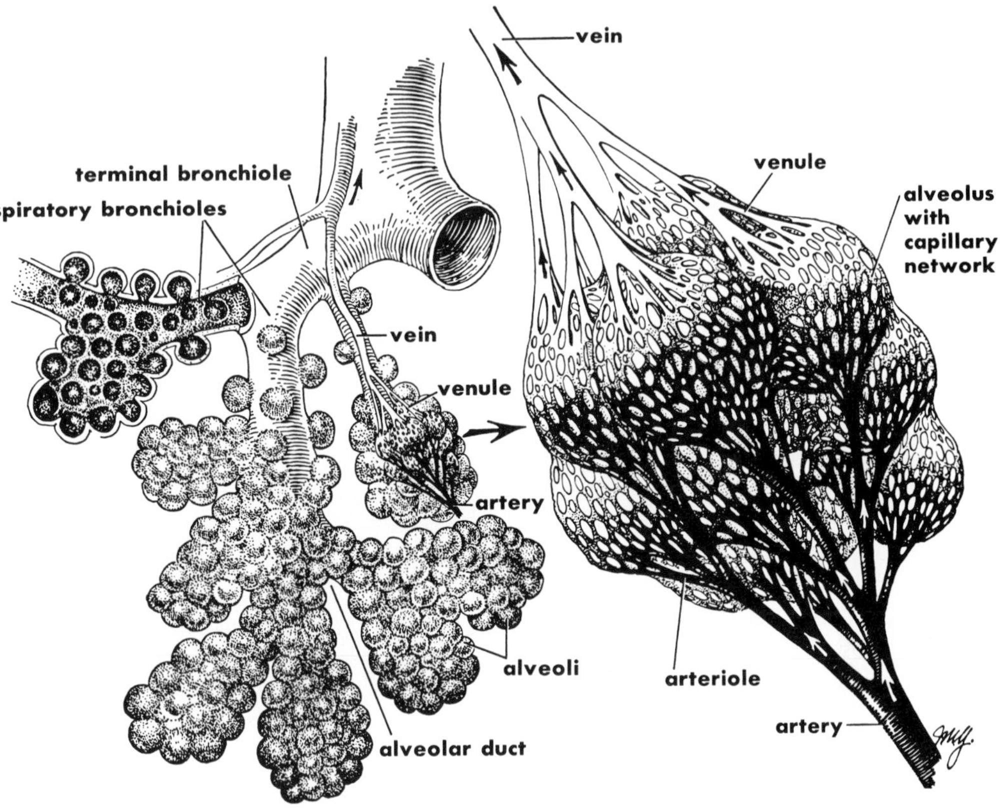

Fig. 5–2. Schematic diagram of the alveoli and alveolar ducts with their blood vessels. (From Crouch, J.E. *Functional Human Anatomy,* 4th Ed. Courtesy of Lea & Febiger, 1985.)

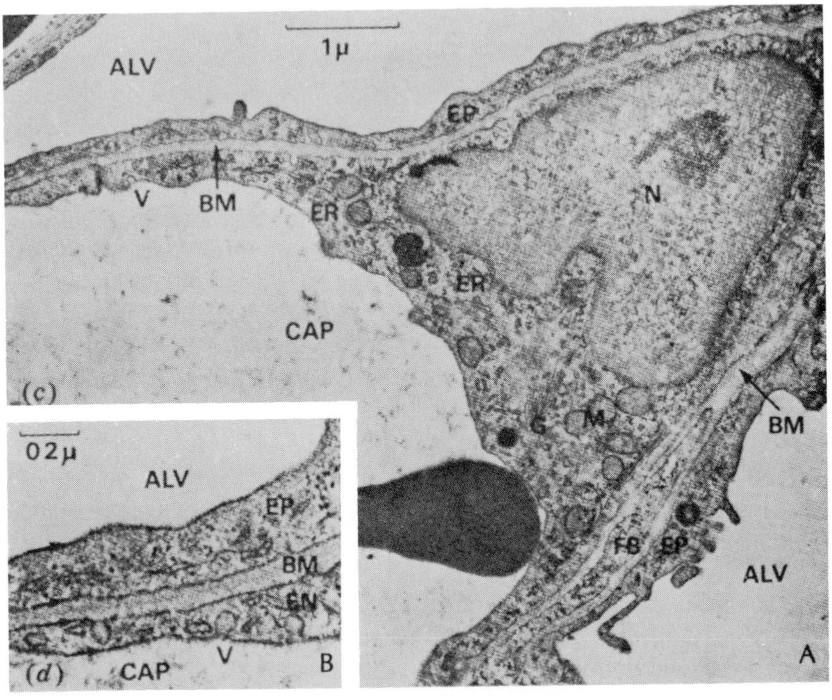

Fig. 5–3. Blood and air are separated by only four thin membranes. (From Astrand, P.O., and Rodahl, K. *Textbook of Work Physiology: Physiological Basis of Exercises,* 2nd Ed. Courtesy of McGraw Hill, 1986.)

intercostal muscles, which increase the thoracic volume. Since the pressure in the lungs is lowered due to the increased volume, outside air rushes in to equalize it. Expiration is caused by a passive relaxation of the diaphragm and a mild contraction of the *internal intercostals.* As the volume inside the lungs gets smaller, the pressure rises and air flows out (Fig. 5–4).

During exercise, the volume of inspired and expired air increases by a larger excursion of the diaphragm (which can descend from 1 to 10 cm) and an increased activity of the intercostals which increase the size of the pulmonary cavity. At intense work loads, even greater inspired volumes can be obtained by involving the scaleni and the sternocleidomastoid. Abdominal muscles can be recruited to help with expiration. The increased volumes associated with high levels of work increase the alveolar size by about 70% which also increases the effective exposure of air to the blood supply.

The lungs maintain their position in the rib cage due to the fluid surface tension between the pleural surfaces covering the lungs and the inside of the thoracic cavity, which allows sliding action, much like two wet panes of glass stuck together. If the surface tension is interrupted by a blow or pneumothorax (air between the pleural surfaces), the lung collapses.

LUNG VOLUMES AND CAPACITIES

During rest, only a small amount of the total usable capacity of the lungs is used during the breathing cycle. This quiet in and out movement of air is called tidal volume (V_T) because of its similarity to the tidal movement of water in the ocean. As exercise begins, the V_T and the frequency of breathing (f) both increase to provide a larger total volume of air to match the increased blood flow through the lungs. The V_T increases by using more of the

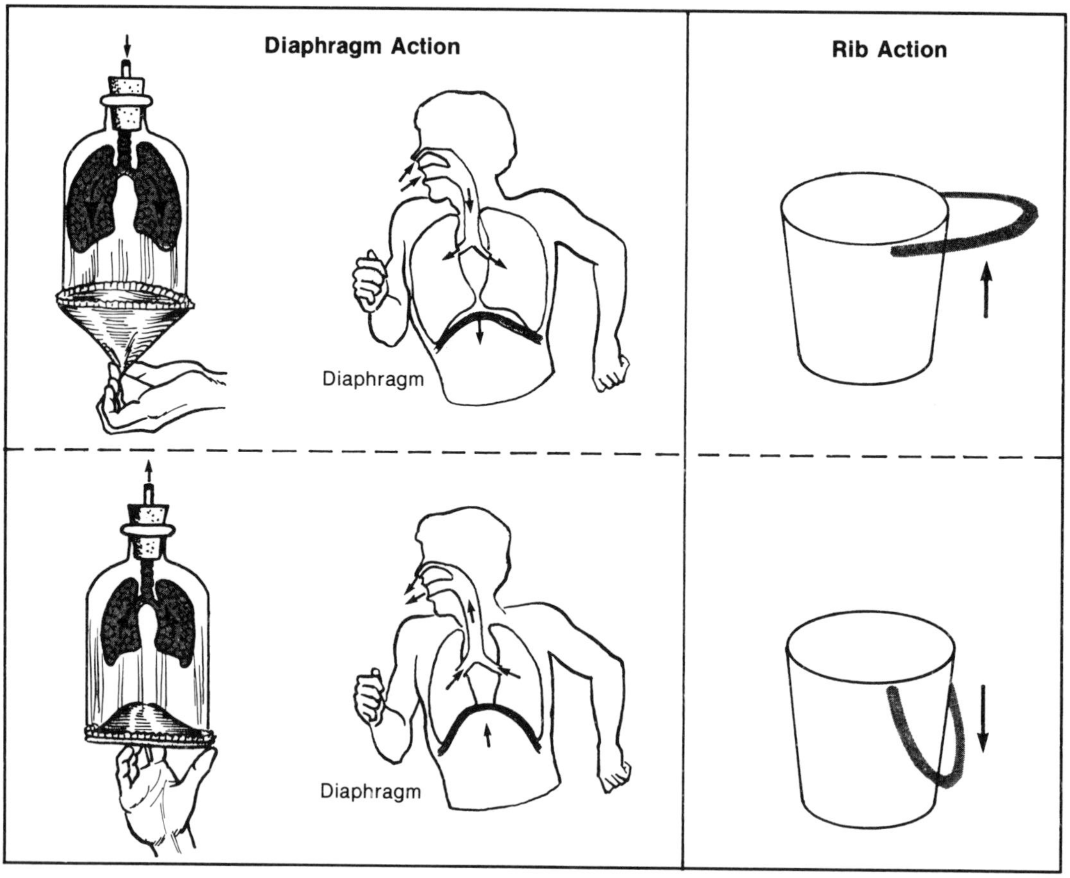

Fig. 5–4. Mechanics of pulmonary ventilation. (From McArdle, W.D., Katch, F.I., and Katch, V.L. *Exercise Physiology*, 2nd Ed. Courtesy of Lea & Febiger, 1986.)

lungs total usable capacity each breath, drawing from both inspiratory and expiratory reserves (ERV and IRV). All but one of these volumes and capacities (residual volume) of the lung can be measured using a simple spirometer (Fig. 5–5).

To measure lung volumes and capacities, a person simply breathes quietly for several breaths, and then inspires and expires as deeply as possible.

Capacities of the lung are by definition, the combination of two or more volumes. Figure 5–6 shows the normal volumes and capacities of the lung that can be measured on a spirometer. Note that total lung capacity (TLC) cannot be measured directly because there is always a "residual" volume (RV) of air that cannot be exhaled. This "buffer" air is important to stabilize the oxygen and carbon dioxide content of the aveoli. Without RV, the oxygen pressure in the alveoli would vary dramatically during each breath being higher during inspiration and lower during expiration and the blood passing the alveoli would not receive a constant supply. Inspiratory capacity (IC) combines VT and IRC, and functional residual capacity (FRC) combines ERV and TV.

The following formula can be used to calculate some estimated lung volume and capacities:

Males:

$$VC = 0.057\,(Ht^*) - 0.0238\,(AGE) - 3.771$$

$$TLC = 0.076\,(Ht) + 0.008\,(AGE) - 7.083$$

$$RV = TLC - VC$$

Females:

$$VC = -3.2457 + 0.04526\,(Ht^*) - 0.01717\,(AGE)$$

$$TLC = -7.9389 + 0.0798\,(ht) - 0.00706\,(AGE)$$

$$RV = TLC - VC$$

*Ht = Height in centimeters

MEASUREMENT OF FUNCTIONAL RESIDUAL CAPACITY (FRC)

Residual volume can be easily measured using a technique called *helium dilution*. To do the test, a small amount of helium (usually about 600 ml) is added to a spirometer containing several liters of air. The percent helium in the spirometer after mixing is called He_1. This value is recorded before the subjects begin the test.

The subject is then placed on the spirometer and begins breathing the air-helium mixture at end tidal volume. End tidal volume is used as the starting point (which leaves FRC in the lungs) because it is quite

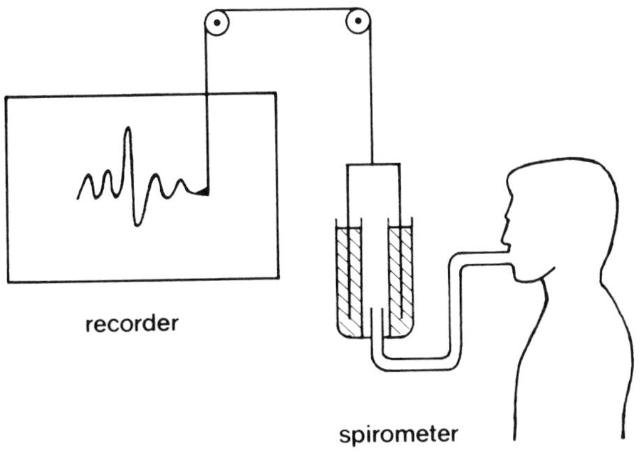

Fig. 5–5. A simple spirometer for measuring lung volumes and capacities.

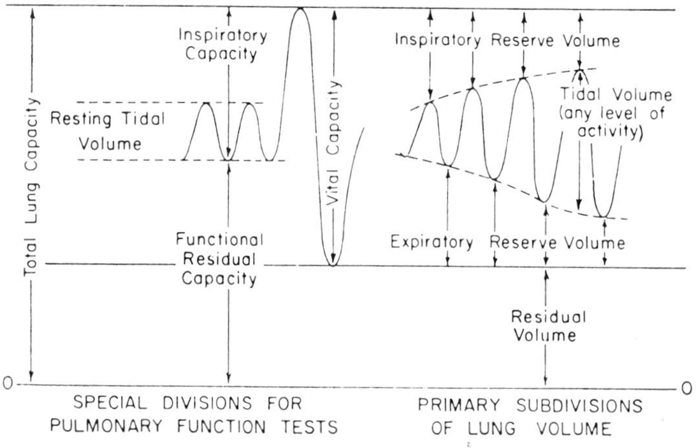

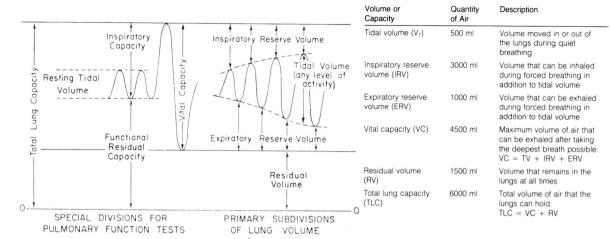

Volume or Capacity	Quantity of Air	Description
Tidal volume (V_T)	500 ml	Volume moved in or out of the lungs during quiet breathing
Inspiratory reserve volume (IRV)	3000 ml	Volume that can be inhaled during forced breathing in addition to tidal volume
Expiratory reserve volume (ERV)	1000 ml	Volume that can be exhaled during forced breathing in addition to tidal volume
Vital capacity (VC)	4500 ml	Maximum volume of air that can be exhaled after taking the deepest breath possible: VC = TV + IRV + ERV
Residual volume (RV)	1500 ml	Volume that remains in the lungs at all times
Total lung capacity (TLC)	6000 ml	Total volume of air that the lungs can hold: TLC = VC + RV

Fig. 5–6. Lung volumes and capacities and a description of each.

repeatable and RV can be easily calculated by subtracting ERV. As the subject breathes normally, O_2 is added to maintain the same spirometer volume and a second % He (He_2) reading is taken after about 6 minutes or when the helium mixture has been completely diluted and stabilized. At the end of the test the subject is asked to breathe out as much as possible to record ERV (Fig. 5–7).

FRC is calculated using the equation:

$$FRC = \frac{He_1 \times (He_1 - He_2)}{He_2}$$

If 600 ml of helium was initially added to the spirometer and He_1 was 8.0% and He_2 5.5%, FRC would be:

$$\frac{600}{.08} \times \frac{8.0 - 5.5}{5.5} = 3409 \text{ ml}$$

To get RV, subtract the measured ERV from the calculated FRC and correct to BTPS. Normal RV values for 20- to 30-year-old males are 1200 ml and for females 1000 ml. These values will increase with age.

A similar technique can be used for healthy subjects by mixing helium in a rebreathing bag and having the subject breathe out completely before breathing the mixture so that only RV is diluted.

PULMONARY VENTILATION

The amount of air breathed each minute is called pulmonary ventilation and is expressed as volume of expired air ($\dot{V}_E$). The dot over the V means volume per unit time (usually one minute). Of course, $\dot{V}_E$ is the product of how much air is moved each breath times the frequency (f) of these breaths or:

$$\dot{V}_E = V_T \times f$$

V_T = Tidal volume (ml or l/breath)
f = Frequency (breaths/min)

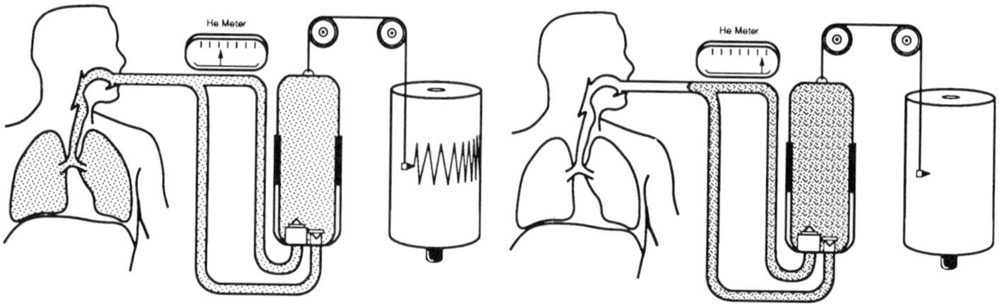

Fig. 5–7. Measuring RV using He dilution. Note that He in the system is diluted into the air of the lungs; the greater the dilution, the larger the FRC.

During rest, V_T is usually about 500 ml and f is 10 to 15 breaths per minute so $\dot{V}_E$ = 5 − 7.5 l/min; (500 × 10 = 5 l/min; 500 × 15 = 7.5 l/min). During work, the breathing rate increases to 40 to 60 breaths/minute, while the tidal volume can increase to about 65% of VC. For a person who has a VC of 6 liters and an f of 50 breaths/minute, the $\dot{V}_E$ would be 195 liters/minute (50 × .65 (VC) or 3.9 liters = 195 l/min). The $\dot{V}_E$ for a healthy athlete at rest and at work is presented in Table 5–1.

The relationship between $\dot{V}_E$ and work is fairly linear to a point about 50 to 80% of max work where it begins to increase out of proportion to the oxidative needs (a process called hyperventilation).

The ratio of the liters of air ($\dot{V}_E$) needed to support the burning of a liter of oxygen ($\dot{V}_{O_2}$) in the metabolic process is called the *ventilation equivalent.* It takes about 20 to 25 liters of $\dot{V}_E$ per liter of $\dot{V}_{O_2}$ at rest and moderate levels of work and 30 to 35 liters $\dot{V}_E$ per liter $\dot{V}_{O_2}$ at higher levels (Fig. 5–8).

$\dot{V}_E$ does not seem to be a limiting factor to increasing work in normal subjects because there is always more capacity to breathe than is used. In world-class athletes $\dot{V}_{O_2}$ can increase from .25 l/min to 5.0 l/min, a 20-fold increase, where $\dot{V}_E$ can increase from 5 l/min to 200 l/min or a 40-fold increase. Normal subjects can always increase their $\dot{V}_E$ during exercise, even at maximum work.

At rest, the muscles of inspiration consume about 1.9 to 3.1 ml of O_2 for every liter of oxygen breathed (about 1% of the total energy requirements of the body). As the rate of respiration and workload increases, the cost of ventilation increases to about 10% of the total energy cost.

MEASURING $\dot{V}_E$ DURING WORK

Measuring $\dot{V}_E$ accurately during work is one of the major challenges facing exercise physiologists. It is critical to use a low resistance breathing valve or mask and large enough tubing (when used) to decrease the internal resistance as much as possible. In addition, measured volumes are always corrected to standard conditions (see "gases" this chapter).

The following techniques for measuring $\dot{V}_E$ during work have been used:

1. Tissot spirometer—a tissot spirometer is a large volume spirometer used by early physiologists to measure $\dot{V}_E$ during work. However, during work, the resistance is large and multiple measurements are difficult to take. The tissot *is* accurate and is often used to measure volumes collected in other bags or balloons after a test is completed.

2. Douglas Bags or meteorologic balloons—a series of collection bags can be used to collect expired air during a graded exercise test. Following the test, the O_2 and CO_2 values are determined and volumes passed into a tissot or through a calibrated gasometer.

3. Gasometer—high speed gasometers allow the computerized measurement of $\dot{V}_E$ during work but are difficult to standardize (partly because of the pulsative flow of respiratory gases) and some have a rather high resistance to flow. Studies have also shown inaccuracies if the gasometer is placed on the expired side of the subject because of the accumulation of moisture in the bellows (Fig. 5–9).

4. Pneumotachs—pneumotachs are probably the most widely used devices for measuring $\dot{V}_E$ during work in the modern research laboratory. They can be accurately standardized to measure both inspired and expired volumes, and can be interfaced with computers for breath-by-breath $\dot{V}O_2$ calculations. They are fairly sensitive in terms of position, and should be heated to prevent moisture accumulation, but have a rather narrow measurement range and labs might need several different sizes of pneumotachs to test large and small subjects.

5. Spinners—a spinner device with almost no mass (to cut down momentum) has been used successfully to measure $\dot{V}_E$ during work. It

Table 5–1. $\dot{V}_E$ At Rest and At Work For a Healthy Athlete

	$\dot{V}_E$	$= V_T \times f$
Rest	5 l/min	= .5 liter × 10 breaths/min.
Maximum Work	200 l/min	= 4.0 liter × 50 breaths/min.

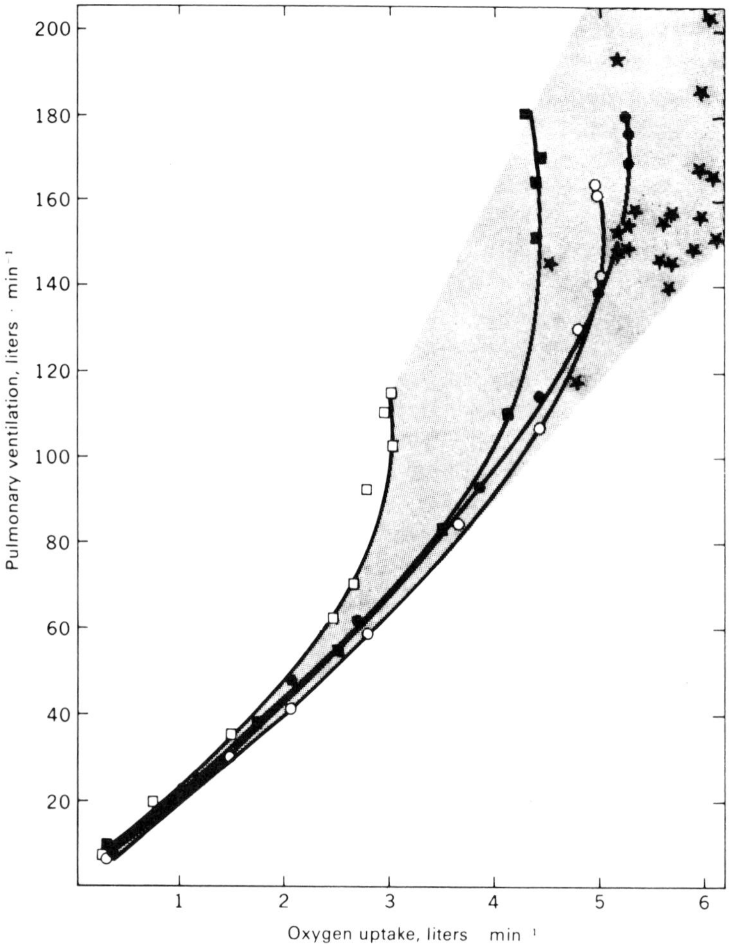

Fig. 5–8. Pulmonary ventilation at rest and during exercise (running or cycling). Four individual curves are present. Several work loads gave the same maximal oxygen uptake. Stars denote individual values for top athletes measured when maximal oxygen uptake was attained. Individuals with maximal oxygen uptake of 3 L/min. or higher usually fall within the shadowed area. Note the wide scattering of high oxygen uptakes. (From Astrand, P.O., and Rodahl, K. *Textbook of Work Physiology: Physiological Basis of Exercises*, 2nd Ed. Courtesy of McGraw Hill, 1986.)

has all the advantages of pneumotachs, but is lighter and easier to use. In addition, there are no hoses or tubes to encumber the test.

CONTROL OF BREATHING

Central Function

The factors that control alveolar ventilation are about the most complex in the body. Although the respiratory centers have a basic rhythmicity, they are adjusted so that the rate and depth of breathing matches the demands of the body, even though blood O_2 and CO_2 change very little during strenuous exercise.

The respiratory center is composed of a group of neurons located in the reticular portions of the medulla oblongata and pons. The neurons in the dorsal medullary area tend to be mostly inspiratory and those in the ventral area mainly expiratory. The basic rhythmicity seems to be in the inspiratory neurons which emit repetitive bursts of activity, even when all incoming signals are blocked (Fig. 5–10). During expiration, the inspiratory neurons are quiet, but after a few seconds they fire automatically, sending signals down the phrenic nerve to the diaphragm and down the intercostal nerve to the external intercostal muscles while at the same time, inhibiting signals to the expiratory neurons.

Two other groups of neurons in the pons

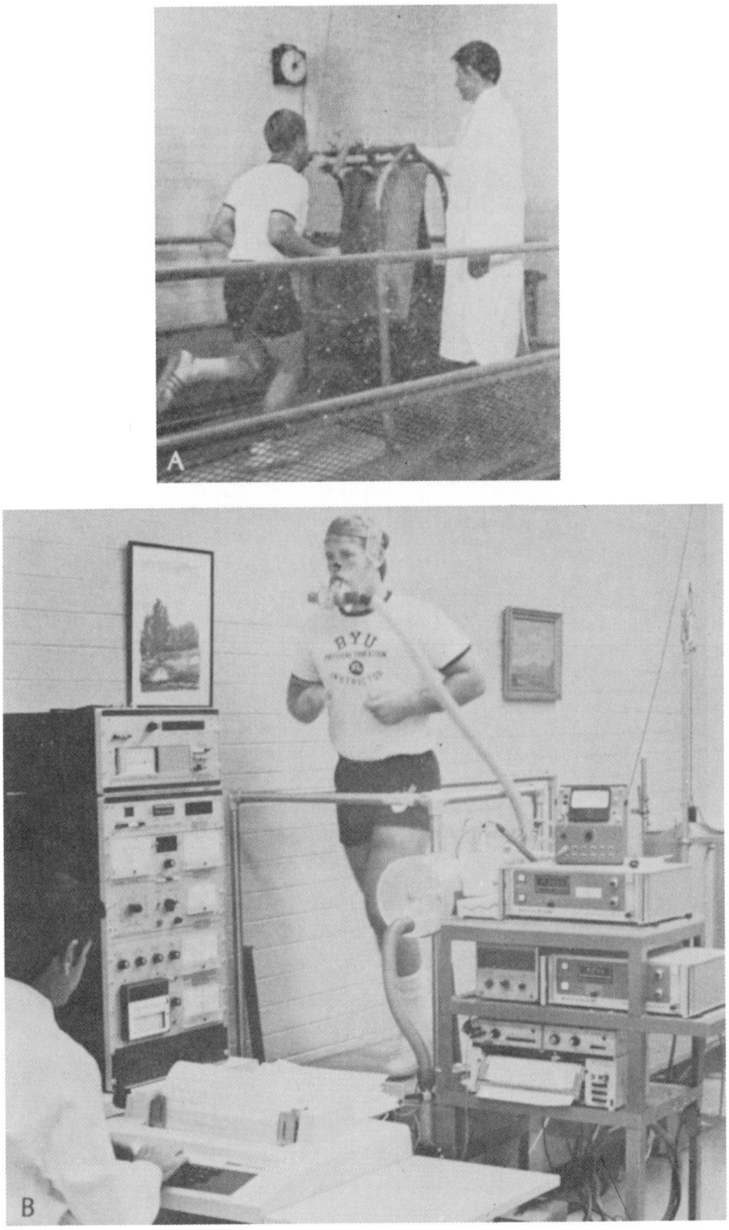

Fig. 5–9. *A.* Collecting expired air in Douglas bags during a max test. *B.* Expired air measured through a pneumotach using an early computerized device. Note tissot in background.

affect the medullary neural activity: the *apneustic center,* which may be involved in the stimulation of inspiration, and the *pneumotaxic center,* whose primary effect is to inhibit or limit inspiration. Strong signals from the pneumotaxic center shorten inspiration, allowing a cycle to occur much more rapidly. Inspiration is also inhibited by stretch receptors in the walls of the bronchi and bronchioles, that protect the lungs from being over extended (the Hering-Breuer reflex).

Central Control. Since the basic purpose of ventilation is to maintain proper blood concentration of oxygen (O_2), carbon dioxide (CO_2), and hydrogen ions (H^+), it is fortunate that respiration is responsive to changes in any of these factors. In fact, there is a chemosensitive area near the respiratory neurons

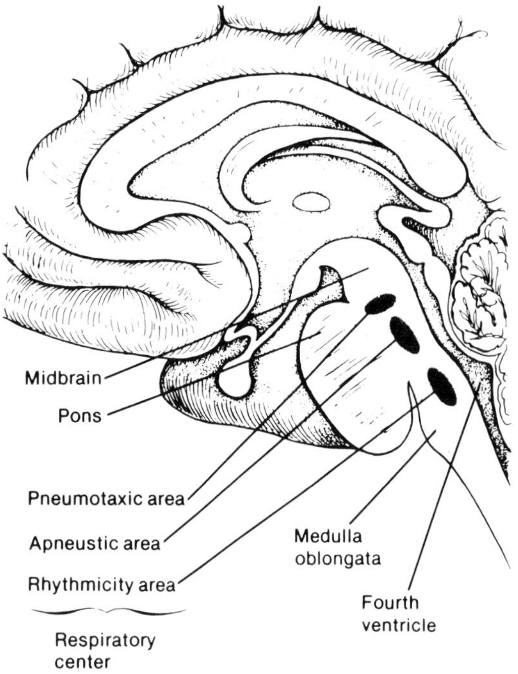

Fig. 5–10. The location of the respiratory center in the medulla and pons of the brain. (From Van De Graaff, K.M. *Human Anatomy.* Courtesy of William C. Brown, 1984.)

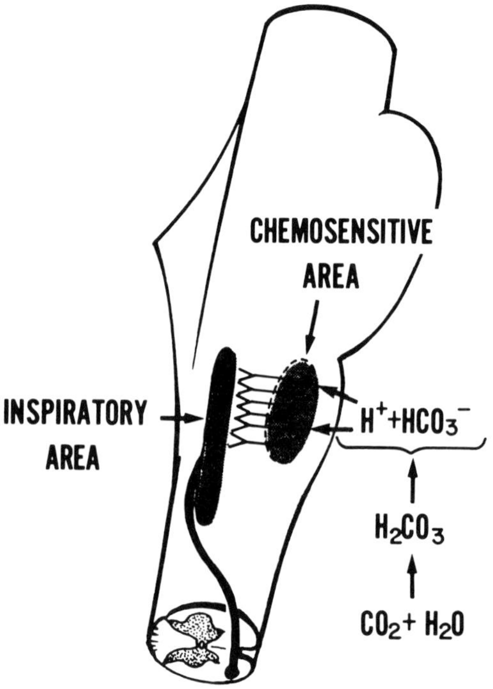

Fig. 5–11. Stimulation of the inspiratory area by the chemosensitive area located bilaterally in the medulla, lying only a few microns beneath the ventral medullary surface. Note also that hydrogen ions stimulate the chemosensitive area, while carbon dioxide in the fluid gives rise to hydrogen ions. (From Guyton, A.C. *Human Physiology and Mechanism of Disease,* 4th Ed. Courtesy of W.B. Saunders Co., 1987.)

that is highly sensitive to changes in either blood CO_2 or hydrogen ions. Interestingly, the neurons are most sensitive to H^+, but H^+ do not easily cross the blood-brain barrier (BBB). Therefore, even though CO_2 has little direct effect on these neurons, it can cross the blood-brain barrier easily, and when it crosses, it reacts with water to form carbonic acid which immediately dissociates to bicarbonate and hydrogen ions. These hydrogen ions then directly stimulate breathing (Fig. 5–11). Of course, breathing can also be controlled from the cortex, which overrides the brainstem for such actions as breath-holding, speaking, blowing musical instruments, and voluntary hyperventilation.

Peripheral

Besides the chemosensitive neurons in the medulla, the body has peripheral chemoreceptors located in the carotid bodies at the bifurcation of the common carotid arteries and in the aortic bodies above and below the aortic arch (Fig. 5–12).

Each of the chemoreceptors receives a special blood supply from a small branch of the nearby arterial trunk. These receptors are sensitive to changes in O_2, CO_2 and H^+ concentrations. Their response to arterial CO_2 is less important than that of the chemosensitive areas in the medulla, accounting for only 20% of the total ventilatory response. However, their response is more rapid and may be important in adjusting ventilation to work. Only the carotid bodies are sensitive to pH (H^+) changes.

The peripheral chemoreceptors are important in that they are almost totally responsible for the increase in ventilation due to decreased oxygen tension (PO_2). However, low blood PO_2 will have little effect on ventilation until it falls to almost one half of normal values. By then the increased CO_2 and H^+ will have clearly stimulated higher breathing levels. The reason O_2 plays such a secondary role in the normal regulation of breathing is that O_2 saturation remains fairly constant whether

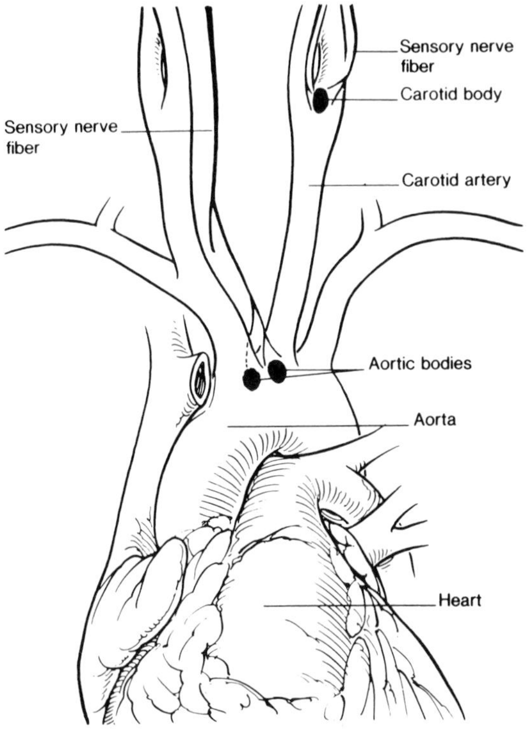

Fig. 5–12. The peripheral chemoreceptors (aortic and carotid bodies) regulate the brainstem respiratory centers by means of sensory nerve stimulation. (From Van De Graaff, K.M. *Human Anatomy.* Courtesy of William C. Brown, 1984.)

alveolar ventilation is 10 times normal or down to ½ normal because of the shape of the oxygen dissociation curve (see section on Oxygen Dissociation Curve later in this chapter). Therefore, ventilation can change rather dramatically without much change in oxygen transport. On the other hand, alveolar ventilation has a large effect on CO_2 concentration and H^+.

Decreases in O_2 do play a major role in regulation of breathing when a person ascends to altitudes (see Chapter 14) or in certain diseases such as pneumonia and emphysema.

Regulation of Breathing During Exercise

Beginning moderate to high levels of work cause a rapid increase in ventilation, probably stimulated by movement of the limbs and the higher centers of the brain controlling respiration. During submaximal exercise, ventilation levels off after reaching steady-state values, while during maximal exercise, ventilation does not level off, but continues to increase until the exercise is terminated. As soon as the exercise is stopped, $\dot{V}_E$ drops quickly with a slower more gradual decline after a few minutes (Fig. 5–13).

In strenuous exercise, ventilation increases rapidly and matches the oxygen uptake and CO_2 production quite accurately. However, little change occurs in blood O_2 and CO_2 levels at any level of work. In fact, blood CO_2 may actually decrease. The H^+ ion concentration remains fairly steady during moderate work, but increases during heavy exercise because of increased lactate production. Since little change in blood levels of these chemicals occurs, none of these factors can account for the large increase in ventilation seen in moderate exercise.

If ventilation does not increase during exercise as a result of chemical changes, what causes the increase? The following ideas have been suggested:

1. *Stimulation of the carotid bodies by increased oscillation of CO_2.* Since arterial CO_2 and pH oscillate with each breath, the change in amplitude and period of these oscillations during exercise may be of sufficient magnitude to stimulate breathing through the carotid bodies.

2. *Stimulation from the motor cortex.* It may be that collateral impulses from motor cortex activity stimulate the respiratory centers causing an increase in ventilation.

3. *Afferent input from exercising muscles.* Limb movement itself may stimulate respiratory centers through joint proprioceptors or mus-

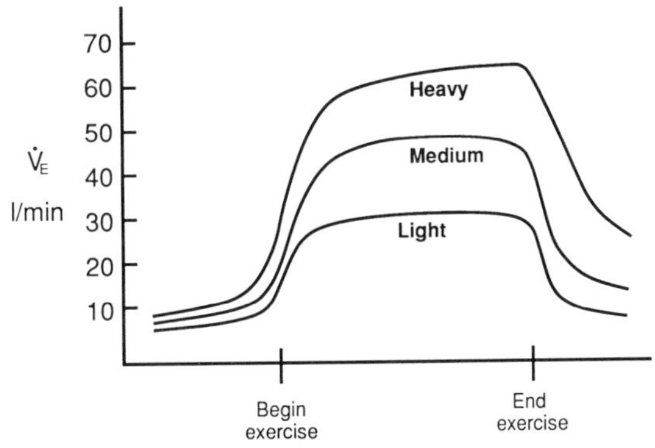

Fig. 5–13. Changes in $\dot{V}_E$ during work of different intensities.

cle spindles. Even passive movements of limbs yield an increase in pulmonary ventilation.

4. *Increased venous return to the heart.* Some researchers have speculated that some mechanism in the heart senses the increased stretch associated with increased venous return and yields an increase in ventilation.

5. *Hypermetabolism.* Since hypermetabolism increases cardiac output, a sensor (a metaboreceptor) could sense pulmonary blood flow, mixed venous CO_2, or some unknown humoral (blood-borne) substance.

In any case, there are probably "feed-forward" mechanisms (the list above may all be feed-forward) that stimulate breathing at the beginning of exercise, and "feed-back" mechanisms that correlate breathing with actual need. The latter mechanisms are probably related to CO_2 production, hydrogen ion concentration, or pH and sensed by the chemoreceptors (Fig. 5–14).

GASES

Gases are quite different from liquids since they are compressible and their volumes are affected by changes in pressure and temperature. When lung volumes are measured or when expired air is collected during an exercise test, these volumes need to be corrected so that comparisons can be made with other standards. Air volumes are normally expressed in one of the following conditions:

1. *Ambient Temperature, Pressure, Saturated (ATPS).* This is the common condition of air collected into some container outside the body. For example, expired air collected during an exercise test in a laboratory is usually about 22°C (room temperature), at the barometric pressure of the laboratory, and completely saturated.

2. *Body Temperature, Pressure, Saturated (BTPS).* This represents the conditions inside the lungs. Typically these values are 37°C (body temperature), ambient pressure (the pressure must be similar both inside and outside the body), and 100% saturated with water. BTPS is used to report all pulmonary lung capacities and volumes. Typically, these volumes are collected in a spirometer (ATPS) and are converted to BTPS.

3. *Standard Temperature, Pressure, Dry (STPD).* Standard conditions are defined as 0°C, 760 mm Hg, and dry (no water vapor). All metabolic gases are converted to STPD for standardization.

Any gas condition can be converted to any other using the following general formula:

$$V_2 = V_1 \times \frac{T_2 + 273}{T_1 + 273} \times \frac{P_1 - P_{H_2O}}{P_2 - P_{H_2O}}$$

Where V_1 is the volume you want to correct. The conditions (temperature, pressure and water vapor) of V_1 are placed in the formula at T_1 and P_1. The conditions of the desired corrections are placed in the formula at T_2 and P_2. For example, what would be the STPD volume (V_2) of a 14 liter sample of expired air collected in a Douglas bag at a room temperature of 22°C and a lab pressure of 645 mm Hg? Enter the pertinent data and solve:

$$V_1 = 14 \text{ liters} \times \frac{0 + 273}{22 + 273} \times \frac{645 - 19.8}{760 - 0}$$

$$V_1 = 10.66 \text{ liters}$$

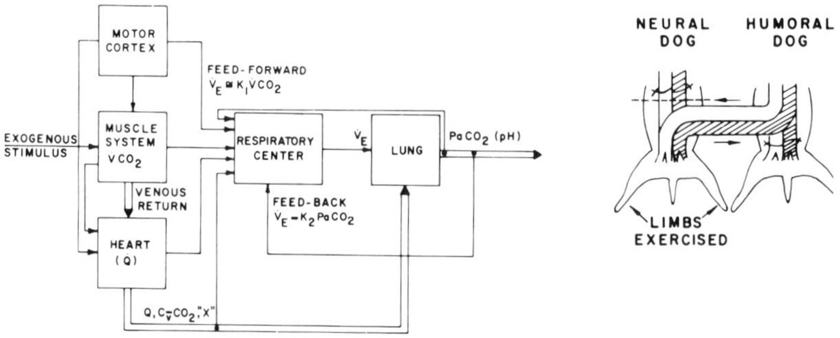

Fig. 5–14. Possible feed-forward/feed back factors relating to the control of $\dot{V}_E$ during exercise. (From Swanson, G.D.: Overview of Ventricular Control During Exercise. Med. Sci. Sports Exerc. *11*:224, 1979.)

The 273 is placed in the formula because gases change 1/273 of their volume for every 1°C change in temperature. Water vapor in the gas (P_{H_2O}) must be subtracted out to get the true volume of the gas itself. The value of the water vapor pressure can be obtained from standard chemistry tables. These values vary with temperature of the gas (warm gas holds more water) and is 47 mm Hg at body temperature (37°C) and about 20 mm Hg at normal room temperature.

Of course, a correction factor can be calculated if the formula is solved for temperature, pressure and water vapor and V_1 is omitted. This correction factor can then be used with any value of V_1. In a typical laboratory setting, a correction factor is calculated every hour or so and all volumes are combined using this factor.

Gas Laws

Boyle's Law. This law states that at a constant temperature, the volume of gas is inversely proportional to its pressure. As the pressure decreases, as in increasing altitude, the gas will expand. As pressure increases, the molecules of the gas are compressed decreasing the volume (Fig. 5–15A). A basketball inflated correctly in Salt Lake City (alt. 5000 ft.) will go flat if taken to California (sea level) because in California, the barometric pressure is greater (760 mm Hg) and compresses the molecules of air more than the barometric pressure of 640 mm Hg in Salt Lake City. A knowledge of Boyle's law is also important for scuba divers. The compressed air a diver breathes at 100 feet underwater will expand as he approaches the surface, and unless the air is released, it may rupture the lungs (see Chapter 14).

Charles' Law. This law states that at a constant pressure, the volume of a gas is directly proportional to its temperature. The volume of a gas increases if the gas is warmed, and decreases if it is cooled (Fig. 5–15B). For example, a car's tires expand while driving across the desert. If the tire pressure is checked and adjusted in that condition, they will be almost flat after sitting all night in the cold. In the 1930s, when tires weren't built as well as they are now, flat tires were common because the rubber in the tires couldn't expand with the increase in gas volume.

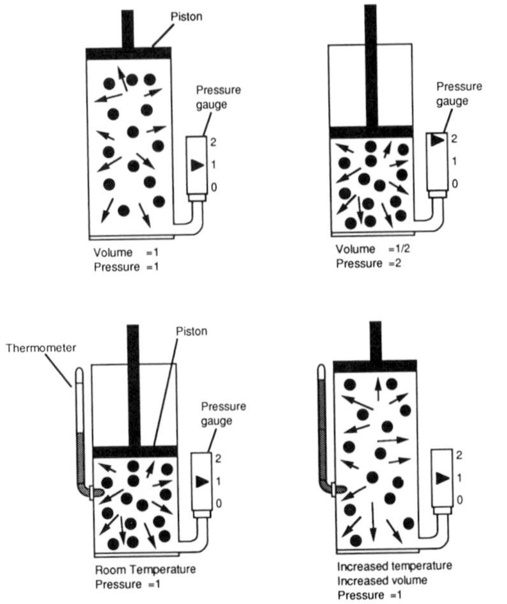

Fig. 5–15. Illustration of *(A)* Boyle's law and *(B)* Charles' law.

Law of Partial Pressure (Dalton's Law). The blanket of air that covers the entire earth has a tremendous weight that is expressed as atmospheric pressure. This pressure varies with the altitude, being greater at sea level and less in mountainous regions. Atmospheric pressure is measured using a *barometer.* If an evacuated tube (the air has been drawn out) is placed upside down in a dish of mercury (Hg), the atmospheric pressure will push Hg up the tube to a point that equals the downward weight of the atmospheric pressure (Fig. 5–16). At sea level, this equalization of pressure is about 760 mm Hg; while in the mountain states, it is about 640 mm Hg. On Mt. Everest, the pressure is less than 200 mm Hg.

Oxygen (O_2) makes up about 21% of the air around us, and that ratio remains constant no matter how low the atmospheric pressure. Therefore, the lower the total pressure, the lower the pressure of O_2 (called partial pressure of O_2 or P_{O_2}). For example, at sea level the total pressure is 760 mm Hg and the P_{O_2} is 159 mm Hg (.21 × 760); at 5,000 feet, the atmospheric pressure drops to 633 and the P_{O_2} to 133. By 20,000 feet, the P_{O_2} has dropped to 74 mm Hg and at 64,000 feet, the

A simplified barometer.

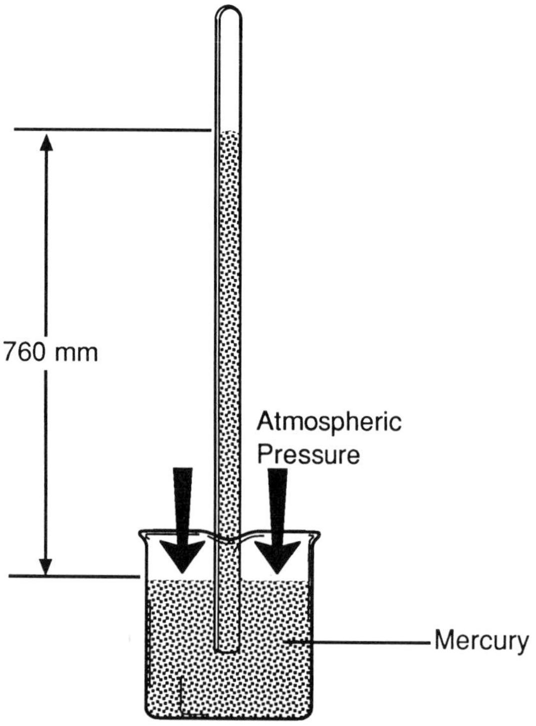

Fig. 5–16. A simplified barometer.

P_{O_2} is lower than the water vapor pressure in the lungs. Obviously, the higher a person goes, the less O_2 is available and the tougher it is to perform well in endurance events.

Gases involved in respiration are usually mixtures of N_2, O_2, CO_2 and water (H_2O), each of which exerts pressure according to its concentration. Of course, the total of the individual gas pressures can never be greater than the total pressure of the gas itself. This means that adding a gas to or increasing the concentration of a gas (such as adding H_2O to air going into the lungs) will decrease the pressure of all the other gases in this mixture. This relationship is described as *the law of partial pressures* and expressed in the formula:

$$P_T = P_1 + P_2 + P_3 + P_4 + \ldots . P_N$$

Where P_T is the total gas pressure and P_{1-N} refers to individual gases. At sea level, atmospheric air has a P_T of about 760 mm Hg. Since oxygen is about 21% (actually 20.94%) of the mixture, it exerts 21% of the pressure. Therefore, the PO_2 is 760 × .21 = 159 mm Hg. If this air is dry, the only other significant gas is N_2 which makes up 79% of the volume. The pressure of N_2 (P_{N_2}) can be determined by multiplying 760 by .79 or by subtracting P_{O_2} from 760. Both calculations will be the same because the total must equal 760 mm Hg.

However, atmospheric air usually contains some water vapor. The *relative humidity* is an expression of how much water is contained in air as compared to how much it will hold. For example, at 22°C, air can hold enough water to exert about 20 mm Hg of pressure. A relative humidity of 50% at 22°C would mean that the P_{H_2O} was 10 mm Hg. In this condition, P_{O_2} would be decreased slightly as shown:

$$\begin{array}{l} 760 \\ \underline{-10} \text{ mm Hg } P_{H_2O} \\ 750 \\ \underline{\times 21\%} \; O_2 \\ 750 \\ \underline{1500} \\ 157.5 \; P_{O_2} \end{array}$$

PARTIAL PRESSURE IN THE CIRCULATORY AND PULMONARY SYSTEM

Gases in the respiratory system move from a higher pressure to a lower pressure by the process of diffusion and the partial pressures of each gas provides the driving force furthering movement from one place to another. As air enters the trachea, it is warmed and saturated with water in the form of vapor, which also contributes to the total pressure of the gas. Water vapor pressure at 37°C (body temperature) exerts a partial pressure of 47 mm Hg. So in order to accurately calculate the partial pressure of oxygen, the partial pressure of H_2O (P_{H_2O}) is subtracted from the atmospheric pressure (760 mm Hg − 47 mm Hg = 713 mm Hg). Therefore, the P_{O_2} of air in the trachea is 149 mm Hg (760 − 47) × 20.94%).

Based on this calculation; the P_{O_2} in the

lungs should be 149 mm Hg but this is not the case. During one ventilatory cycle, only a fraction (⅓) of the air in the lungs is totally expelled, leaving behind used air and carbon dioxide to dilute the inspired air. As a result, the P_{CO_2} that should only equal 0.3 mm Hg mixes with the carbon dioxide that is produced by the cells, and increases the P_{CO_2} to about 40 mm Hg. With the increased P_{H_2O} and P_{CO_2} the pressure of oxygen in the lungs is decreased to 105 mm Hg and the P_{N_2} to 568 mm Hg (Fig. 5–17). Interestingly, the P_{O_2} in arterial blood is about 5 mm Hg lower than alveolar P_{O_2}. This occurs, not because blood flows too rapidly to become saturated, but because some blood flows past alveoli that are either not inflated or have not been exchanged. This blood is not oxygenated fully and decreases the total saturation of arterial blood somewhat.

The P_{O_2} of venous blood reflects the average of all the tissue needs and is usually about 46 mm Hg. The partial pressure of various tissues varies according to their demands. For instance, the P_{O_2} in venous blood taken directly from muscles can be almost normal (if inactive) or almost completely depleted. P_{CO_2} can be high or low depending on metabolic activity.

It is interesting that P_{O_2} drops from 100 mm Hg in the arterial system to 46 mm Hg in the veins (a 60 mm Hg drop) while CO_2 changes from 40 to 46 mm Hg even though the production of CO_2 is similar to the use of O_2. The reason for this seeming discrepancy relates to the relative solubility of the two gases in solution. Partial pressure of gases is a function of the molecules in solution. Oxygen is very insoluble and only 3% of the total gas is carried in solution, CO_2 is much more soluble and nearly 30% is carried in solution. Because of this difference, a similar change in the number of molecules exchanged will result in quite different pressure changes.

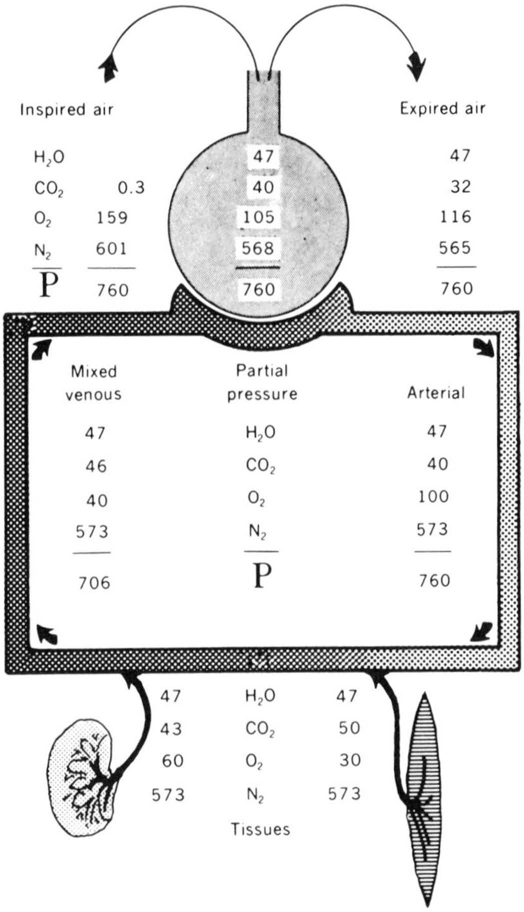

Fig. 5–17. Typical values of gas tension in inspired air, alveolar air (encircled), expired air, and blood at rest. Barometric pressure, 760 mmHg; for simplicity the inspired air is considered free from water (dry). Tension of oxygen and carbon dioxide varies significantly in venous blood from different organs. In this figure, gas tensions in venous blood from the kidney and muscle are presented. (From Astrand, P.O., and Rodahl, K. *Textbook of Work Physiology: Physiological Basis of Exercises*, 2nd Ed. Courtesy of McGraw Hill, 1986.)

TRANSIT TIME

As blood enters the capillary beds surrounding the alveoli, five "barriers" separate the red blood cells and the alveolar sacs. These barriers are: (1) the alveolar epithelium, (2) the alveolar basement membrane, (3) the capillary endothelium, (4) the capillary basement membrane, and (5) the interstitial space (see Fig. 5–3).

At rest, blood passes entirely through the capillaries in less than 1 second. Because the blood is in the capillary such a short time, there needs to be a rapid exchange of gases for the blood to totally release its carbon dioxide and pick up oxygen. Within 0.1 second after the blood has entered the capillaries, the P_{CO_2} has reached equilibrium, while after .30 second, the P_{CO_2} is at equilibrium (Fig. 5–18). The reason for such a difference in the speeds

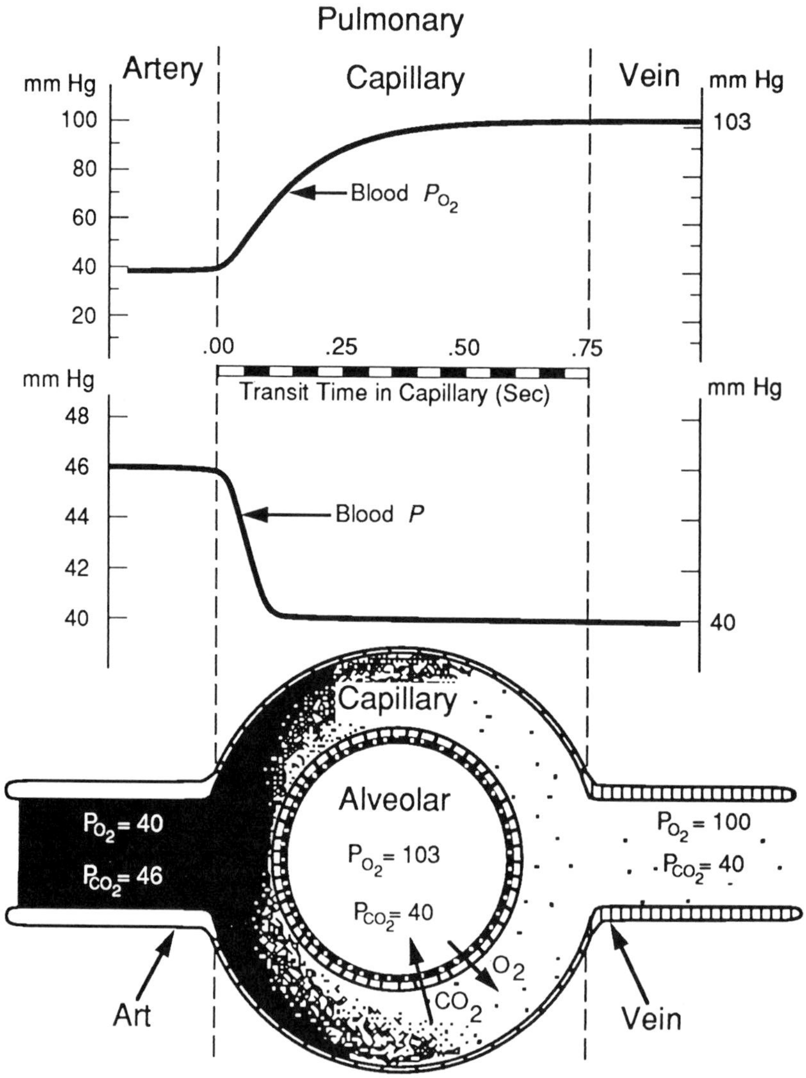

Fig. 5–18. Change in the partial pressures of oxygen and carbon dioxide as blood passes along the pulmonary capillary. Note that in the first part of the capillary the blood is already equilibrated with the alveolar gas. (From Cherniak, R.M.: *Respiration in Health and Disease,* 2nd edition. Courtesy of W.B. Saunders, 1972.)

of exchange is that the carbon dioxide molecule is about 25 times more soluble in liquid than the oxygen molecule, resulting in a CO_2 diffusion rate 20 times faster than O_2. During maximal exercise, the average transit time of RBCs through the pulmonary capillary is maintained within about half of the resting time because more capillaries open up in the lungs. In addition, the ventilation of the alveoli matches closely the flow of blood so that arterial P_{O_2} is maintained at resting values.

OXYGEN TRANSPORT

Since oxygen does not readily dissolve in water, only a fraction of the oxygen transported from the lungs is dissolved in the plasma. Most of it (97%) is combined with hemoglobin to form a complex called *oxyhemoglobin* (HbO_2). Four oxygen molecules can bind to one hemoglobin molecule at any one time. Since there are about 280 million hemoglobin molecules in each red blood cell, each carrying four oxygen molecules, just one erythrocyte can carry over one billion molecules of oxygen. When you think that every cubic millimeter of blood contains 5 million red blood cells, the oxygen carrying capacity of the blood is substantial. Approximately 200 ml of oxygen is transported with every liter of blood. Normal hemoglobin levels are 15.8 g per 100 ml of blood in men and about 14 g per 100 ml of blood for women. Each gram of hemoglobin can carry 1.34 ml of O_2. Therefore, the average male with a hemoglobin level of 15.8 g Hb/100 ml of blood carries 21.17 ml of O_2 (15.8 × 1.34) and his female counterpart 18.86 ml O_2 per 100 ml of blood.

O_2 DISSOCIATION CURVE

The shape of the oxygen dissociation curve contributes greatly to the effectiveness of the Hb molecule in terms of loading and unloading oxygen. The curve is relatively flat in the range of P_{O_2} experienced routinely at most elevations on the earth's surface. At sea level, Hb is about 97% saturated; in mountainous regions, saturation may drop as low 90%, but the blood still carries enough oxygen for normal activity.

Under normal circumstances, the saturation curve dips rather rapidly as the partial pressure decreases below about 60 mm Hg. This enhances the ability of the body to unload oxygen at the cell. Of course, the lower the P_{O_2} at the cellular level (indicating higher metabolic activity and greater oxygen need) the less O_2 can be held by the Hb and the more O_2 will be available for the metabolic processes of that group of cells. In addition, factors associated with high work (heat, CO_2 production, H^+, 2 3-DPG, and acidity of the blood) effectively reduce the strength of the bond between Hb and O_2 and allow a greater O_2 unloading at the same P_{O_2}. This effect is called the Bohr effect (Fig. 5–19).

In 1967, researchers found that red blood cells, as part of their energy production, produced large amounts of 2, 3-diphosphoglycerate (2,3-DPG). 2,3-DPG reduces the hemoglobin affinity for oxygen by a factor of 26, meaning that with higher levels of 2,3-DPG, oxygen is released more freely from the blood. Production of 2,3-DPG is inhibited by oxyhemoglobin. When the amount of oxyhemoglobin drops (as with high altitudes), it stimulates an increase in production of 2,3-DPG.

The increase of 2,3-DPG is one of the many adaptations the body undergoes at higher altitudes. Residents in the Andes mountains have been observed to have extremely high levels of 2,3-DPG and elevated hematocrits, all adaptations which aid in increased oxygen transport to the muscle cells.

Interestingly, although moderate altitudes have little effect on normal activity, world records for distance running are never set at those altitudes. In fact, a major track at 4500 feet has recorded only one sub 4-minute mile even though many world class athletes have competed there.

TRANSPORT OF CARBON DIOXIDE

The processes involved in carbon dioxide transport are complex as compared to those of the transport of oxygen. However, they are every bit as important since the production of CO_2 matches the use of O_2 closely. As CO_2 is produced by the cell, it diffuses to the capillaries (an area of lower concentration) where it is carried using one of the following schemes:

1. Dissolved CO_2. About 5 to 8% of all the CO_2 produced is carried by the blood as dissolved carbon dioxide.

2. Bicarbonate ion. Most of the CO_2 produced is carried as bicarbonate ion (HCO_3^-). CO_2 produced in the cell diffuses into the blood and then into the RBC where it joins with water under the influence of an enzyme in the RBC called *carbonic anhydrase* and forms carbonic acid (H_2CO_3) according to the following reaction:

$$CO_2 + H_2O \longleftrightarrow H_2CO_3$$

Carbonic acid is unstable and proceeds to break down almost immediately into a *bicarbonate ion* (HCO_3^-) and a hydrogen ion (H^+), according to the following reaction:

$$H_2CO_3 \longleftrightarrow HCO_3^- + H^+$$

Of course, as the concentration of HCO_3^- increases, it begins to diffuse into the plasma

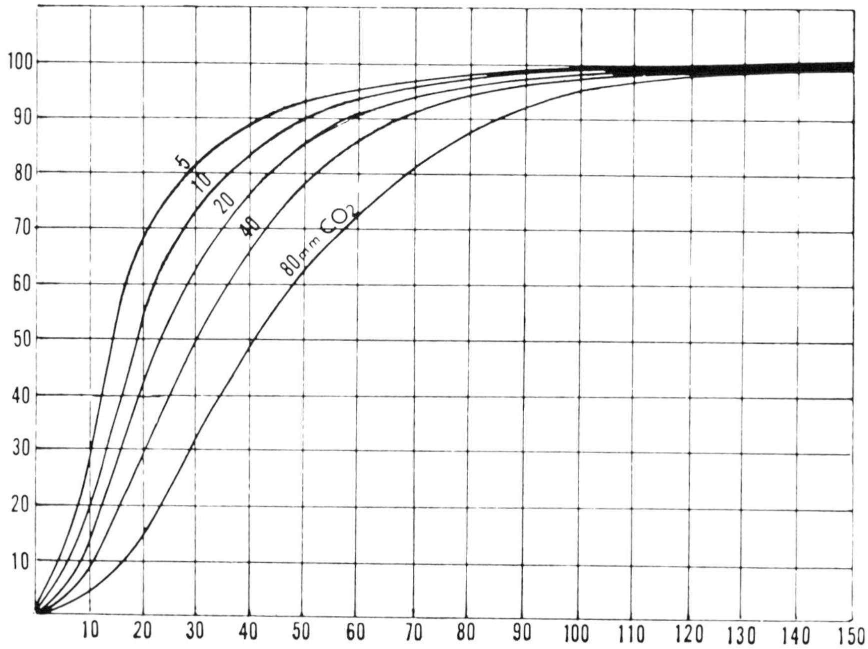

Fig. 5–19. An increase in blood P_{CO_2} will decrease the affinity of hemoglobin for oxygen. (From DeVries, H.A. *Physiology of Exercise for Physical Education and Athletics.* Courtesy of William C. Brown, 1967.)

causing the negative chloride ion (Cl^-) to "shift" into the RBC to balance the charge.

The H^+ from the above reaction is almost immediately picked up by the hemoglobin molecule. When Hb loses its oxygen to the cell, it becomes an excellent buffer and can easily buffer the H^+ produced as a result of carbonic acid degradation. Almost 70% of all CO_2 is carried as HCO_3^- as described in this section.

3. Carbamino Hemoglobin. Some of the CO_2 that enters the blood stream (about 20 to 25%) is carried by the heme molecule of the RBC as carbamino Hb. Of course, there is a CO_2 dissociation curve for CO_2 just as there is for O_2, but since such a small percentage of the CO_2 is carried by Hb, it is not as important as the O_2 dissociation curve (Fig. 5–20).

The processes used to carry CO_2 can be reversed at the lungs to reform CO_2. This CO_2 is then released into the alveoli and from there into the air.

The Bohr effect was described earlier as the effect of CO_2 and H^+ on the dissociation of O_2 from the RBC. Oxygen has a similar effect on the release of CO_2 from the Hb of the RBC. This reverse process is called the *Haldene effect.*

a-$\bar{v}O_2$ DIFFERENCE

In an earlier section of this chapter (O_2 transport), it was seen that arterial blood carries about 20 ml O_2 per 100 ml (dl) of blood. This volume was calculated using a Hb level of 15 g/dl and a loading capacity of 1.34 ml per g. After circulating past the tissues, the oxygen content of the mixed venous blood is still about 15 ml O_2/dl of blood. The difference in oxygen content between the arterial and venous blood (5 ml O_2 in this example) represents the amount of oxygen unloaded or extracted by the tissue. This difference in oxygen content is referred to as the *arterio-venous oxygen difference* or *a-$\bar{v}O_2$* difference.

At rest, the a-$\bar{v}O_2$ difference averages between 4 to 5 ml of O_2/dl of blood. The remaining oxygen bound to the hemoglobin acts as an oxygen reserve. For example, during strenuous exercise, the arterial blood still supplies 20 ml O_2/dl of blood, but the venous side drops to 5 ml O_2/dl of blood, meaning that the amount of oxygen extracted by the tissues or a-$\bar{v}O_2$ difference increased to 15 ml O_2/100 ml. Of course, the total cardiac output ($\dot{Q}$) increases, so oxygen is supplied by both increased pumping and increased extraction.

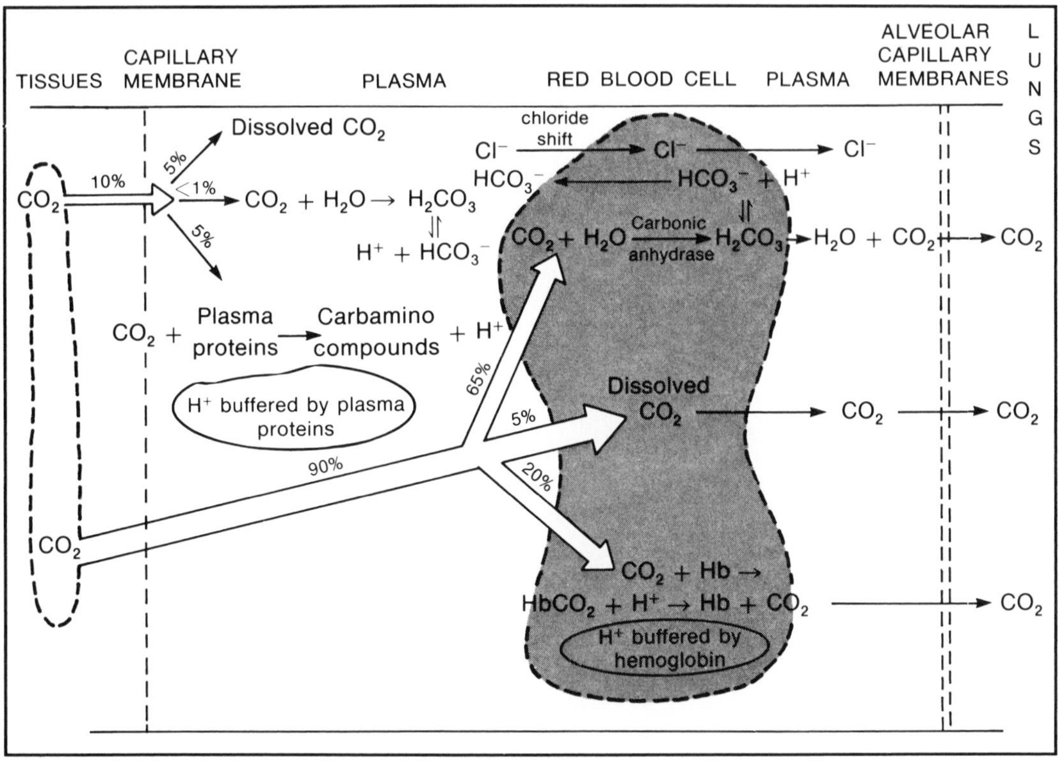

Fig. 5–20. Schematic diagram showing the ways that CO_2 is carried by the blood. (From McArdle, W.D., Katch, F.I., and Katch, V.L. *Exercise Physiology,* 2nd Ed. Courtesy of Lea & Febiger, 1986.)

Figure 5–21 shows the changes in a-$\bar{v}O_2$ difference as work increases for both men and women subjects.

Note that even though the alveolar P_{O_2} goes up at maximal work, the amount of oxygen carried goes down because of the Bohr effect which decreases the amount of O_2 that can be carried. However, this effect is modified somewhat by the increased concentration of RBCs as the plasma loses some of its fluid.

The ability of the body to increase its extraction of oxygen from the blood is extremely important from the standpoint of performance and allows us to do much higher levels of aerobic work than would be possible if no such adjustments were available.

a-$\bar{v}O_2$ Difference in the Heart

Unlike skeletal muscle which at rest extracts only 25% of the oxygen (5 ml O_2/100 ml) from the blood, cardiac muscle extracts 65 to 70% of the available oxygen even at rest. During work, skeletal muscle can increase its extraction rate dramatically, whereas cardiac muscle does not enjoy this luxury. Therefore, any increase in cardiac metabolism must be met by a proportional increase in coronary blood flow. The resting coronary blood flow is approximately 260 ml/min representing 4 to 5% of the total cardiac output. During strenuous exercise, this value increases to a maximum value of 900 ml/min which still represents 4 to 5% of the total cardiac output.

BUFFERING SYSTEMS

One of the most important functions of the body is the regulation of acid-base balance because only slight deviations in this balance can cause changes in cellular activity that are harmful to the organism. The by-products of cellular activity, such as carbon dioxide, lactic acid, phosphoric acid, and the like, tend to drive the pH down to a more acidic level, whereas certain illnesses tend to move the pH toward a more alkaline level.

The pH scale extends from 0 to 14.0, with a low number indicating an acidic condition,

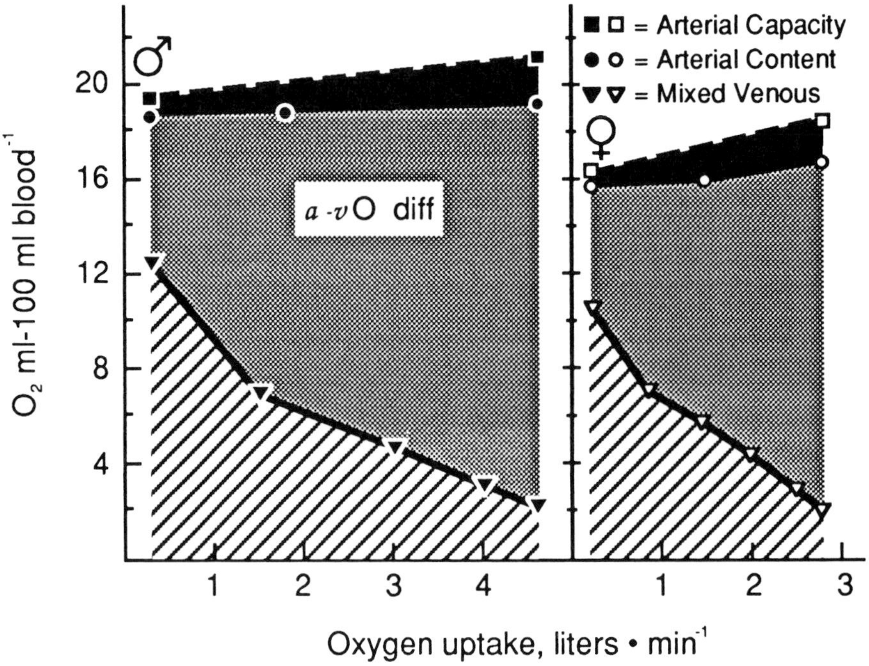

Fig. 5–21. Oxygen-binding capacity and measured oxygen content of arterial blood and calculated oxygen content of mixed venous blood at rest and during work up to maximum on bicycle ergometer. Note changes in a-$\bar{v}_{O_2}$ difference with work. (From Astrand, P.O., and Rodahl, K. *Textbook of Work Physiology: Physiological Basis of Exercises,* 2nd Ed. Courtesy of McGraw Hill, 1986.)

and a high number indicating an alkaline condition. A neutral solution would have a pH of 7.0. The pH of the blood is normally about 7.4, or slightly toward the alkaline side of the scale.

To prevent acidosis or alkalosis, several systems are available: (1) the blood buffer systems, (2) the respiratory system, and (3) the kidneys. The buffer systems of the blood act within a fraction of a second to prevent a drastic change in pH, and they are important to the maintenance of homeostasis. The respiratory system is stimulated by an increase in carbon dioxide to increase the rate of removal of carbon dioxide through the lungs. The kidneys can excrete either an acidic or alkaline urine to help adjust the hydrogen ion concentration (the pH).

Blood Buffer System

A strong acid dissociates almost completely to form many hydrogen ions (H^+). When many hydrogen ions are released into a solution without a buffer, the pH drops drastically. The buffer systems of the body contain chemicals which absorb the excess hydrogen ions so that little change occurs in pH. A typical buffer system in the blood is the bicarbonate system. This system contains a mixture of carbonic acid (H_2CO_3) and sodium bicarbonate ($NaHCO_3$). If a strong acid such as hydrochloric acid (HCl) were added to this buffer system, the following reaction would take place:

$$HCl + NaHCO_3 \text{ ------> } H_2CO_3 + NaCl$$

Of course, the carbonic acid (H_2CO_3) would then dissolve to form H^+ and HCO_3^- and the H^+ would be buffered by one of the other buffers. From this you can see that the strong HCl would be converted to a weak acid (H_2CO_3) which causes little change in the pH of the solution. In the blood there are other bicarbonate salts such as potassium bicarbonate, calcium bicarbonate, and magnesium bicarbonate which perform the same function as sodium bicarbonate. There is also a *phosphate* buffer system that acts in almost the same manner as the bicarbonate system. This system is important in the tubular fluids of the kidneys and in the intracellular fluids.

The most powerful buffer system in the

blood is probably the protein buffer system. This system is similar to the bicarbonate system, because there are free radicals on the amino acids which can combine with hydrogen ions to buffer them. Although the protein buffers are not as efficient as other systems, it is extremely powerful because of the great quantity of protein in the body.

The Respiratory Buffer System

Carbon dioxide is continually being formed by the metabolic process of the body. Under the influence of carbonic anhydrase in the RBC, CO_2 forms carbonic acid, which dissociates to hydrogen ions and bicarbonate ions. As metabolic activity increases as in exercise, more hydrogen ions are formed and the pH of the blood tends to decrease. Because of the ability of the body to react to hydrogen ion concentration by increasing ventilation and because alveolar ventilation can decrease the concentration of hydrogen ions (by blowing off CO_2), the respiratory system is a typical feedback regulatory system for controlling hydrogen ion concentration. In fact, it may be the hydrogen ion system that triggers the hyperventilation response seen in maximal work.

The Renal System as a Buffer

The kidneys are the final and long-term adjustment mechanism for maintaining proper pH. They do this by increasing or decreasing the bicarbonate ion concentration in the body fluid and by excreting excess hydrogen ions into the urine using the phosphate system.

SELECTED REFERENCES

Astrand, P.O., and Rodahl, K.: *Textbook of Work Physiology.* New York: McGraw-Hill Book, Co., 1970.

Bloom, W., and Fawcett, D.W.: *A Textbook of Histology,* 9th Ed., Philadelphia: W.B. Saunders Co., 1968.

Comroe, J.H.: *Physiology of Respiration.* Chicago, Year Book Medical Publishers, Inc., 1968.

Davis, J.S.: Symposium on ventilatory control during exercise. Med. Sci. Sports, *11*:2, 190, 1979.

Dempsey, J.A. and Pelligrino, D.A.: The brain's role in exercise hyperpnea. Med. Sci. Sports, *11*:2, 213–220, 1979.

Dempsey, J.A.: Is the Lung Built for Exercise? Med. Sci. Sports Exerc., *18*:2, 143–155, 1986.

DeVries, H.A.: *Physiology of Exercise,* 2nd Ed., Dubuque, Wm. C. Brown Co., 1974.

Falls, H.B. (ed.): *Exercise Physiology.* New York: Academic Press, 1968.

Guyton, A.C.: *Textbook on Medical Physiology,* 4th Ed., Philadelphia, W.B. Saunders Co., 1971.

Kao, F.F.: *Introduction to Respiratory Physiology.* New York: American Elsevier Publishing, Co. Inc., 1974.

Karpovich, P.V., and Sinning, N.E.: *Physiology of Muscular Activity.* 7th Ed., Philadelphia, W.B. Saunders Co., 1971.

Lahiri, S., et al.: Relative Responses of Aortic Body and Carotid Body Chemoreceptors to Carboxyhemoglobinia. J. Appl. Physiol.: Resp. Environ. Exer. Physiol., *50*:580, 1981.

Lahiri, S., et al.: Comparison of Aortic and Carotid Chemoreceptor Responses to Hypercapnia and Hypoxia. J. Appl. Physiol: Resp. Environ. Exer. Physiol., *51*:55, 1981.

Loke, J., D.A. Mahler, and J.A. Virgulto: Respiratory Muscle Fatigue after Marathon Running. J. Appl. Physiol.: Resp. Environ. Exerc. Physiol., *52*:821, 1982.

Mahler, M.: Neural and humoral signals for pulmonary ventilation arising in exercising muscle. Med. Sci. Sports, *11*:2, 191–197, 1979.

Morehouse, L.E., and Miller, A.T.: *Physiology of Exercise,* 7th Ed., St. Louis: C.V. Mosby, Co., 1976.

Ruch, T.C., and Patton, H.E.: *Physiology and Biophysics,* 19th Ed., Philadelphia: W.B. Saunders Co., 1966.

Sutton, J.R., and Jones, N.L.: Control of pulmonary ventilation during exercise and mediators of the blood: CO_2 and Hydrogen Ion. Med. Sci. Sports, *11*:2, 198–203, 1979.

Swanson, G.D.: Overview of ventilatory control during exercise. Med. Sci. Sports, *11*:221–224, 1979.

Whipp, B.J., and Davis, J.: Peripheral chemoreceptors and exercise hyperpnea. Med. Sci. Sports, *11*:2, 204–212, 1979.

Whipp, B.J., and S.A. Ward: Ventilatory Control Dynamics during Muscle Exercise in Man. Int. J. Sports Med., *1*:146, 1980.

6

Physiology of Energy Use

In the preceding chapters, you have learned that movement occurs only when muscles contract, that muscles cannot contract unless stimulated by motor neurons and that contraction can occur only if energy is available. We discussed the source of the energy used for muscle contraction in some detail, noting that (1) some energy is immediately available to muscles in the resting state, (2) that some energy can be produced rapidly from glucose without oxygen availability, and (3) that sooner or later, all of the energy production depends upon the oxidative pathways of the body. Since oxygen is ultimately necessary for energy production, we discussed the cardiovascular system's role in carrying oxygen to the cells (Chapter 4) and the role of the lungs in providing oxygen to the red blood cells (Chapter 5). The purpose of this chapter is to more fully explain the relationship between the factors discussed in the preceding chapters and their application to the physiology of energy use in the body.

MEASURING METABOLIC RATE

In Chapter 3 we saw that the breakdown of energy resulted in heat and that we could estimate the metabolic rate or energy production of the body by measuring the amount of heat that was produced using a process called *direct calorimetry.* Measuring the heat of metabolism directly is a complex process requiring more sensitive and expensive equipment than is routinely available in the exercise physiology laboratory. Luckily, metabolic rate (or the heat produced by these processes) can be estimated much more easily by measuring the amount of oxygen used to support the metabolic processes. Since all metabolic processes of the body ultimately use oxygen and produce carbon monoxide, the energy production of the body is related directly to the quantity of oxygen used and the relative amount of carbon dioxide produced.

There are two basic ways to measure metabolic rate indirectly: *closed-circuit calorimetry and open-circuit calorimetry.*

Closed-Circuit Calorimetry

The closed-circuit system is so named because the subject breathes directly into and out of a tank through a two-way valve with no access to outside air. The expired air passes through a container of soda lime, which absorbs all of the CO_2 produced. As the CO_2 is absorbed, the total volume of the tank decreases, and the amount of decrease is recorded on a revolving drum (Fig. 6–1). If the base of the recording rises 400 ml/minute and the STPD correction factor is .70, the total metabolic rate would be 280 ml/minute. *Basal metabolic rate* (BMR) is most often expressed in Kcals/hour. To calculate Kcals/hour, first calculate total oxygen use for an hour (280 ml/min × 60 min = 16,800 ml/hour or 16.8 liters/hour). Since there about 5 Kcals/liter, there would be a total of 84 Kcal/hour of heat produced for the person in this example.

The "average" BMR is about 70 Kcals/hour. However, there are many factors that affect this value. To decrease the chance of error, the following conditions should be observed when measuring BMR: (1) No food for at least 12 hours before the test; (2) A night of restful sleep prior to the test; (3) No exercise between

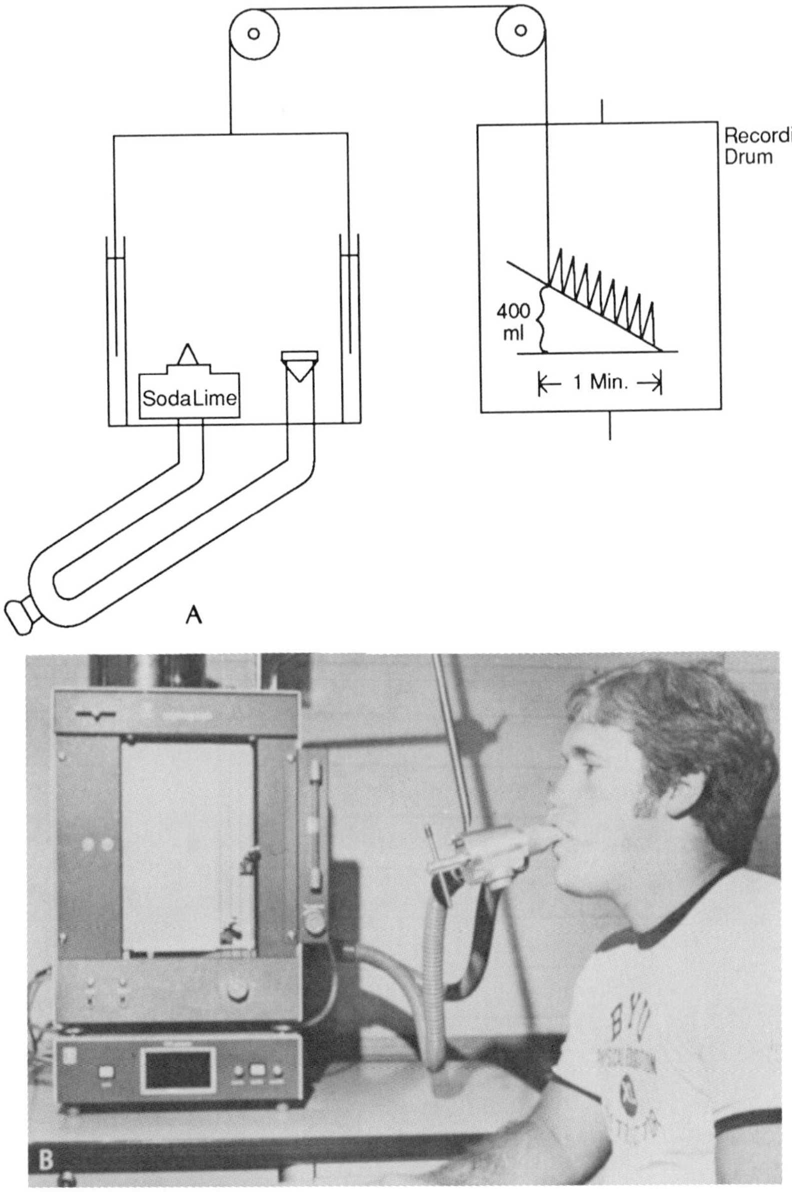

Fig. 6–1. *A*. Drum drops as CO_2 is absorbed, causing a rising line on the recorder. The amount of this rise is related to the metabolic rate. *B*. Subject being tested for RMR using a closed-circuit calorimeter. (From Jensen, C.R., and Fisher, A.G. *Scientific Basis of Athletic Conditioning,* 2nd Ed. Courtesy of Lea & Febiger, 1979.)

the night of sleep and the test: (4) Complete rest in a reclining position for at least 30 minutes immediately prior to the test; (5) Elimination of all physiologic and psychologic stressors (coffee, smoking, sex, etc.). If these conditions cannot be met, the resulting value might more properly be called resting metabolic rate (RMR).

Closed-circuit calorimetry has been used routinely for evaluating resting metabolic rate especially in physicians' offices and small hospitals. However, this system cannot be used effectively for exercise metabolic measures because of the following problems: (1) the volume of the drum is usually too small to be used during any kind of vigorous exercise, (2) the resistance to higher breathing rates can be a problem, (3) the accuracy of the system is not all that good, especially since it is difficult to absorb the amount of CO_2 produced during even moderate work, and (4) CO_2 volumes are not measured (just absorbed) so no information concerning R is available (see next section).

Open-Circuit Calorimetry

Open-circuit calorimetry is the most commonly used method for determining metabolic cost during work. The standard open-circuit system requires breathing through a one-way, low resistance type valve into a Douglas bag or meteorologic balloon so that the volume of expired air and the concentration of expired gases can be measured (Fig. 6–2). Usually the volume of expired air contained in a bag is measured through a tissot spirometer (see Chapter 5, measuring expired air), or through some other type of gas meter). The concentration of the physiologic gases can be analyzed using a mass spectrometer, one of the electronic gas analyzers on the market or (less often) by chemical analysis using a Scholander gas analyzer. Once these data are collected, oxygen consumption can be calculated.

The calculation of oxygen consumption ($\dot{V}O_2$) using the standard open circuit system is fairly simple except that in "real life" there are several correction factors that must be considered. Figure 6–3 shows the basic calculation. If the volume of expired air ($\dot{V}_E$) was 60 liters/min. (after correcting it for STPD) and the percent oxygen in the expired air was 16%, the total volume of oxygen in the expired air would be 9.6 liters (60 l/m × .16). Since the inspired volume must be similar to expired volume (when burning pure carbohydrates they are exactly the same), and since the percent oxygen in the air around us is about 21 (really 20.94%), the amount of oxygen coming into the body each minute can also be computed. In this example, the vol-

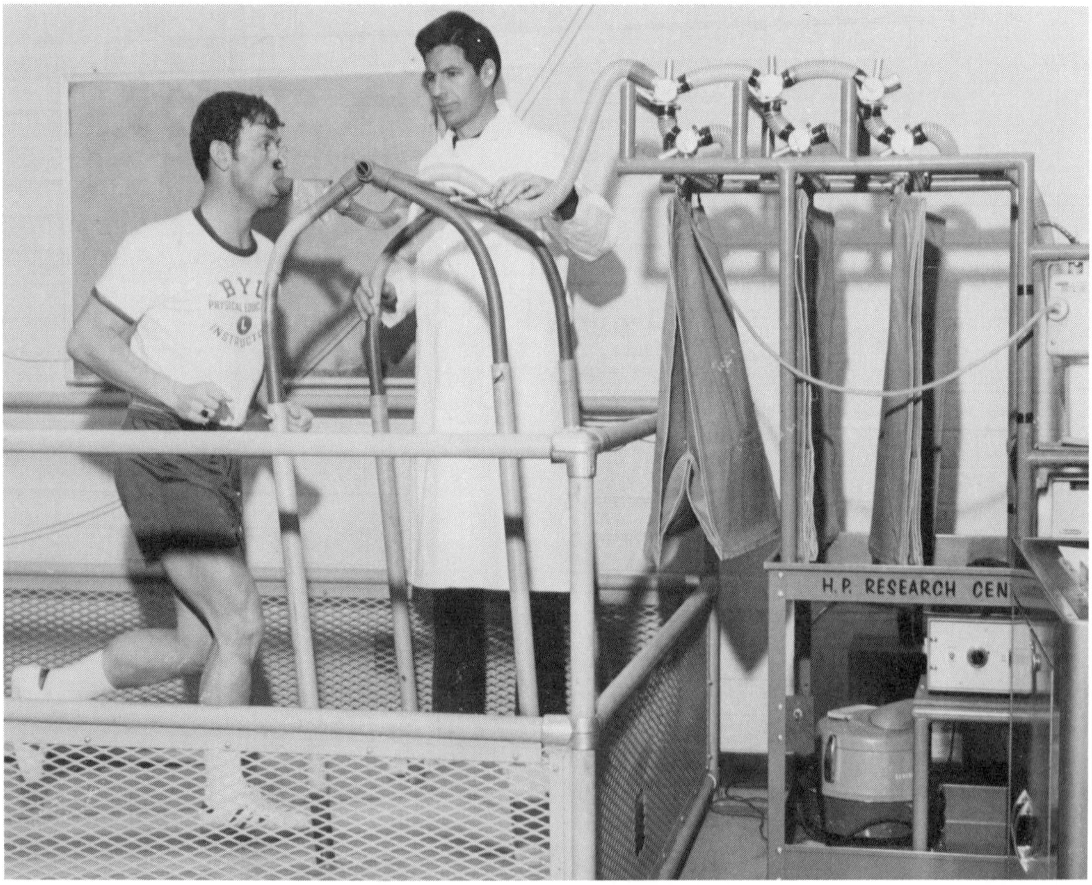

Fig. 6–2. Collecting expired air into a series of Douglas bags. A different bag would be collected during the last 30 sec. of each stage.

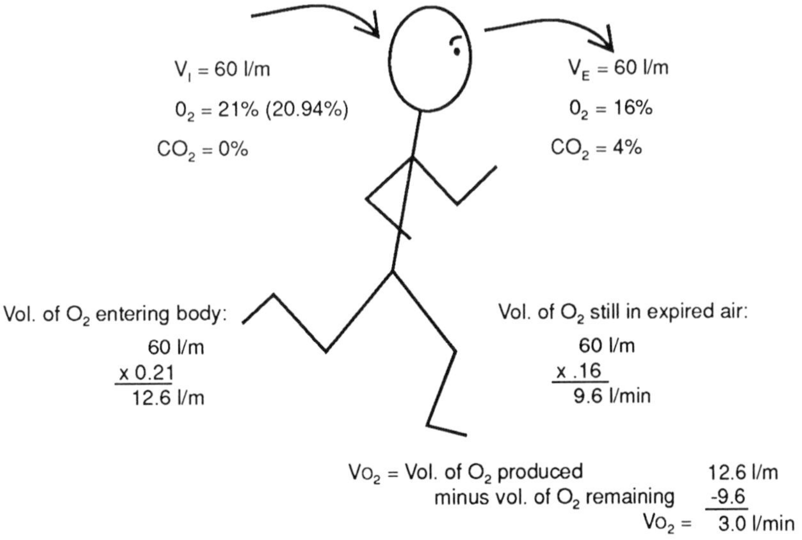

Fig. 6–3. The difference between the amount of oxygen coming into the body each minute (60 l/min. × .04% = 2.4 l/min.) and the amount going out (60 l/min. × 16% = 9.6 l/min.) is oxygen consumption of $\dot{V}O_2$. (From Jensen, C.R., and Fisher, A.G. *Scientific Basis of Athletic Conditioning,* 2nd Ed. Courtesy of Lea & Febiger, 1979.)

ume of oxygen in the inspired gas is 12.6 liters/min. (60 liters/min. × .21 = 12.6 liters/min.). The difference between the amount of oxygen that comes into the body each minute (12.6 liters/min.) and the amount that comes back out (9.6 liters/min.) is 3.0 liters/min. Therefore, oxygen consumption or $\dot{V}o_2$ in this example equals 3.0 liters/min.

The amount of carbon dioxide produced ($\dot{V}CO_2$) can also be calculated (Fig. 6–4). Using the same volumes as before, if the expired air contains 4% CO_2, there would be about 2.4 liters of CO_2 produced (60 × .04 = 2.4 liters/min.). Since the air around us contains almost no carbon dioxide (about .03%), we can ignore any CO_2 in the inspired air so $\dot{V}CO_2$ (or carbon dioxide production) is about 2.4 liters per minute.

The ratio of CO_2 production ($\dot{V}CO_2$) and O_2 usage ($\dot{V}O_2$) is called the respiratory quotient (RQ = $\dot{V}CO_2/\dot{V}O_2$) and tells what kind of food is being burned in the metabolic pathways. With carbohydrates (a 6-carbon glucose molecule), there are six CO_2's produced for every six O_2's used so the RQ is equal to 1.0. With fats, there are more "oxidizable" carbons so there is less CO_2 produced relative to O_2 used. For example, with a 57-carbon fat called trioleate, only 57 CO_2's are produced as opposed to 80 O_2's used. The RQ for fat then is about .71 (57/80 = .71). Although the RQ for protein is about .8, there is such a small amount used for energy (about 5 to 10%), that the effect of protein on RQ is usually ignored.

Using the earlier example (Figs. 6–3 and 6–4) we can calculate RQ by dividing the volume of CO_2 produced by the volume of O_2 used (2.4/3.0) to get a ratio of 0.80. Using this information, the total number of calories per liter of oxygen can be calculated by entering Table 6–1. Note that about 4.8 Kcals of heat are produced per liter of oxygen at an RQ of .80. If more carbohydrates were being used, the amount of energy per liter would go up (remember that the RQ for carbohydrates is 1.0).

NOTE: Do not get confused about the term "kilocalorie." This is the proper way to express heat as it relates to the metabolic systems of the body. This term is often changed to "Calorie" with a capital C, or simply written as "calorie." However, as it is expressed, it means kilocalorie, or the amount of heat needed to raise 1 kg water 1°C.

At high work levels, the ratio of CO_2/O_2 sometimes exceeds 1.0. This is caused by: (1) hyperventilation, where excess blood levels of CO_2 are blown off into the expired air, and (2) the reconversion of hydrogens from lactate to form CO_2 at the lungs. Because RQ is

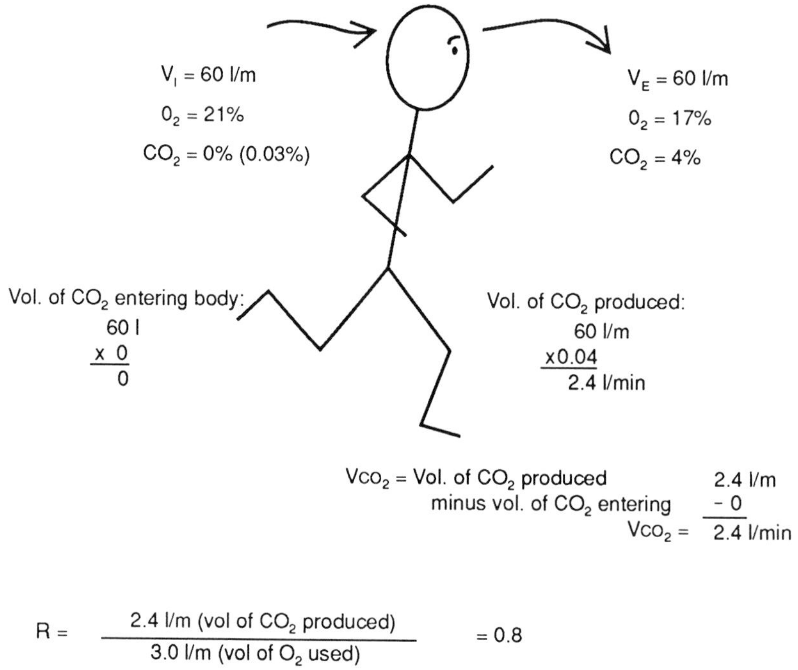

Fig. 6–4. The difference between the amount of CO_2 coming into the body (only about .03%) and the amount produced by the body each minute (60 l/min. × .04% = 2.4 l/min.) is called V_{CO_2}. (Courtesy MCG Corporation.)

Table 6–1. Caloric Values for Nonprotein *R*

R.Q.	*Calories/Liter O_2*
0.707	4.686
0.71	4.690
0.72	4.702
0.73	4.714
0.74	4.727
0.75	4.739
0.76	4.751
0.77	4.764
0.78	4.776
0.79	4.788
0.80	4.801
0.81	4.813
0.82	4.825
0.83	4.838
0.84	4.850
0.85	4.862
0.86	4.875
0.87	4.887
0.88	4.899
0.89	4.911
0.90	4.924
0.91	4.936
0.92	4.948
0.93	4.961
0.94	4.973
0.95	4.985
0.96	4.998
0.97	5.010
0.98	5.022
0.99	5.035
1.00	5.047

a real calculation representing the actual conditions at the cell, the ratios of CO_2/O_2 measured at the mouth during work are called "R."

The "standard" open circuit system is seldom used in the modern exercise physiology laboratory any more, except to standardize the new computerized systems. These newer systems use rapid oxygen and carbon dioxide analyzers or mass spectrometers to analyze gases and pneumotachs or spinner devices for volumes. The analysis is so rapid that many of these computer analyzers actually calculate oxygen consumption ($\dot{V}O_2$) each breath and plot the data for an entire test right while the test is being run. These machines take the tediousness away from doing $\dot{V}O_2$'s and allow the exercise physiologist to "see" the dynamic changes related to a variety of different work tests (Fig. 6–5).

OXYGEN CONSUMPTION THEORY

It will be easier to understand the meaning and value of $\dot{V}O_2$ measurements if you understand something about the basic physiology associated with oxygen consumption in the body. These concepts have been presented

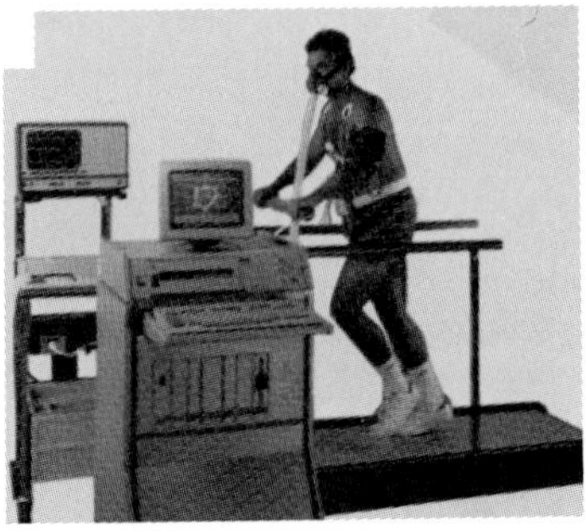

Fig. 6–5. A typical commercial computerized system for measuring $\dot{V}O_2$. (Courtesy MCG Corporation.)

before, but in separate sections. If you have questions about any of the individual concepts, go back to the chapter where that concept is discussed and study that section again.

The amount of oxygen used by the body is related to two major factors; the amount of blood that is pumped by the circulatory system (pumping factors), and the amount of oxygen removed by the cells as the blood flows by (extraction factors). This relationship can be expressed in the following formula:

$$\dot{V}O_2 = \dot{Q} \times \text{a-}\bar{v}O_2 \text{ difference}$$

$\dot{Q}$ is a symbol used to describe the cardiac output, or total volume of blood pumped by the heart through the circulatory system. Since O_2 is carried by the blood, the more blood pumped, the more O_2 available to the cells (see Chapter 4 if a review of cardiac output is needed). The second term, a-$\bar{v}O_2$ diff, refers to the amount of oxygen removed from the blood as it circulates through the body. The amount of oxygen removed is limited by the number of mitochondria and their oxidative capacity since this is where most oxygen use occurs.

The small "a" is arterial oxygen saturation. Since blood contains about 15 g of hemoglobin (Hb) per deciliter (dl), and since each gram Hb can carry about 1.34 ml of O_2, arterial blood usually carries about 20 ml O_2 per dl or about 200 ml O_2 per liter of blood. The small "v" with a line over it refers to the O_2 content of mixed venous blood. At rest, when mixed venous blood returns to the heart from all the different areas of the body, there is still 15 ml O_2/dl blood (150 ml/l) left in it, so the difference is about 5 ml/dl. As work increases, muscle cells need more energy, so more oxygen is extracted. At maximum work, the oxygen content of mixed venous blood decreases to only about 5 ml O_2/dl (50 ml/l) so the a-$\bar{v}O_2$ diff increases (more oxygen is extracted) to about 15 to 17 ml/dl. An analogy may help. The total steel production of a steel mill ($\dot{V}O_2$) may be related to the amount of ore carried to the furnace ($\dot{Q}$) in little ore cars and how much of this ore is unloaded so it can be "burned" in the furnace (a-$\bar{v}O_2$ diff) as it is carried by. If the cars moved slowly and only 1 of the 4 dumped its ore into the furnace, the steel production would be low (like resting metabolic rate in the body). If the train speeds up and more cars dump ore, the production would increase. With the train at full speed, and 3 of the 4 cars dumping ore, maximum steel production ($\dot{V}O_2$) occurs. Further, if either the ore cars quit carrying ore or the furnace quits burning ore, steel production stops. So it is with metabolism. Cardiac patients may have restricted activity levels because the heart is too weak to circulate blood properly—or, a person breathing carbon monoxide (which ties up the oxygen carrying sites on Hb so there is no room to carry oxygen) will die because his arterial blood carries too little oxygen for the metabolic processes of the cell, even though his $\dot{Q}$ may be normal (at least for a while).

Measuring Cardiac Output Using $\dot{V}O_2$

The basic formula for $\dot{V}O_2$ can be rearranged and used to measure cardiac output. The problem is that arterial and venous oxygen concentrations must be measured, and most exercise physiology laboratories are not equipped to do this type of work. These values are routinely measured, however, in the cardiac catheterization laboratory. With catheters placed in the heart to evaluate coronary artery blockage, a-$\bar{v}O_2$ diff can be easily measured from the left and right heart. Expired air is then analyzed to measure $\dot{V}O_2$ and $\dot{Q}$ can be calculated using the Fick equation shown below:

$$\dot{Q} = \dot{V}O_2/\text{a-}\bar{v}O_2 \text{ diff.}$$

An example of typical values might help.

What is the cardiac output if $\dot{V}O_2$ = 250 ml/min. and a-$\bar{v}O_2$ = 50 ml/liter?

$$\dot{Q} = \frac{250 \text{ ml}}{\text{min}} \times \frac{\text{liters}}{50 \text{ ml}} \text{ (invert and multiply)}$$

$$\dot{Q} = 5 \text{ liters/min}$$

Submaximal Work and $\dot{V}O_2$

At rest, the average person uses about 3.5 ml of O_2/kg body wt./min. This value represents 1 *MET*, a shorthand way of saying resting metabolic rate. The total $\dot{V}O_2$ in liters per min. will vary depending on body size. For instance, a 70-kg person will burn about 245 ml/min. ($3.5 \times 70 = 245$). A 110-kg person with normal metabolic rate would burn 385 ml/min. ($3.5 \times 110 = 385$). When exercise begins, the metabolic rate goes up rapidly to a higher level depending on the intensity of exercise and total body weight. The $\dot{V}O_2$ of walking at some given speed will be very similar if expressed in ml/kg/min., but since a larger person weighs more, the total oxygen cost, and therefore the total caloric cost will be greater.

During a given submaximal work bout, two people who are the same size will use approximately the same amount of oxygen. Why is it then, that an untrained person has so much trouble running with a trained person? The most important reason is that $\dot{V}O_2$ is related directly to $\dot{Q}$. Since cardiac output equals heart rate times stroke volume ($\dot{Q}$ = HR × SV), the person with the largest stroke volume (the trained person) will need fewer beats of the heart to pump the same amount of blood. Therefore, the untrained person will have a much higher heart rate than the trained at any given work load and will be tired because there is relatively more effort involved in the work (Fig. 6–6).

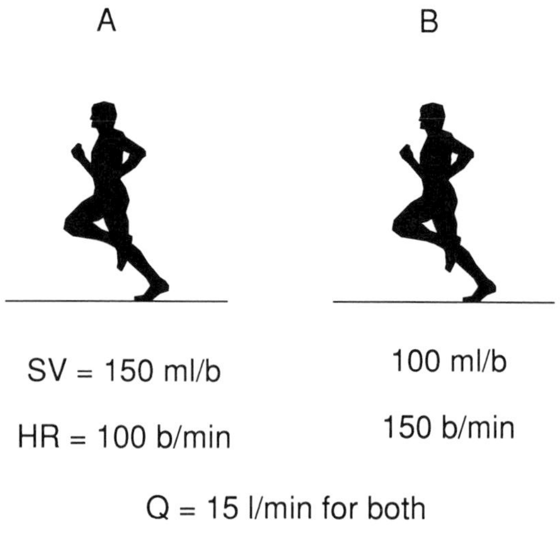

Fig. 6–6. A and B are about the same size, so the oxygen needs and cardiac output are similar. Because A has a larger SV, his heart rate is much lower at the same workload than B's.

Maximum Oxygen Uptake

Maximum oxygen uptake (abbreviated $\dot{V}O_2$max) refers to the maximal amount of oxygen that can be used during an all-out work test. Tests for $\dot{V}O_2$max should involve a significant amount of the total muscle mass and usually increase on a "graded" basis from low level of work to high. In fact, when subjects ask how long they are to continue the test, the answer is "until you can't do any more."

Treadmills are often used because walking and running use such a large amount of muscle, and maximum involvement of muscle gives the best test of $\dot{V}O_2$max. Bicycle ergometers use less total muscle mass and usually result in a lower value (by 10 to 15%). With arm exercises, the value may be decreased by 30%.

There are several criteria for determining if $\dot{V}O_2$max has been achieved: (1) the respiratory exchange ratio (R) must be greater than 1.0. This means that the lungs are hyperventilating and the person is working hard enough to produce significant lactate. (2) Heart rate should be at or near the maximum predicted heart rate. This point can be calculated by subtracting age from 220. For instance, the max predicted heart rate for a 35-year-old subject would be 185 ($220 - 35 = 185$). (3) The $\dot{V}O_2$ should level off near the end of the test and not increase even with increasing work loads. Most young, healthy people can work above their $\dot{V}O_2$max for short periods of time. If work load is increased, but $\dot{V}O_2$ levels off, there is good evidence that the person has reached his/her max. (4) If you measure lactic acid, the blood levels should be greater than 140 mg/dl. If lactate levels are not increased, the person simply has not worked hard enough to be to max.

If a maximum test fails to meet the criteria above, it is best to call the oxygen consumption measured, $\dot{V}O_2$peak. Untrained persons often stop well before maximum levels are reached because they are unaccustomed to the physical feelings associated with high work levels. If a fitness study pretest was done to a "peak" level of $\dot{V}O_2$ and then a training program was prescribed, the post test may show a much greater gain in $\dot{V}O_2$ than really occurred since it could easily be a true $\dot{V}O_2$max test.

Standardizing $\dot{V}O_2$max

There is some discussion concerning the meaning of $\dot{V}O_2$max. For instance, who is the most fit, a person with a $\dot{V}O_2$max of 5 l/min. or a person whose $\dot{V}O_2$max is 3.5 l/min. There is a tendency to choose the higher value since larger is often considered better. However, with $\dot{V}O_2$, the higher value may only reflect a larger total muscle mass. If the 5-liter person weighs 100 kg, and the 3.5-liter person weighs only 60 kg, the amount of oxygen available for each kg of muscle would be greater for the second person (this is calculated by multiplying liters by 1000 to get ml, and then dividing this number by kg). Thus the 5-liter person has 50 ml/kg/min. (5000 ml/100 kg) and the 3.5-liter person has 58.3 ml/kg/min. (3500 ml/60 kg) (Fig. 6–7). Since the ability to do endurance work relates more to the ml/kg/min. than just l/min., $\dot{V}O_2$max is most often expressed as a function of body weight. Highly trained male endurance athletes often have $\dot{V}O_2$max values between 70 and 90 ml/kg/min., and female endurance athletes are between 60 and 70 ml/kg/min. Untrained adults may have values of only 20 to 30 ml/kg/min., and most college students have $\dot{V}O_2$max levels between 40 and 60 ml/kg/min (Fig. 6–8).

Even when $\dot{V}O_2$max is standardized for body weight, there are questions about its meaning. For instance, is a person whose $\dot{V}O_2$max is 40 ml/kg/min. more highly trained than one with 35 ml/kg/min.? The son of a great long distance runner, a non-runner himself, was tested at about age 20 and had a $\dot{V}O_2$max of over 60 ml/kg/min. Although his $\dot{V}O_2$max was high, he was not "fit" because he never trained. On the other hand, some adults who train religiously have marginal levels of $\dot{V}O_2$max. Obviously, the results of a max test cannot tell us how "trained" a person is. There is much evidence to indicate that heredity and natural endowment play a role in determining a person's maximal aerobic capacity, or $\dot{V}O_2$max. Therefore, a person who has never trained may have a larger $\dot{V}O_2$max than a person who has trained daily for years.

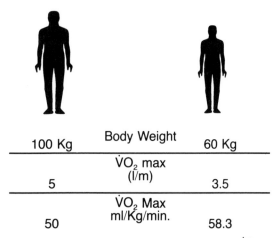

100 Kg	Body Weight	60 Kg
5	$\dot{V}O_2$ max (l/m)	3.5
50	$\dot{V}O_2$ Max ml/Kg/min.	58.3

Fig. 6–7. The 100-kg subject has a much larger $\dot{V}O_2$ in l/min., but when standardized for body weight, the 60-kg person has the larger value.

Does a higher $\dot{V}O_2$max mean that a person can run faster or longer than another? The maximal oxygen consumption in ml/kg/min. does indicate the maximal potential to produce energy using the aerobic processes and is indicative of the effectiveness of the cardiovascular system. However, the person with the highest $\dot{V}O_2$max does not always win. Some people can work at a much higher percentage of $\dot{V}O_2$max than others and may win a race because of this characteristic. Frank Shorter, one of America's best marathon runners of the past, often outran competitors who had a much higher $\dot{V}O_2$max than his. Another interesting fact is that running speed can often be increased without a change in $\dot{V}O_2$max. This is true because training can increase $\dot{V}O_2$max by only about 25%, but can increase muscle mitochondrial content by 100%. Specificity of training may also be a factor. $\dot{V}O_2$max measured on a treadmill may not accurately tell the story if the person trained on a bicycle, and someone who has trained aerobically in a swimming pool may not measure as high using a bicycle test.

With all of these factors, what is the use of $\dot{V}O_2$max? In spite of all the problems, $\dot{V}O_2$max is still the best measure of *functional oxidative capacity,* and as such, indicates *potential* for events demanding great endurance. As a general rule, great athletes have to have a great aerobic capacity to be great, and as a group, will have much higher levels of $\dot{V}O_2$max than the average. Figure 6–8 clearly shows that individuals participating in events related to endurance have a higher $\dot{V}O_2$max than those participating in less demanding events. Interestingly, many track coaches ignore $\dot{V}O_2$max data. Their reply when asked why is "who cares what his $\dot{V}O_2$max is if he can run 1500 meters in 3:50?"

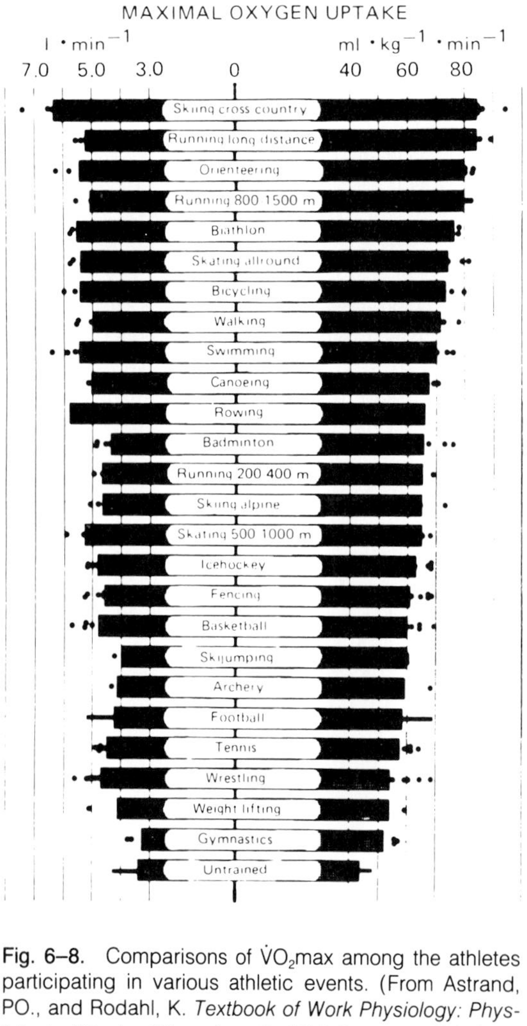

Fig. 6–8. Comparisons of $\dot{V}O_2$max among the athletes participating in various athletic events. (From Astrand, PO., and Rodahl, K. *Textbook of Work Physiology: Physiological Basis of Exercises*, 2nd Ed. Courtesy of McGraw Hill, 1986.)

Perhaps the most important reasons to measure $\dot{V}O_2$max relate to basic research. This measure has been used routinely to evaluate the effectiveness of training programs used to develop cardiovascular endurance and literally thousands of studies have been published using $\dot{V}O_2$max data to substantiate certain treatments or findings. Surely, $\dot{V}O_2$max is a mainstay in the exercise physiology laboratory. Another important use relates to determining aerobic impairment in cardiac and other patients. Levels of $\dot{V}O_2$max compared to "normal" levels give the physician information regarding the ability of a patient to return home or to work safely.

It should be pointed out that there is no significant difference between boys and girls in $\dot{V}O_2$max before puberty, but after that, women's aerobic capacity is only about 70 to 75% that of men. Also, the maximal aerobic capacity decreases steadily with age, after about 25 years old. Of course, this decline can be slowed by consistent training. Many 65-year-olds have levels as high or higher than untrained younger persons.

ESTIMATING ENERGY COST

Physiologists have measured the energy cost of many activities and have developed tables showing these costs (Table 6–2). The cost of activity can be expressed in liters per min., kilocalories per min. or hour, or in METS. The relationship between liters and calories is shown scientifically in Table 6–1. However, for most calculations, a standard 5 kcals per liter can be used to get caloric cost. The cost in METS can be calculated by dividing the cost in ml/kg/min. by 3.5.

METS are a useful tool for the average person because they are so easy to use. As mentioned before, the resting metabolic cost is equal to 1 MET (3.5 ml/kg/min.). A three MET activity would then be one using 3 times the resting energy cost. This activity would cost about 10.5 ml/kg/min. (3 METS × 3.5 = 10.5 ml/kg/min.). Table 6–2 shows the costs of various activities in METS. This table is useful for choosing an activity for a post car-

Table 6–2. Leisure Activities in METS: Sports, Exercise Classes, Games, Dancing

	Mean	*Range*
Archery	3.9	3–4
Back Packing	—	5–11
Badminton	5.8	4–9+
Basketball		
Gameplay	8.3	7–12+
Non-game	—	3–9
Billiards	2.5	—
Bowling	—	2–4
Boxing		
In-ring	13.3	—
Sparring	8.3	—
Canoeing, Rowing and Kayaking	—	3–8
Conditioning Exercise	—	3–8+
Climbing Hills	7.2	5–10+
Cricket	5.2	4.6–7.4
Croquet	3.5	—
Cycling		
Pleasure or to work	—	3–8+
10 mph	7.0	—
Dancing (Social, Square, Tap)	—	3.7–7.4
Dancing (Aerobic)	—	6–9
Fencing	—	6–10+
Field Hockey	8.0	—
Fishing		
from bank	3.7	2–4
wading in stream	—	5–6
Football (Touch)	7.9	6–10
Golf		
Power cart	—	2–3
Walking (carrying bag or pulling cart)	5.1	4–7
Handball	—	8–12+
Hiking (Cross-country)	—	3–7
Horseback Riding		
Galloping	8.2	—
Trotting	6.6	—
Walking	2.4	—
Horseshoe Pitching	—	2–3
Hunting (Bow or Gun)		
Small game (walking, carrying light load)	—	3–7
Big game (dragging carcass, walking)	—	3–14
Judo	13.5	—
Mountain Climbing	—	5–10+
Music Playing	—	2–3
Paddleball, Racquetball	9	8–12
Rope Jumping	11	—
60–80 skips/min	9	—
120–140 skips/min	—	11–12
Running		
12 min per mile	8.7	—
11 min per mile	9.4	—
10 min per mile	10.2	—
9 min per mile	11.2	—
8 min per mile	12.5	—
7 min per mile	14.1	—
6 min per mile	16.3	—
Sailing	—	2–5
Scubadiving	—	5–10
Shuffleboard	—	2–3
Skating, Ice and Roller	—	5–8
Skiing, Snow		
Downhill	—	5–8
Crosscountry	—	6–12+
Skiing, Water	—	5–7
Sledding, Tobogganing	—	4–8
Snowshoeing	9.9	7–14
Squash	—	8–12+
Soccer	—	5–12+
Stairclimbing	—	4–8
Swimming	—	4–8+
Table Tennis	4.1	3–5
Tennis	6.5	4–9+
Volleyball	—	3–6

diac patient or someone whose fitness level is extremely low.

Again, a larger person, having more total metabolic tissue, would have a larger total cost than a smaller person. An example might help:

What is the total caloric cost at rest (1 MET) and at 3 METS work (about like walking 3 mph)? Since each kg requires 3.5 ml of oxygen a minute, a 60-kg person would use 210 ml/min. (60 kg × 3.5 ml = 210 ml/min.). 210 ml/min. is = .21 l/min. and at 5 kcals/ liter, the cost is 1.05 kcals/min. At 3 METS, a 60-kg person would use 3 × 3.5 ml/kg/min. or 10.5 ml/kg/min. Multiplying this by kg (60) = 630 ml/min. To find the caloric cost, change ml to liter (multiply by 1000) and multiply by 5 (since there are about 5 kcals/liters). In ths example, .63 l/min × 5 kcal/liter = 3.15 kcal/ min.

The average cost of walking from a review of several different studies came out to 1.3 kcals/kg/mile; for running, 1.6 kcals/kg/mile. Using these figures, a 70-kg person would use about 91 kcals to walk a mile (70 kg × 1.3 kcals/kg = 91 kcal/mile) and about 112 kcal to run a mile (70 kg × 1.6 kcal/kg = 112). Many physiologists use 100 kcal a mile as a ball-park calculation for predicting energy cost for either walking or running. But it is clear that running (since it involves being clear of the ground between steps) costs slightly more than walking.

The American College of Sports Medicine has published formulas for predicting the energy cost of walking, running, grade walking and running, and ergometry. The simplified formulas are listed below (for more complete information concerning these formulas[2]):

Walking (ml/kg/min.) = (Speed (m/min) × 0.1) + 3.5

Running (ml/kg/min.) = (Speed (m/min) × 0.2) + 3.5

Additional cost of grade work (ml/kg/min.) = speed (m/min.) × percent grade (decimal fraction) × 1.8 (for treadmill running, multiply this number by .5). NOTE: This calculation is to be added to the costs of level of work from the preceding formulas).

Ergometer (ml/min.) = (work load (kgm/ min.) × 2) + (3.5 × body weight in kg)

NOTE #1: multiply miles per hour by 26.8 to get meters per minute in the equations for walking and running

NOTE #2: ergometer costs are in ml/min. (not ml/kg/min.) because the subject's weight is carried by the ergometer seat.

An example may help. Calculate the cost of running on a treadmill at 7 mph up a 4% grade. First, convert 7 mph to meters per minute (7 × 26.8 = 187.6 m/min.), then multiply by 2 to get 37.52 ml/kg/min.; add 3.5, and you are left with 41.02 ml/kg/min.—this is the cost of level running at 7 mph. To get the grade cost, multiply meters per minute (187.6) by 1.8, then multiply this by .04 (the grade as a decimal fraction). This equals 13.51 ml/kg/ min. This number is multiplied by .5 when calculating grade costs for running on a treadmill, for a total grade cost of 6.75 ml/kg/min. The total cost is the level cost (41.02) plus the grade cost (6.75), or 47.77 ml/kg/min.

Now calculate the cost of riding a cycle ergometer at 600 kgm·min.$^{-1}$ for a 70-kg subject. First, multiply the workload by 2 (2 × 600 = 1200) to get the cost of work. Then, multiply body weight by 3.5 (70 × 3.5 = 245 ml/min.) to get the resting cost. The total cost is 1445 ml/min. (1200 ml/min. + 245 ml/min. = 1445 ml/min.).

ENERGY DYNAMICS DURING EXERCISE

It is clear that the changes in metabolic rate associated with activity have a certain amount of inertia; that is, they often change less rapidly than the work load itself. For instance, if a person were standing on a treadmill and the treadmill suddenly began moving at 8 mph, the cost of the activity would immediately go from about 3.5 ml/kg/min. to about 45 ml/kg/ min. The metabolic rate would rise, but nowhere near rapidly enough to meet the need for energy. This discrepancy between need and production of energy at the beginning of work has been called the *oxygen deficit*.

If the treadmill is increased in speed or grade until the cost of work is significantly above the subject's ability to supply energy, the deficit is much greater and there is no way the body can supply enough energy for the work it is being asked to do. In this case, the VO_2 levels off at its maximum (Fig. 6–9) and

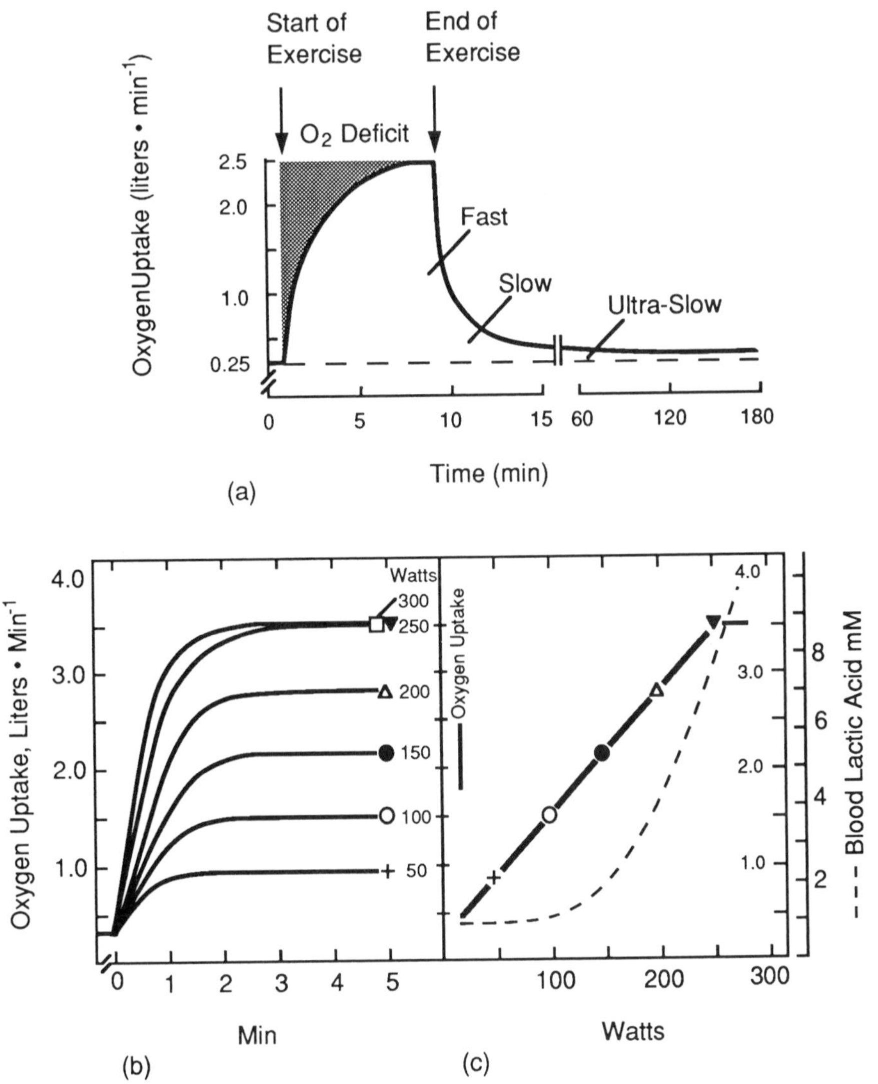

Fig. 6–9. *A.* During the first minutes of exercise, there is an oxygen deficiency while the oxygen uptake increases to a level adequate to meet the oxygen demand of the tissue. At the cessation of exercise, there is a gradual decrease in the oxygen uptake and several components can be identified. Note the change in time scale. *B.* Schematic demonstration of the increase in oxygen uptake during exercise on cycle ergometer with different intensities (noted within shadowed area) performed during 5 to 6 min. *C.* Oxygen uptake in the above-mentioned experiments, measured after 5 min. and plotted in relation to rate of exercise. Note that 250 watts did not further increase the oxygen uptake; the increased rate of exercise was possible thanks to anaerobic processes. Maximal aerobic power = 3.51 × min.$^{-1}$. (For simplicity, the work rate that is sufficient to bring the oxygen uptake to the subject's maximum, in this case 250 watts, may be written WL_{max} $\dot{V}O_2$.) Peak lactate concentrations in the blood at each experiment have been included (blood samples secured immediately after exercise and every second min. up to 10 min. of recovery). (From Astrand, P.O., and Rodahl, K. *Textbook of Work Physiology: Physiological Basis of Exercises,* 2nd Ed. Courtesy of McGraw Hill, 1986.)

the energy is supplied by anaerobic mechanisms and lactate production will be high. If the change in work load is small, the metabolic rate of the body adjusts rapidly to meet the need and the deficit is small and can probably be "paid off" by a slightly increased metabolic rate for the first few minutes of the activity. When work is stopped, the cost of activity again returns immediately to resting values, but the metabolic rate returns at a much slower pace (Fig. 6–9A). This excess metabolic activity following work has been called *oxygen debt.*

It has been clear for a number of years that

the elevated oxygen consumption after exercise (the so-called oxygen debt) is more than merely replacing oxygen that was somehow "borrowed" during the exercise bout. Actually, during maximal exercise, depletion of the oxygen stores of the muscle and blood could account for only about 0.5 liters of oxygen. Because of this, other terms such as "recovery oxygen" or "excess post-exercise oxygen consumption (EPOC)" have been suggested to describe this phenomenon.

In Figure 6–9A, it is clear that the recovery oxygen consumption decreases exponentially with time. During the first minute or two, the decrease in oxygen consumption is rapid, then it decreases more slowly until a constant rate is reached. The rapid recovery phase was called the "alactacid" portion of the oxygen debt because it was not thought to be related to the reconversion of lactate. This phase is now called the "fast" component or "rapid-recovery phase." The slow recovery phase was called the "lactacid" portion of the oxygen debt because it was thought to be related to the removal of the lactate accumulation following exercise. It is now called the "slow" component or "slow-recovery phase."

The question is, what causes the fast and slow components of the recovery oxygen curve? It was clear from the discussion in Chapter 3 that there were two important sources of energy that could be used during intense exercise—the ATP-PC system for immediate use, and the lactate system for slightly longer bouts of intensive exercise. Several studies have shown that the ATP and PC stores depleted during short, high intensity exercise are restored rapidly during the first 30 seconds or so of recovery (70%) and then more slowly until they are completely restored within a few minutes following the exercise bout. If blood flow is restricted to a muscle following the exercise bout, this recovery does not occur. This experiment indicates the need for oxygen in the restoration of the ATP-PC stores. It is important to remember that PC cannot be directly restored by oxidative means, but must be restored from ATP that is produced by oxidation. The excess oxygen during the fast phase not only helps restore the ATP-PC stores, but also helps replace the small amount of oxygen depleted from myoglobin stores (about .5 liters). The total amount of oxygen during the fast recovery phase is of course related to the intensity and volume of anaerobic work. However, estimates are usually between 2 to 3 liters.

The cause of the slow phase of the recovery oxygen curve is a little more difficult to explain. Early scientists tried to quantitatively relate the removal of lactate with the amount of recovery oxygen. However, there was much variability in these calculations. It is clear that lactate does account for some of this extra oxygen consumption (about 20%) as a small amount is reconverted by the liver to new glucose (gluconeogenesis). However, the major contributors to the slow phase probably relate to the "winding" down of the metabolic processes after work. Of these factors, elevated body temperature resulting from the previous exercise plays a major role. Temperature not only increases metabolic rate directly, but could "uncouple" the oxidative phosphorylation process causing a use of oxygen, but no ATP production, similar to the process used by the body (nonshivering thermogenesis) to produce heat in cold environments. There is also an extra oxygen cost needed to meet the needs of the heart and respiratory muscles because heart rate and respiration remain elevated during recovery. Another possible factor relates to the circulating catecholamines (epinephrine and norepinephrine) following exercise. These substances increase metabolism directly and could, in addition, affect cell membranes, making them more "leaky" which would increase the metabolic cost of maintaining the membrane potential. Increased calcium uptake by the mitochondria may be another factor to explain the slow component of the excess oxygen consumption following exercise. The important point is that lactate is probably not the primary *cause* of the extra oxygen used after heavy work as previously speculated. More likely, lactate is used as a fuel to supply energy for the recovery process. The amount of excess recovery oxygen during the slow phase relates to the amount and intensity of work and ranges between 5 and 10 liters. It can be larger in athletes, particularly those who train for and participate in power type sports. The slow component is indeed slow, and may take up to an hour to complete.

Anaerobic Threshold

Another controversial issue related to energy use involves the production and removal of lactic acid during exercise. At rest and during low level exercise, blood lactic acid levels are fairly stable. As exercise increases, there is a slow rise in blood lactate until a certain point where lactate levels rise dramatically (see Fig. 6–9C). This point has been called the "anaerobic threshold" and refers, in this sense, to a point in exercise where anaerobic work begins to be done. It was thought to be some magical point where suddenly the anaerobic mechanisms were forced to begin producing energy. However, more recent research indicates that lactate production is continuous and related linearly to work. That is, as work increases, so does lactate production. However, increased production of lactate stimulates increased removal. As long as the removal rate can keep up with production, no significant lactate shows up. At a certain point in exercise, production outstrips removal and the blood lactate rises dramatically. This point could more properly be called the "lactate threshold" (Tlact).

There are several reasons for the lactate threshold. (1) As exercise gets heavier, more white, fast-twitch muscle fibers are recruited. These muscles are low in oxidative machinery but good at supplying energy anaerobically but produce lactate in the process. The more of these fibers that are recruited, the more lactate is produced. (2) As exercise intensity increases, more and more of the blood flow is shunted to muscles. This makes less flow available to tissues that normally remove lactate. (3) Higher workloads tend to increase sympathetic output to the body. This, in turn, tends to trigger glycolytic pathway activity. All of these factors come into play as work loads increase and can account for the increased lactate seen at some point in work.

It should be noted that the lactate threshold occurs at a different intensity for different people. In untrained, overweight adults, the threshold may be as low as 40 to 50% of their maximum aerobic capacity. Moderately trained people may be in the range of from 50 to 80%, and highly trained athletes may work at around 90% of their capacity without triggering a significant lactate load. Working above this threshold can be detrimental to performance. Coaches who encourage their athletes to "keep contact" with other performers regardless of how fast they must go may cause their athletes to fail during the later stages of the contest. The better approach is to run at a constant "best speed" without significant lactate load until the final stages of the race, even if competitors are several hundred yards ahead. The best times will occur when an athlete runs a consistent speed that will result in his best time during the initial stages of the contest, and then increases the pace past the lactate deflection point during the final sprint.

SELECTED READINGS

1. Ahlborg, F., R. Hendler, and P. Felig: Lactate Production by Resting Muscle during and after Prolonged Exercise: Mechanism of Redistribution of Muscle Glycogen. Clin. Physiol., *1*:608, 1981.
2. American College of Sports Medicine: *Guidelines for Graded Exercise Testing and Prescription.* 3rd Ed., Philadelphia: Lea & Febiger, 1985.
3. Asimov, I.: *Life and Energy.* Garden City, N.Y.: Doubleday and Co., 1962.
4. Astrand, I., P.-O. Astrand, I. Hallback, et al.: Reduction in Maximal Oxygen Uptake with Age. J. Appl. Physiol., *35*:649, 1973.
5. Astrand, I.: Aerobic Work Capacity in Men and Women with Special Reference to Age. Acta Physiol. Scand., *49*(Suppl. 169): 1960.
6. Astrand, P.-O., and B. Saltin: Oxygen Uptake during the First Minutes of Heavy Muscular Exercise. J. Appl. Physiol., *16*:971, 1961.
7. Astrand, P.-O., and B. Saltin: Maximal Oxygen Uptake and Heart Rate in Various Types of Muscular Activity. J. Appl. Physiol., *16*:977, 1961.
8. Astrand, P.-O., and K. Rodahl: *Textbook of Work Physiology,* 3rd Ed., New York: McGraw-Hill Book Co., 1986.
9. Bergh, U., I.-L. Kanstrup, and B. Ekblom: Maximal Oxygen Uptake during Exercise with Various Combinations of Arm and Leg Work. J. Appl. Physiol., *41*:191, 1976.
10. Bleich, H.L., and Boro, E.S.: Fuel homeostasis in exercise. N. Engl. J. Med., *293*:1078–1084, 1975.
11. Brooks, G.A., Brauner, K.E., and Cassens, R.G.: Glycogen synthesis and metabolism of lactic acid after exercise. Am. J. Physiol., *224*:1162–1166, 1973.
12. Brooks, G.A., and G.A. Gaesser: End points of lactate and glucose metabolism after exhausting exercise. J. Appl. Physiol., *49*:1057–1069, 1980.
13. Brooks, G.A., K.E. Brauner, and R.G. Cassens: Glycogen Synthesis and Metabolism of Lactic Acid after Exercise. Am. J. Physiol., *224*:1162, 1973.
14. Brooks, G.A.: Anaerobic threshold: review of the

concept and directions for future research. Med. Sci. Sports Exerc., *17*:22–34, 1985.
15. Brooks, G.A.: Response to Davis' manuscript. Med. Sci. Sports Exerc., *17*:19–21, 1985.
16. Davis, J.A., M.H. Frank, B.J. Whipp, et al.: Anaerobic threshold alterations caused by endurance training in middle-aged men. J. Appl. Physiol., *46*:1039–1046, 1979.
17. Davis, J.A., P. Vodak, J.H. Wilmore, et al.: Anaerobic threshold and maximal aerobic power for three modes of exercise. J. Appl. Physiol., *41*:544–550, 1976.
18. Davis, J.A.: Anaerobic threshold: review of the concept and directions for future research. Med. Sci. Sports Exerc., *17*:6–18, 1985.
19. di Prampero, P.E., U. Boutellier, and P. Pretsch: Oxygen Deficit and Stores at Onset of Muscular Exercise in Humans. J. Appl. Physiol.: Resp. Env. Exer. Physiol., *55*:146, 1983.
20. Ehrsam, R.E., G.J.F. Heigenhauser, and N.L. Jones: The effect of respiratory acidosis on metabolism in exercise (Abstract). Med. Sci. Sports, *13*:85, 1981.
21. Green, J., B. Daub, D. Painter, et al.: Anaerobic threshold and muscle fiber type, area and oxidative enzyme activity during graded cycling. Med. Sci. Sports, *11*:113–114, 1979.
22. Hagberg, J.M., E.J. Coyle, J.M. Miller, et al.: Ventilatory threshold without increasing blood lactic acid levels in McArdle's disease patient anaerobic threshold? Med. Sci. Sports, *13*:115, 1981.
23. Harris, R.C. et al.: The Time Course of Phosphocreatine Resynthesis During Recovery of the Quadriceps in Man. Pflugers Arch., *367*:137–142, 1976.
24. Jones, N.L., and R.E. Ehrsam: The Anaerobic Threshold. Exerc. Sport Sci. Rev., *10*:49–83, 1982.
25. Kasch, F., J.P. Wallace, R.R. Huhn, et al.: VO^2 max during Horizontal and Inclined Treadmill Running. J. Appl. Physiol., *40*:982, 1976.
26. Margaria, R., H.T. Edwards, and D.B. Dill: The possible mechanisms of contracting and paying the oxygen debt and the role of lactic acid in muscular contraction. Am. J. Physiol., *106*:689–715, 1933.
27. Orr, G.W., H.J. Green, R.L. Hughson, et al.: A computerized technique for determination of anaerobic threshold (Abstract). Med. Sci. Sports, *12*:86, 1980.
28. Saltin, B.: Aerobic Work Capacity and Circulation at Exercise in Man. Acta Physiol. Scand., *62*(Suppl. 230), 1964.
29. Stenberg, J., P.-O., Astrand, B. Ekblom, et al.: Hemodynamic Response to Work with Different Muscle Groups, Sitting and Supine. J. Appl. Physiol., *22*:61, 1967.
30. Vogel, J.A., M.U. Ramos, and J.F. Patton: Comparison of Aerobic Power and Muscle Strength between Men and Women Entering the U.S. Army. Med. Sci. Sports, *9*:58, 1977.
31. Yeh, M.P., et al.: "Anaerobic threshold": problems of determination and validation. J. Appl. Physiol.: Resp. Exer. Env. Physiol., *55*:1178–1186, 1983.

Part II

Applying Physiologic Principles to Performance

World records have improved steadily since the time records were kept. Athletes jump farther and higher, run faster and longer, and propel objects with more force and skill. What are the factors that affect this improvement in performance? Obviously, muscle strength and endurance play a major role as does the ability to produce energy through either the anaerobic or aerobic energy systems. Performance also includes the neural pathways, muscle fiber types and other genetic factors. It also includes the desire to excel and the skill developed through proper practice. Obviously, to excel in a certain sport or activity, the athlete, young or old, male or female, must do everything possible to maximize all of the factors related to that sport or activity. This section is included to help the student apply the physiologic principles learned in the preceding section to the more practical requirements of training athletes. You have looked at each system of the body separately and in some detail. It is now time to apply that knowledge to more specific training principles, for knowledge of systems may be of little value unless made applicable to the individual athlete.

7

Muscular Strength and Endurance

The importance of muscular strength and endurance to performance in certain activities has been known for years. Before coaches used strength training to any great degree, football teams from areas where hard physical work was a way of life always had winning records. Successful field athletes were usually men who worked on farms or in factories and had developed great strength from the type of work they did. From observation, it became clear that increased strength was an important factor for many athletic events, especially those involving contact or where large, heavy objects were thrown. Watching modern day professional basketball convinces the viewer that strength is also important even in so-called "non-contact" sports. In fact, as time goes by, more coaches are using strength training as a means of improving performance, even in sports such as golf, tennis, and distance running.

The definition of strength, the ability to apply force, implies its importance to performance. Even though nearly all movements are performed against some resistance, athletes perform movements against much greater resistance than usual. For example, in the shot put, discus throw, pole vault, gymnastics, jumping, running, swimming and leaping, the body segments must exert maximal force. All else being equal, greater strength will result in better performance than normal in most athletic events. In certain events, strength is the primary contributor and is therefore fundamental to excellence (Fig. 7–1).

In addition to being an important trait by itself, strength is important to performance because of its relationship to other factors. For example, strength contributes to *power* because power is equal to force times velocity, and increased strength results in more force. Strength is also a factor in *muscular endurance*, which is the ability of the muscles to resist fatigue while doing work. A stronger muscle has the ability to move a given amount of resistance through a range of motion more times than a weaker muscle. Strength contributes to *agility* because adequate strength is required to control the weight of the body against the force of inertia when the athlete changes direction rapidly. Strength is even a factor in *rapid acceleration* and *running speed*, where great force is required to accelerate the body and to keep it in motion.

In addition to its importance in athletic performance, muscular strength also plays an important role in protecting athletes from injury. Strong muscles not only increase body control, and thus the ability to avoid injury, but they also increase joint stability. Several studies have found the lack of strength or an imbalance in strength to be a factor in the high incidence of injury. It could be said that strength is fundamental to athletic success.

HOW TO INCREASE STRENGTH

One of the most impressive aspects of muscle is its ability to adapt to loads placed on it.

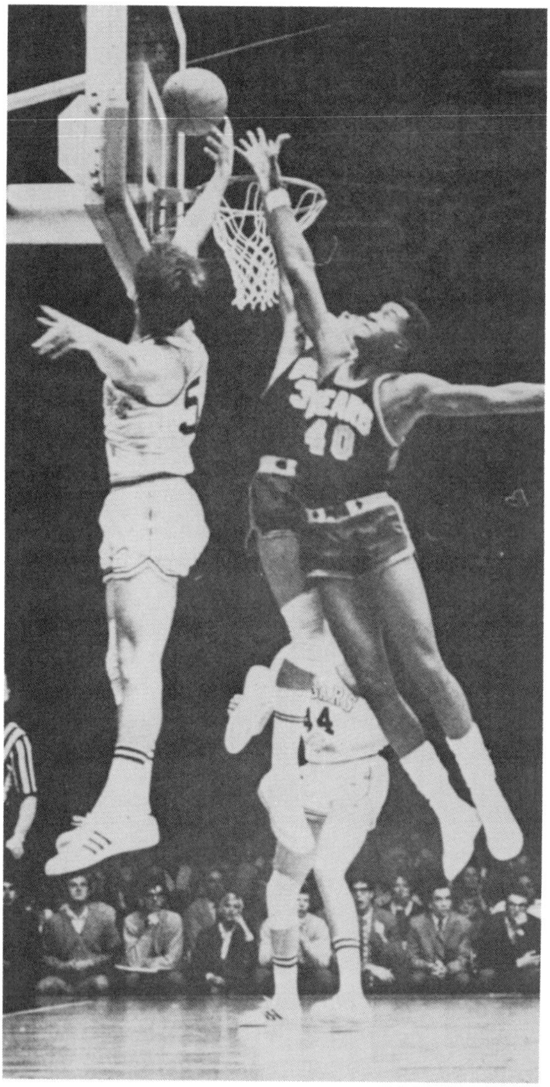

Fig. 7–1. Strength is important for developing maximum force. (From Jensen, C.R., and Fisher, A.G. *Scientific Basis of Athletic Conditioning,* 2nd Ed. Courtesy of Lea & Febiger, 1979.)

If a person lifts more than normally lifted for a period of time, the muscle gets stronger. This principle is called the *overload principle.* As the muscle gets stronger, the load must be increased to maintain the overload and continue to make gains. This principle is called *progressive resistance.*

There are many approaches to develop strength. In fact, any form of activity that applies heavier than usual resistance to muscles will stimulate an increase in strength. Strength building stimuli may be provided by:

1. Hard physical labor or vigorous athletic performance (work)
2. Specific exercises against body weight (calisthenics)
3. Heavy resistance exercises using weights with either shortening or lengthening contractions (weight training)
4. Application of muscle force against an immoveable object (isometrics)

The first three methods of building strength all result in *dynamic* contractions, meaning that the muscles change length, and movement of the body segment occurs. The fourth method results in a *static* contraction, in which the muscles apply tension but do not shorten, and do not move a body segment. Neither hard physical labor nor calisthenics will result in maximal strength gains because maximum overload cannot be applied. Although maximum overload can be applied with isometrics, strength gains occur at the specific angle trained so this method has limited applicability. The four basic types of contractions used for increasing strength are summarized in Table 7–1.

As with all training programs, the principle of *specificity* must be recognized and used if maximum benefits are to be realized from strength training programs. This principle implies that a training program must be implemented for each individual athlete and must be relevant to the demands of the event or sport for which the athlete is being trained. It is necessary to consider the predominant energy system and the muscle groups in-

Table 7–1. Types of Contractions Used for Increasing Strength

Type of Contraction	*Definition*
Dynamic or Isotonic	
Concentric	The muscle develops enough tension to exceed the resistance
Eccentric	The resistance exceeds the amount of tension the muscle applies
Static or Isometric	Tension develops but there is no change in muscular length
Isokinetic	The muscle applies tension against a resistance that moves at a constant speed through the full range of motion

volved. Gains in muscular strength and endurance will have their greatest effect on performance when the training program consists of progressive resistance exercises that stimulate the muscles and include movement patterns used during the actual performance. Weight resistance exercises should focus on those muscles associated with a particular movement in the execution of the event so that the specific fibers involved are trained. Training must also be specific to the joint angle at which the muscle group is trained. Therefore, muscles should be moved through the full range of motion required in the performance of a certain skill. Training programs should also be specific to the mode of training, i.e., isotonic training will best increase isotonic strength, isometric training will best increase isometric strength, etc. Interestingly, even the type of training program appears to be specific. For instance, simultaneously training for muscular strength and aerobic endurance will interfere with reaching the same potential that could be attained by training for strength or endurance alone.

PROGRAMS FOR DEVELOPING STRENGTH

Many different programs for developing strength are used by athletes and coaches. The following are the most common of the structured programs.

Static Strength Training

Early studies by Hettinger and Muller of Germany proved the effectiveness of static overload or isometrics. They reported that static contractions of two-thirds maximum contractile strength held for 6 seconds once a day, 5 days a week were effective in producing a 5% strength increase per week. Although more recent studies support the use of isometrics to increase strength, few have shown increases in strength of the same magnitude. Subsequent research has not been consistent in reporting the optimal frequency and duration of isometric contractions for maximal strength gains. One of Muller's later studies reported that 5 to 10 maximal isometric contractions 5 days per week was best for increasing maximal strength. Other studies have shown that a variety of combinations of tension (% maximal contraction), duration, frequency, and number of contractions all produced strength gains. However, the information available on isometric training probably does not support its routine use for strength development in athletes. This type of training can be useful when other training equipment is not available or for special purposes (i.e., rehabilitation).

Earlier it was mentioned that the development of strength and endurance is specific to the joint angle at which the muscle group is trained. If using isometrics, it is necessary to train any muscle group at several different joint angles.

Equipment. No specific equipment is needed for static strength training. Some facilities build racks to provide resistance for certain muscle groups or for certain angles, but little commercial equipment is available (Fig. 7–2).

Advantages. Static strength training is simple and inexpensive and there is little danger in terms of weights dropping or muscle injury. This type of training can be done at home, in the office, or even in a car (for example, tightening the abdominal muscles or pushing one arm against the resistance of the other).

Disadvantages. The major disadvantage relates to the specificity of strength gains to the angle of training. To train a muscle through its full range of motion requires using several different angles. It is also difficult to train certain areas and movements with static resistance. Other disadvantages relate to the difficulty of knowing the amount of force being applied and the lack of feedback regarding strength gains.

Eccentric Strength Training

Eccentric strength training is often termed "negative resistance" training because the load is so heavy that it cannot be moved in a "positive" direction without help. To perform a lift, the athlete is helped into the intermediate position by spotters. He then resists the load while it returns to the starting position. For example, in the bench press, spotters help the athlete lift the bar to an extended (intermediate) position over the chest. They then stand by in a ready position while the athlete returns the superheavy bar to the chest.

a

b

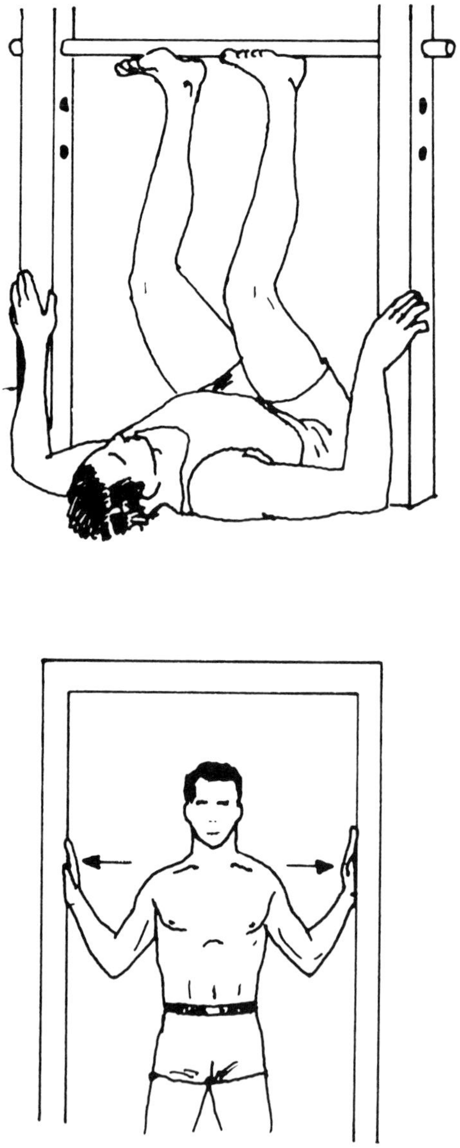

Fig. 7–2. Examples of a setup for static or isometric training. (From Jensen, C.R., and Fisher, A.G. *Scientific Basis of Athletic Conditioning,* 2nd Ed. Courtesy of Lea & Febiger, 1979.)

Weight training programs structured around eccentric contractions are not common and have not been fully accepted by coaches and trainers. There are two reasons for this lack of acceptance. First, eccentric programs have not proven to be better than isotonic or isokinetic programs. Johnson and associates compared concentric and eccentric strength training, using concentric exercises that were 80% of 1 RM* for 2 sets of 10 repetitions, and eccentric exercises that were 120% of the concentric 1 RM for 2 sets of 6 repetitions. Both routines produced significant gains in strength but neither training procedure produced dynamic or static strength gains significantly greater than the other. Second, there seems to be much more delayed muscle soreness following eccentric exercises. These two factors place eccentric programs at a definite disadvantage.

A review of the literature on this topic revealed the following:

1. The energy costs of performing against a constant amount of resistance are much less using eccentric contractions than using concentric contractions. This means that in order to apply the same amount of overload, eccentric contractions must be performed against considerably greater resistance than that for concentric contractions.

2. At practically all angles of pull, measured muscle tension is consistently greater (about 32%) for eccentric movements than for concentric movements or isometric contractions. This means that eccentric strength measures cannot logically be compared to concentric or isometric measures.

3. The amount of strength that can be developed through eccentric exercise is not statistically different from the amount that can be developed with concentric exercise.

4. Concentric exercises are often preferred because they relate more closely to the movement patterns involved in performance. Most athletic events require positive work, and only rarely are muscles called upon to do heavy resistance negative work.

Equipment. Any strength training equipment that can be used for isotonic training can be used for eccentric training. The only difference relates to the amount of the load.

Advantages. Since research has not shown an advantage in terms of strength gains, this is not an advantage. However, some trainers use this technique to "speed up" the gain. In addition, changing the type of lift, especially when the load is so much greater, can have a positive psychologic effect on athletes and

*RM means repetition maximum. A 10 RM is a weight that can be lifted 10 times but no more.

help them avoid the boredom sometimes associated with training.

Disadvantages. The greatest disadvantages relate to the increase in muscle soreness and the potential dangers of lifting much heavier weights.

Plyometrics. Eccentric exercises are sometimes used in areas other than the weight room. For example, in jump training, the athlete steps from a bench, absorbing the force of the landing within his legs by flexing at the ankles, knees, and hips. The energy developed in the landing is thus stored in the elastic structures of the muscles and tendons. He then converts the stored energy to kinetic energy by jumping back into the air. This action is much like a compressed spring being relieved of the downward force that originally compressed it. In addition, the sudden stretch of the stretch reflexes is thought to facilitate the recruitment of additional motor units.

Plyometrics is often used for track and field, volleyball, and basketball and coaches in other areas are applying the principles. There are several benefits of plyometric training. First, the athletes may learn timing of muscular contractions which would be helpful in sports such as gymnastics and volleyball. Second, plyometric movements are similar to those movements of actual performance. Plyometrics can also be modified for progressive increases in intensity and duration (Fig. 7–3).

There are problems associated with this type of training, however. Several well-known world class athletes have sustained joint and tendon injuries and other athletes have complained of increased muscle soreness. Because of the benefits, plyometrics can probably be used but the following precautions may help prevent problems: (1) Be sure that each athlete has a good strength base from regular strength training programs prior to using plyometrics. (2) Work on flexibility as part of the training to avoid injury. (3) Begin at a low level and progress slowly. With jump training, start with a 12-inch box and increase in 6-inch increments. There is surely a maximum effective height for this type of training. In one study, the height of the center of gravity (cg) following the jump for men volleyball players began to decrease at about 2 feet; for women gymnasts and physical education students, it

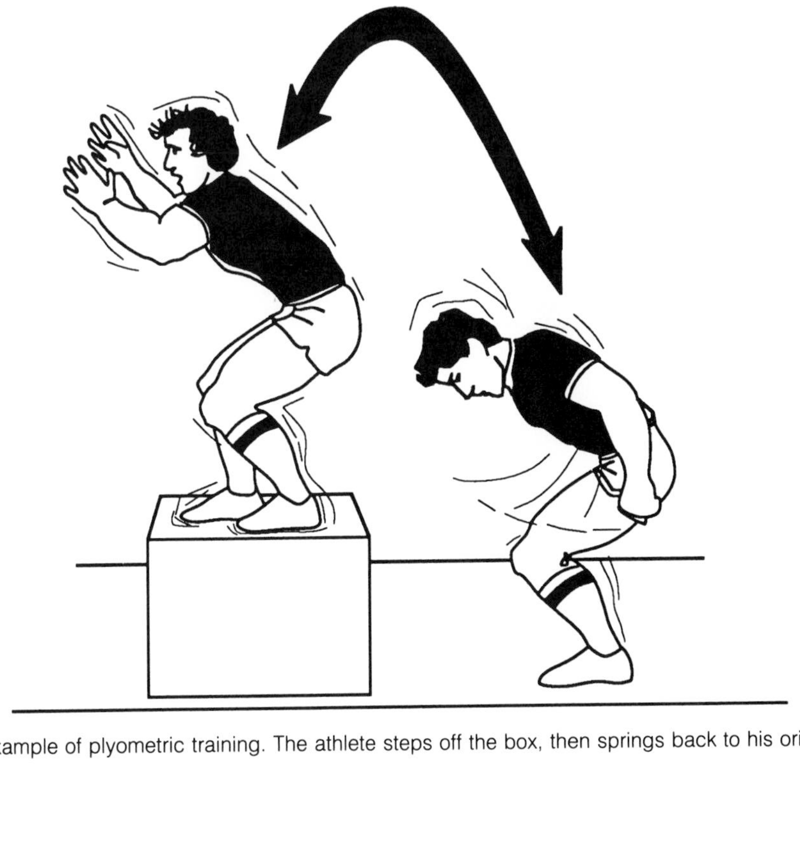

Fig. 7–3. An example of plyometric training. The athlete steps off the box, then springs back to his original position.

was between 16 to 20 inches. This may indicate that the most effective training occurs in these ranges.

Isokinetic Strength Training

Isokinetic exercise is a form of isotonics performed with equipment that moves at a constant speed regardless of the force exerted. This is usually accomplished using some hydraulic device which essentially has an infinite range of resistance. The harder one pushes, the greater the resistance. This may allow the resistance to more closely match the force exerted against it than with regular barbells or other isotonic devices. A distinct disadvantage of conventional strength training is that the muscle being trained is not stressed evenly through the full range of motion. This is due to changes in leverage combined with changes in the direction of movement of the resistance in relation to the line of gravity. Only at certain points in the range of motion does a muscle contract at maximum.

Since the resistance is matched more closely to the strength of the muscle, the muscles can contract maximally through all points, regardless of the mechanical advantage. Because muscles are maximally contracting, there is a greater recruitment of motor units and a greater overload.

Thistle and associates compared isokinetic training with isotonic and isometric training and found that, after 8 weeks of training, the isokinetic group had gained approximately 35% quadriceps strength as compared with 27.5% for the isotonic group, and 9.2% for the isometric group. Other studies have not been so positive. One reported no differences in strength gains between isokinetic and isotonic or isokinetic and isometric training programs.

Equipment. Isokinetic equipment is still in the developmental stage in some regards. It is fairly expensive and there have been nagging problems with maintaining some training devices. However, the isokinetic testing devices (Fig. 7–4) have been extremely dependable and are used regularly by athletic trainers, especially for rehabilitating athletes after injury.

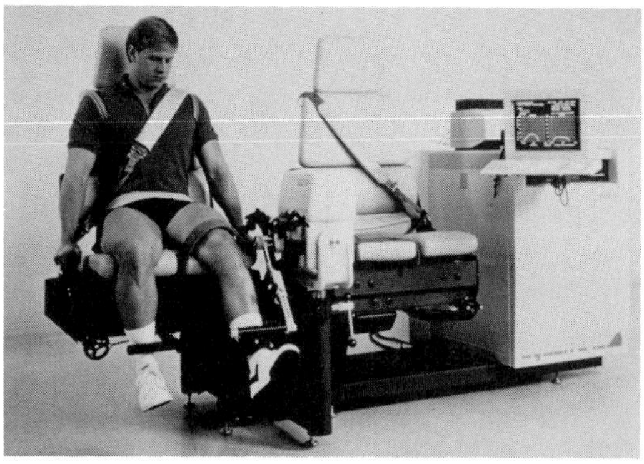

Fig. 7–4. Isokinetic testing (and training) device. (Photograph by Barry Axelrod. Courtesy of Cybex.)

Advantages. (1) A unique feature of some isokinetic machines is that the speed of the movement can be controlled, so the maximal contraction through the entire range of motion occurs at any specified speed. Being able to control speed raises the question of what speed to use during training. Again the concept of specificity applies. Studies have indicated that isokinetic training produces strength gains at velocities of movement equal to or slower than the training velocity. If the training velocity was 120 degrees per second, strength gains would result at speeds of 120 degrees per second or less, but not greater than 120 degrees per second. This may not be helpful since performance speeds are typically much higher than speeds available on isokinetic devices. (2) Since there is so little ballistic component in isokinetic training, higher speeds can be used more effectively. (3) Some studies have found that the total training time for effective isokinetic training is less than with isotonic, suggesting that the same volume of training may not be necessary with isokinetics. (4) There is little danger from using isokinetic machines relating to weights or strains.

Disadvantages. The one major drawback with isokinetic training is that the resistance can be moved easily and athletes sometimes fail to work at maximal intensities. A second problem has to do with seeing progress. Unless the device has a recorder or gauge, it is difficult to see the week to week strength gains that are so easy to see using conventional devices. With all of these problems, isokinetics has a bright future as a training method and should probably be used in athletic programs training today, at least as a supplemental program.

Isotonic Strength Training

Isotonic training refers to the more traditional systems of lifting a heavy weight through a range of motion. It is termed isotonic because the weight or resistance remains the same during the range of movement (Fig. 7–5).

Prior to World War II, strength training was not used routinely for conditioning athletes. In fact, it was believed that "muscle-boundness" resulted from such programs, and they were taboo to those seeking to improve athletic performance. During World War II, Thomas DeLorme and his co-workers experienced great success with heavy resistance exercises in the rehabilitation of hospital patients. Following his work, much research was done to determine the effects of this kind of training on athletic performance. Increased strength was found to be highly beneficial to athletic performance, and heavy resistance exercise using weights was the most expedient method for increasing strength.

It is now clear that strength can be increased rapidly by exercising against heavy resistance for a few repetitions. Early programs by DeLorme and Wilkins recommended the following:

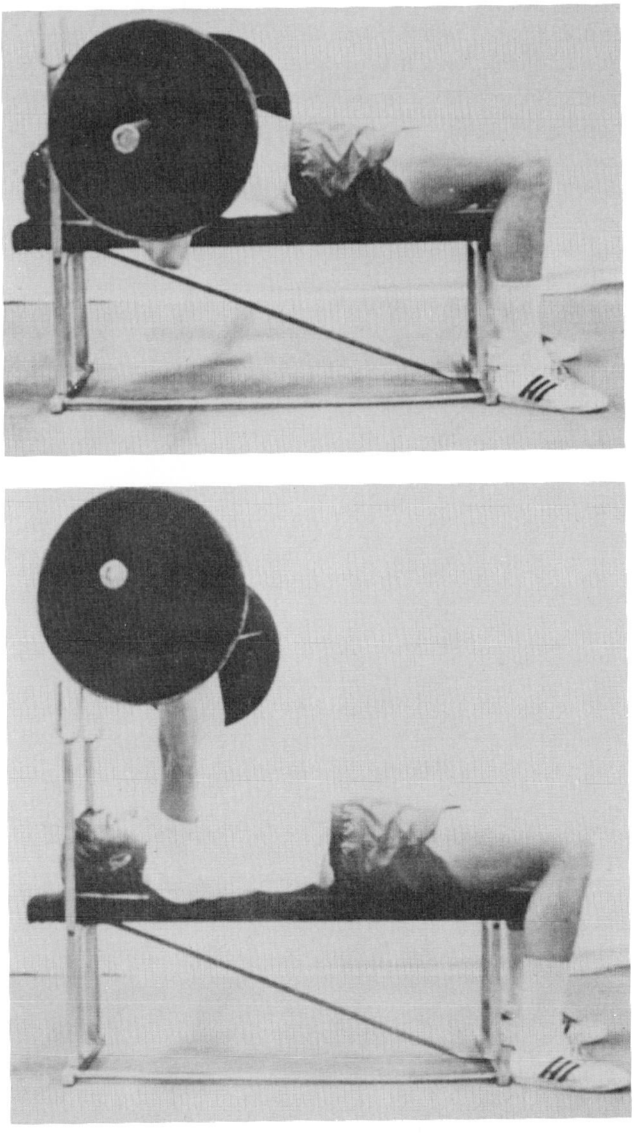

Fig. 7–5. Bench press using an olympic bar.

Set 1 = 10 repetitions with 1/2 10 RM
Set 2 = 10 repetitions with 3/4 10 RM
Set 3 = 10 repetitions at a load of 10 RM

The most important set was the third, for it represented the greatest resistance for the muscle group. Variations in the warm-up sets (sets 1 and 2) probably do not effect the results appreciably. DeLorme's original recommendations were to train 4 consecutive days. A fifth day was thought to interfere with recovery.

Berger studied the effects of various combinations of sets and repetitions on strength gains. With 3 sets of 6 to 8 RM, subjects made similar strength gains whether lifting 2 days per week or 3 days per week. It is now common practice to recommend that progressive resistance exercises be performed 3 to 4 days per week on alternating days rather than consecutive days. Research has also shown that 3 sets of each exercise results in greater strength gains than does 2 or 1, and the optimum number of repetitions is between 3 and 9.

Even though DeLorme and Wilkins' method is still considered effective, more recent evidence supports the use of fewer repetitions and heavier weight for developing strength. However, there is still some lack of agreement among experts about the exact number of sets and repetitions that is best for building strength. Very likely, there is no single combination of sets and repetitions that yields optimum strength for everyone. The underlying principle is to work in the overload zone on a regular basis using exercises selected to work the specific muscles relating to performance.

The old rule that a person should use low repetitions and high resistance for strength and high repetitions and low resistance for endurance appears to be valid. However, it may not be quite that simple because of the relationships between strength and endurance. Programs that work well for strength also increase muscular endurance because stronger muscles can lift any given load more times. The old rule should be extended based on the fact that both strength and absolute muscular endurance have been shown to be equally developed from either a low repetition/high load program or a high repetition/low load program. However, absolute endurance is related more strongly to strength programs than strength is related to endurance programs. Since athletes require strength, power, and absolute endurance more so than relative endurance, it makes sense that athletes train for strength using higher loads and lower repetitions. Even when training specifically for endurance, athletes should lift to exhaustion because prolonged "underloaded" repetitions have little effect on endurance.

Because fixed weights (barbells or machines) cannot match the force available through the entire range of motion, manufacturers have developed *variable resistance* machines that vary the resistance to more closely match the strength curve of the various muscle groups of the body. These machines work by using an elliptical lever arm arrangement or by varying the length of the lever arm of the weight rack. Entire rooms of these machines are now available at larger universities. Whether better than conventional barbells or not, they make an impressive sight for prospective athletes who visit the campus (Fig. 7–6).

Advantages. There are several advantages associated with using isotonic strength training: (1) The athlete can see work being done. With bar bells, there is a feeling of great strength associated with the size and massiveness of the weight being lifted. With machines, the setting is the goal. (2) Progress can be easily seen. When another plate is added or another setting is reached, the athlete, and other athletes in the facility, knows about the change. (3) With bar bells, there is a great use of accessory muscles. Just getting bar bells into position for some lifts is a workout. Machines tend to diminish this advantage since they are stabilized and work specifically on one muscle group. (4) Cost is a definite advantage for bar bells. A high school teacher recently supplied his weight room with used weights by advertising in a local newspaper and picking up the weights from the homes around the school. By welding these weights together in ascending weight levels, he had an inexpensive and effective addition to his training program.

Disadvantages. The major disadvantage falls to the machines and is related to cost. As good

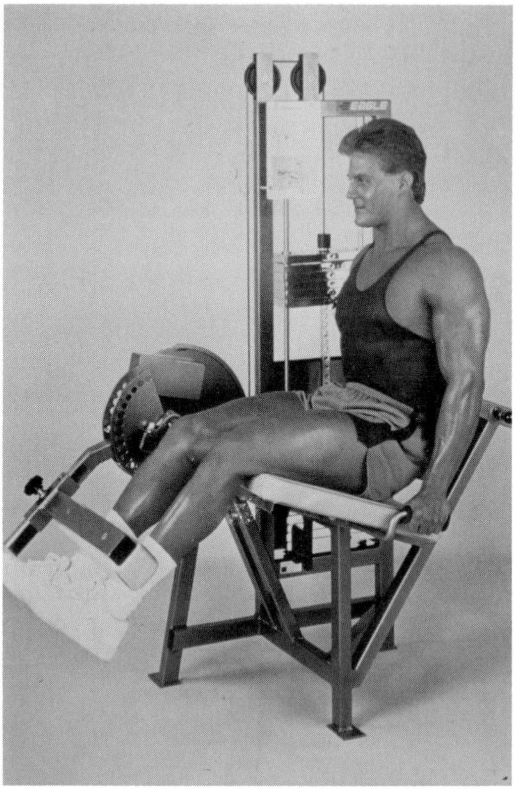

Fig. 7–6. A variable resistance Cybex Eagle machine for leg extensions. (Photograph by Barry Axelrod. Courtesy of Cybex.)

as many of these machines are, they are expensive and may be out of reach for the average high school or junior college budget. Another disadvantage, for free weights, relates to safety. Using free weights can be a worrisome task with a large group of inexperienced, exuberant boys. Even athletes who have used weights for some time can injure themselves. Correct lifting techniques and safety precautions are a must.

Other Strength-Building Methods

A limited amount of research supports the claim that strength can be gained at a rapid rate by *combining isometrics* and *isotonics*. This is done by contracting the muscles isometrically against a rope or a cable arrangement for about 10 seconds, then reducing the resistance to allow a slow motion isotonic contraction to occur. Several mechanical devices for use with this approach have been developed and sold commercially. With this method it is recommended that each exercise be repeated 8 to 10 times daily.

A less effective and seldom used method is *functional overload* where the activity itself is performed under resistive conditions. Weighted vests, ankle weights, and other weighted objects and implements have been used in the past. Throwing weighted baseballs and swinging weighted bats are still used by some. These methods have the advantage of closely coordinating the strength gains into the movement patterns, but some experts think it reduces coordination and timing. Only mild strength gains result from this method, because typically the resistance is too little to provide a strong stimulus for strength.

In addition to the different programs for developing strength, there are different approaches to make strength training more interesting and to avoid some of the problems of overtraining and boredom associated with simply using the same daily routines. Both *circuit training* and *periodization* are used as alternative approaches for applying the basic principles of weight training. These two approaches are discussed in more detail below.

Circuit Training. Circuit training is a popular method of applying isotonic strength training techniques. A number of "stations" are set up in a logical sequence allowing the athlete to move from one station to the next until the "circuit" is completed. "Stations" usually involve some type of weight training exercises, but stretching, calisthenics, or aerobic activity may also be included. Therefore, circuit training programs may be designed to work rather specifically to develop muscular strength and endurance, or on such components as flexibility or cardiovascular endurance as well. In most cases the circuit is repeated several times.

The physiologic effects will depend upon the type of circuit that is designed. The primary role of circuit training is to improve strength. Only minimal changes in cardiovascular fitness have been reported even when the circuit was done continuously and at fairly constant intensity.

The circuit should include exercises that will develop the specific muscles and movements pertinent to the sport for which the athlete is training. The advantage of circuit training is that the principle of progressive training can be implemented for an entire team of athletes, where all are performing exercises at the same relative workload. The amount of overload can be assigned by manipulating the time for performing each circuit, increasing the load at each station, or a combination of both.

The circuit can be simple, composed of minimal equipment and involving calisthenics or it can involve an elaborate arrangement of weight training equipment. It should consist of 6 to 15 stations. At each station, athletes can perform either a given number of repetitions, or do as many repetitions as possible in a given amount of time (e.g., 30 seconds). If cardiovascular endurance is of interest, rather than having a 15- to 30-second rest between stations, there can be a period of running or bicycling. Two consecutive stations should not emphasize the same muscle group (Fig. 7–7).

Periodization. One of the most difficult tasks facing any coach is to prepare his athletes optimally, without overtraining and staleness. Periodization is a technique of varying the training workload into cycles to optimize the training effect, but still keep interest in training. If there were only one competition or event a year, training programs would be simplified. The athlete would begin at a low level of work several months prior to the event and increase his workload until he peaked in strength just before competing. However, most athletes compete for a significant part of the year, and have many major events.

There are differences in training emphasis depending on the sport. For instance, if the win/loss ratio is important, coaches must prepare the team so they are near their peak performance at the beginning of the season. Teams with poor season records will not even qualify for important games at the end of the season. In other sports, especially certain track and field events, athletes must do well enough to qualify, but they must be prepared optimally for the championship at the end of the season.

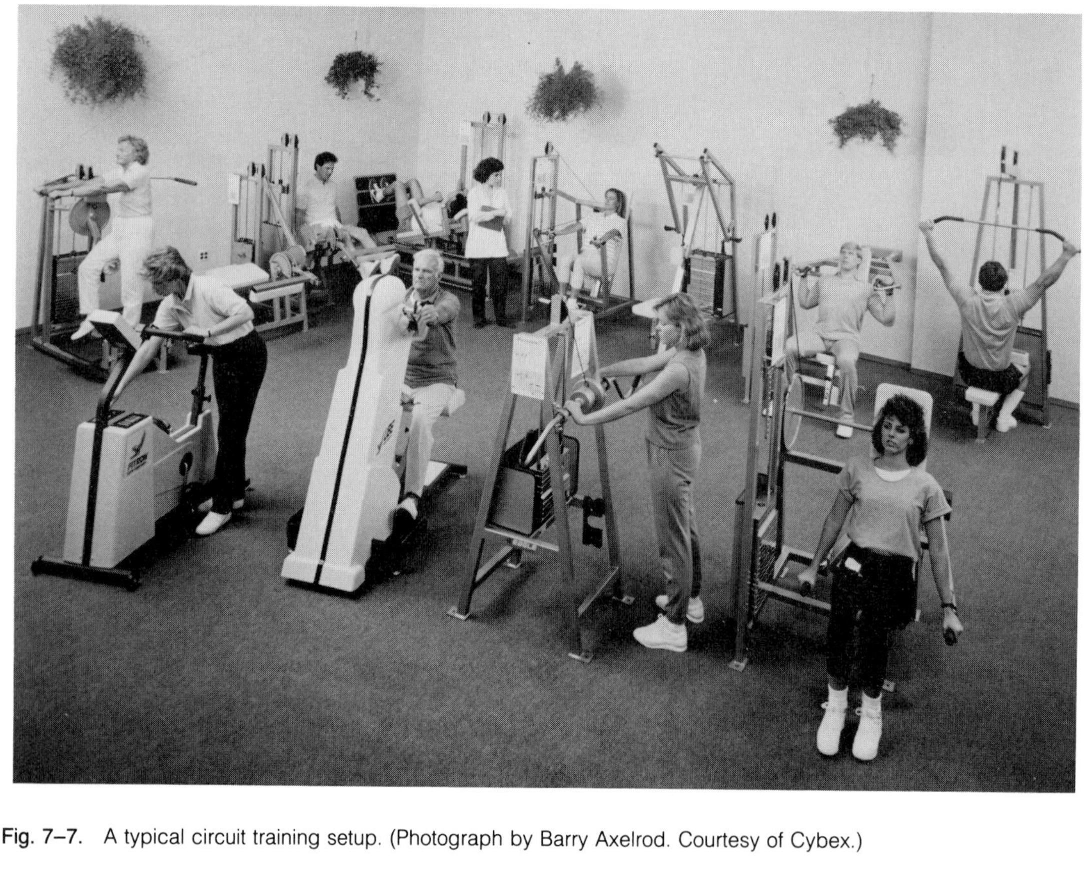

Fig. 7–7. A typical circuit training setup. (Photograph by Barry Axelrod. Courtesy of Cybex.)

In sports such as football, where every game is critical, the ideal is to keep the team and individual athletes at optimal performance levels throughout the season. These athletes must train hard in the pre-season to be at peak performance at the start of the season. The problem is to keep their peak for the entire season and also be ready for post season play.

Realistically, it is difficult for athletes to maintain 100% performance, especially if they continue to train hard throughout the season. Periodization allows for a change in pace called tapering to overcome this problem. *Tapering* is the slowing down of the intensity and duration of training to allow maximal performance. If peak performance is reached several weeks prior to a major competition, it is necessary for the athlete to reduce the work load to avoid over-stressing his body. Workouts may be 80 to 90% of normal so rest can occur without a sacrifice in strength.

It is essential that coaches and trainers plan a year-a-round training program so each athlete peaks at the right time. Manipulation of intensity and volume of workouts, and the recovery periods are the basis for periodization. *Volume* refers to the quantity of training performed in a period of time. *Intensity* refers to the strength of the stimulus (%VO_2max, repetitions, %RM, etc.) or concentration of work per unit of time. Volume and intensity are integrally related and dependant upon each other and are not increased simultaneously. Intensity of exercise is progressed to a peak just prior to competition. Volume is peaked as intensity is on the uprise, and decreases as intensity peaks (Fig. 7–8).

In periodization the training year is divided into major periods, the preparation period (the longest of all three), a competition period, and a transition period. The first phase of the preparation period is characterized by increasing intensity and volume of exercise with an emphasis on general training. In phase two of the preparation period, the volume and intensity rise to their greatest level and an increase in competition specific training occurs (still maintaining general training). During the competition period, the volume of training decreases to allow for the added stress of regular practice, but intensity increases. During the second phase of the competition period (phase 4), if competition is continuing (as during a football season), there are several *cycles*, where the volume, load, and intensity of the workouts are altered to avoid staleness where there is a taper to allow for good performance as during weekly game situations. For special events (bowl games, olympics, etc.) there is a phase 5 of the competition period where the athlete(s) is in a peak condition for performance. Following the competitive season, the transition period allows for recuperation from the stress of training

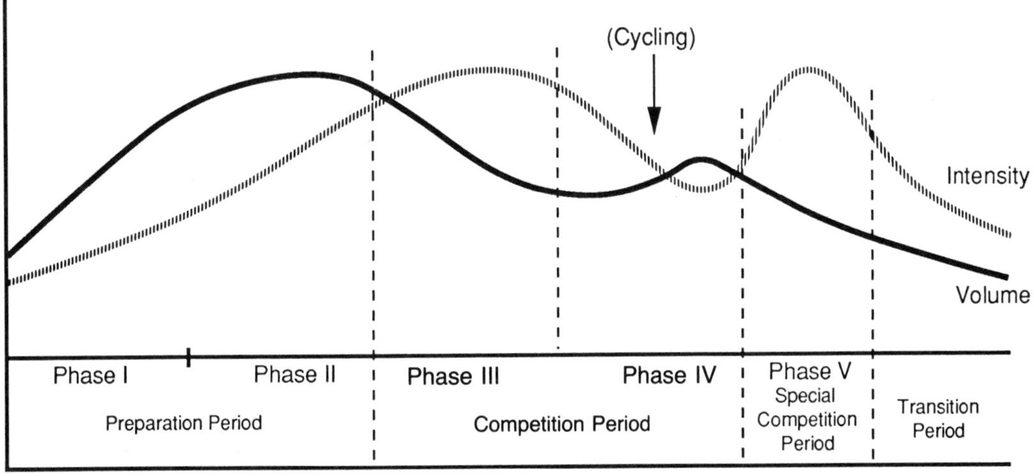

Fig. 7–8. Intensity follows volume until competition phase.

and competition. Complete rest is not advised. Active rest with activity other than that normally done in training is best. This period should be long enough to restore the athletes, both in mind and body.

Because an athlete is unlikely to maintain 100% performance throughout the season, training can be peaked and tapered on a weekly basis (mesocycles). During these mesocycles, there is a weekly change in training volume and intensity followed by a short transition period. On a 7 day/week training period, progression continues until a peak workout occurs on the 4th day. The 5th day is a minimal workload followed by two days of progression with a 2nd peak on the 7th day. This allows the athlete to "stairstep" to higher and higher levels of performance throughout the season (Fig. 7–9). If competition occurs on the weekend, the cycle may be completed on the third or fourth day and the athlete would use light workouts, emphasizing skill, on the day immediately preceding the competition.

A beneficial feature of periodization is that the athlete is either physically active or training year-round. Year-around conditioning helps maintain fitness levels and helps prevent injuries, especially at the beginning of the sports season. The athlete who is active year-around will have a less stressful transition into intense practices and be less prone to injury.

Periodization applies to many or all sports and requires planning and structure. These principles can also be used for both strength and endurance training. Some tips to remember if using periodization are:

1. The longer the season the longer the preparation before season. The ratio for preparation is about 2:1. If the season lasts 12 weeks, the pre-season preparation should be 24 weeks.

2. Peaking at the right time is the objective of periodization.

3. During the season, strength and conditioning workouts should be reduced in intensity and duration to accommodate the extra stress of practice and competition.

4. Tapering for a whole season is complex. The team cannot go all out for just two games. The taper and workload must be spread out for all games.

For more information on periodization, see the books by Bompa and Freeman cited in Selected Readings.

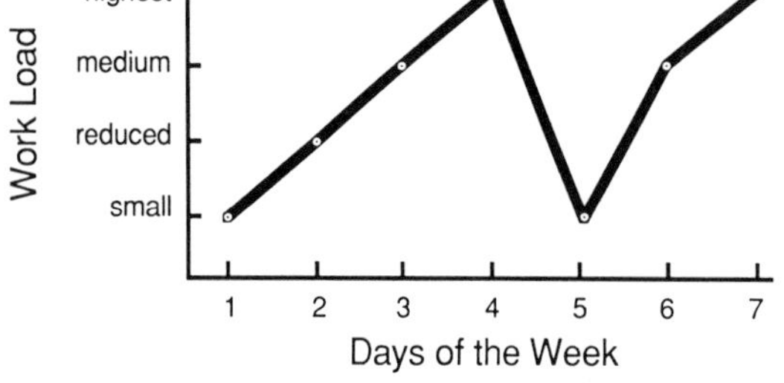

Fig. 7–9. Changes in volume and intensity during weekly training cycle.

TRAINABILITY OF MUSCLE

There is a great deal of variation in the strength increases reported by different researchers under varying conditions. Large, rapid increases in strength should not be expected even though reports have indicated 160% increase in strength in 1 week of training. A 5% gain per week over a period of several weeks should be considered extraordinary. After several weeks of training, strength gains will plateau, beyond which additional strength gains are slow.

There are several interesting points about strength trainability:

1. Some persons are more responsive to training than others. Mesomorphs (those who are naturally muscular) seem to gain strength more rapidly and to a greater extent than ectomorphs (tendency towards thinness) or endomorphs (people with a tendency toward a "pearshape").

2. The same person responds differently to training as he becomes more highly trained. Generally, muscles in poor condition respond rapidly, whereas already trained muscles respond more slowly. Gains in strength become increasingly more difficult as the strength level approaches maximal.

3. People gain strength less rapidly as they get older. Men are the most responsive during the formative years, up to about age 25, after which they become less and less responsive. Women are the most responsive to strength gains up to about age 21. However, as long

as people are healthy and normal, they will respond to strength stimuli, regardless of age.

4. Not all muscles respond at the same rate even when optimal strength stimuli are provided. This may be due to the fact that some muscle groups are more trainable than others, and each muscle group in the body differs in its level of condition.

Will training a muscle group on one side of the body have effects on the same muscle group on the opposite side of the body? Research suggest that there may be slight electrophysiologic transfer (cross training) between muscle groups. Training one muscle group may result in slight but measurable increases in strength in other muscle groups. Some research has concluded that cross training in strength occurs only when isotonic methods are used. Other researchers have found no cross training effects regardless of the training mode. Underloading will not result in increased strength or cross training effects. During strength training, the untrained muscle group demonstrates isometric contractions and increased EMG activity (muscle electrical activity) during contraction of the trained muscle group. This may be due to factors in the central nervous system rather than in the muscles themselves. There may be an overflow of neural stimulus from the motor cortex to the untrained muscles while the trained muscles are contracting. It should also be pointed out that research investigating cross training often utilized strength tests at various intervals throughout the study. Maximal contractions of the untrained muscles may have contributed to the reported strength gains.

MUSCULAR ENDURANCE

Endurance is defined as the ability to withstand a resistance for a period of time. It can also be thought of as resistance to fatigue and quick recovery after fatigue. A high level of endurance implies that a given level of performance (or resistance) can be continued for a relatively long time. Increased endurance postpones the onset of fatigue. Endurance improves performance in instances in which fatigue is a limiting factor. Endurance may apply to the body as a whole or to a particular body system, or to specific areas of the muscular system.

Muscular endurance is closely related to strength and is dependent upon (1) the type of muscle, (2) blood supply to the muscle, and (3) the nervous intervention. It has been well established that strength contributes to muscular endurance. In fact there is a high correlation (.75 to .97) between strength and absolute muscular endurance (the amount of time an individual can work against a given resistance unrelated to his strength). As an athlete becomes stronger he/she will be able to lift a given weight more times. For example, a person who can bench press 300 pounds could lift a 100-pound weight many more times than a person who can bench only 125 pounds. If the weight is adjusted to correspond to his/her strength (e.g. one-third of 1 RM for each person), the difference is diminished.

There is a strong positive relationship between isotonic strength and absolute isotonic endurance and between isometric strength and absolute isometric endurance.

MUSCULAR FATIGUE

Since endurance often implies resistance to fatigue, it is necessary to discuss the possible causes of muscular fatigue. It is important to note that because of the biochemical and physiological differences between fast and slow twitch fibers, fast twitch fibers are more easily fatigued than slow twitch fibers.

There are four potential sites of muscular fatigue. Failure of any one of these neuromuscular mechanisms will result in muscular fatigue: (1) the synapses in the central nevous system, (2) the motor neuron, (3) the myoneural junction, and (4) the contractile mechanism of the muscle tissue.

There is recent evidence which suggests that recovery from local muscular fatigue is influenced by a central nervous system factor that is independent of local blood flow. Use of diverting activities during recovery periods has been shown to increase the amount of work performed during repeated work periods. Diverting activities were those physical activities performed with non-fatigued muscles. How exactly the central nervous system offsets the effects of muscular work is unknown. The central nervous system itself, in theory, may become fatigued. Even though repeated voluntary contractions results in eventual fatigue, in situ muscle stimulated with similar loads and frequencies endure the workloads for much longer periods of time. The precise mechanism for CNS fatigue is not understood, but may be linked to peripheral nerve transmission.

Although a potential site of fatigue, it is unlikely that fatigue occurs within the motor neuron. Fatigue is much more likely to occur at the neuromuscular junction where a decreased release of acetylcholine from the nerve endings may inhibit the impulse from the brain. This may be one of the reasons that fast twitch fibers are more fatiguable than red.

There is evidence to suggest that the muscle itself is the most likely site of muscular fatigue. The contractile mechanism may be most vulnerable to fatigue because of either the accumulation of lactic acid or the lack of ATP-PC. Lactic acid causes the H+ concentration to increase and lowers pH. A decrease in pH hinders the excitation-coupling process by decreasing the amount of Ca^{++} released from the sarcoplasmic reticulum and interferes with Ca^{++}-troponin binding capacity. The decrease in pH also inhibits the activity of phosphofructokinase, a key enzyme involved in anaerobic glycolysis. This would slow glycolysis and reduce the amount of ATP available for energy. Since fast twitch fibers produce more lactic acid than slow twitch fibers, they would fatigue more rapidly from this potential problem.

A second possible reason for contractile mechanism fatigue is lack of ATP and PC (phosphagen) stores. Depletion of these substances would result in fatigue. However, studies with humans have not substantiated this theory. Even when muscle was fully fatigued there was still 76% of the resting concentration of ATP in it. ATP and PC stores regenerate rapidly during recovery while muscular force changes very little during the same time period. These and other possible causes of fatigue are summarized in Table 7–2.

Table 7–2. Summary of Possible Sites and Mechanisms of Muscular Fatigue

Site of Fatigue/Possible Mechanisms

1. Neuromuscular Junction
   decreased release of acetylcholine at the nerve endings
2. Central nervous system
   local disturbances caused by contractile fatigue results in inhibitory signals being sent to the motor units, reducing work output
3. Contractile mechanism
   a. decreased Ca^{++} released from sarcoplasmic reticulum and reduce Ca^{++}-troponin binding capacity
   b. increased lactic acid results in an increase in pH
   c. decreased ATP and PC stores
   d. decreased muscle glycogen
   e. lack of oxygen and inadequate blood flow

FACTORS AFFECTING THE APPLICATION OF STRENGTH

The tension developed by muscles as they shorten lever systems is affected by several important factors: (1) the initial length of the muscle fibers, (2) the angle of pull of the muscle on the skeleton, (3) the speed of contraction, (4) coordination of accessory muscles, (5) muscle size, and (6) muscle type.

Muscle Length

The initial length of the muscle is important because stretched fibers exert more force. Apparently, in the stretched state, cross-bridges are more effectively aligned with active sites and maximal force can be generated. Muscle fibers stretched beyond 120% of resting length begin to decrease their tension. This condition seldom exists in the human body, however, because muscle length is limited by joint movement, and many fibers are about 120% of resting length when joints reach their full extension. When fibers are less than fully extended, there begins to be an overlap of actin filaments which interferes with the coupling potential of the cross bridges.

Angle of Pull

From the discussion above, it could be concluded that a person can lift the heaviest load when the muscle is at or above its resting length. This is not always true because the human body utilizes muscle for developing force, and bones for providing leverage, and the combined effect of both muscles and levers determines the outcome in terms of applied strength. Although the contractile force of a muscle is greatest in its extended resting position, the mechanical advantage is most often less than optimal in this position. For example, in the fully extended arm, the bicep muscle can apply maximum force because of its structural position, but the angle of pull is not optimal. As the elbow joint moves through its range of motion, the mechanical advantage increases and the force the muscle needs to apply decreases yielding a rather stable "strength curve" for that particular joint and muscle group. During elbow flexion the greatest force is exerted between 80 and 140 degrees (180 degrees is full extension). At its strongest point in terms of length, the force at the hand was only 74% of maximum. In reality, the heaviest resistance that can be moved through a full range of motion is not the load that can be lifted at the optimal angle but the much smaller load at the point of mechanical disadvantage when the muscle is contracting maximally. Manufacturers have tried to compensate for this effect by developing machines which provide variable resistance so that maximal tension is being developed throughout the range of motion (Fig. 7–10).

Speed of Shortening

The relationship between muscular force and speed of shortening is important to athletes, especially in limb movements such as kicking and throwing. The faster a muscle is contracted, the less time there is for cross-bridge coupling (see Fig. 1–11). The force generated by a muscle is greatest at the slowest speeds of movement and decreases as the speed of movement increases. Likewise, for any given force, the greater the contribution of fast twitch fibers, the greater the velocity of movement. Physiologically, fast twitch fibers have a greater capacity for calcium release and uptake from the sarcoplasmic reticulum which allows for faster tension development. This information has practical application in the sense that athletes with a high genetic distribution of fast twitch fibers will probably perform better in power type events compared to those with predominantly slow twitch fibers.

Coordination of Accessory Muscles

Strength is also related to the coordination of the antagonistic muscles and the action of the neutralizer and stabilizer muscles. These factors can be improved through appropriate training which allows more efficient application of muscular force.

Muscle Size

The contractile force of a muscle is related to the muscle's cross-sectional measurement (4 to 6 kg/cm^2). As strength increases, the size of the individual muscle fibers increase, resulting in a greater cross-sectional area of the muscle. The increase in size relates fairly well with the increase in strength. Other factors may influence this relationship, such as (1) the fat around the muscle, (2) the proportion of active fibers, and (3) the efficiency of contraction. Nevertheless, muscle size and strength are closely related and an increase in muscle size will result in a significant increase in strength.

Muscle Type

Fast and slow fibers are recruited selectively depending on the force required. Training programs for strength emphasize high resistance/low repetition movements to stimulate recruitment of fast twitch fibers. For muscle endurance, the resistance is decreased and the number of repetitions are increased to allow slow twitch fibers to be recruited. There may also be selective hypertrophy in fast and slow fibers. Fast twitch fibers are much larger in power athletes than in cross country runners.

Relationship of Strength to Age

Research, combined with practical experience, indicates that under normal conditions boys increase in strength rather consistently until the age of 25. After this age, strength increases at a slower rate. Maximal strength is attained at the age of 25. Soon after the maximal strength is attained, strength begins to diminish. After the age of 25, it is speculated that a person loses 1% of his strength each year. At age 65 most persons are 65 to 70% as strong as they were at age 20 to 30. The rate of strength loss is influenced considerably by one's activity level throughout life.

As a child grows from infancy to adulthood, strength increases in approximate proportion to the increase in muscle size. Apparently there is no change in muscle quality, because

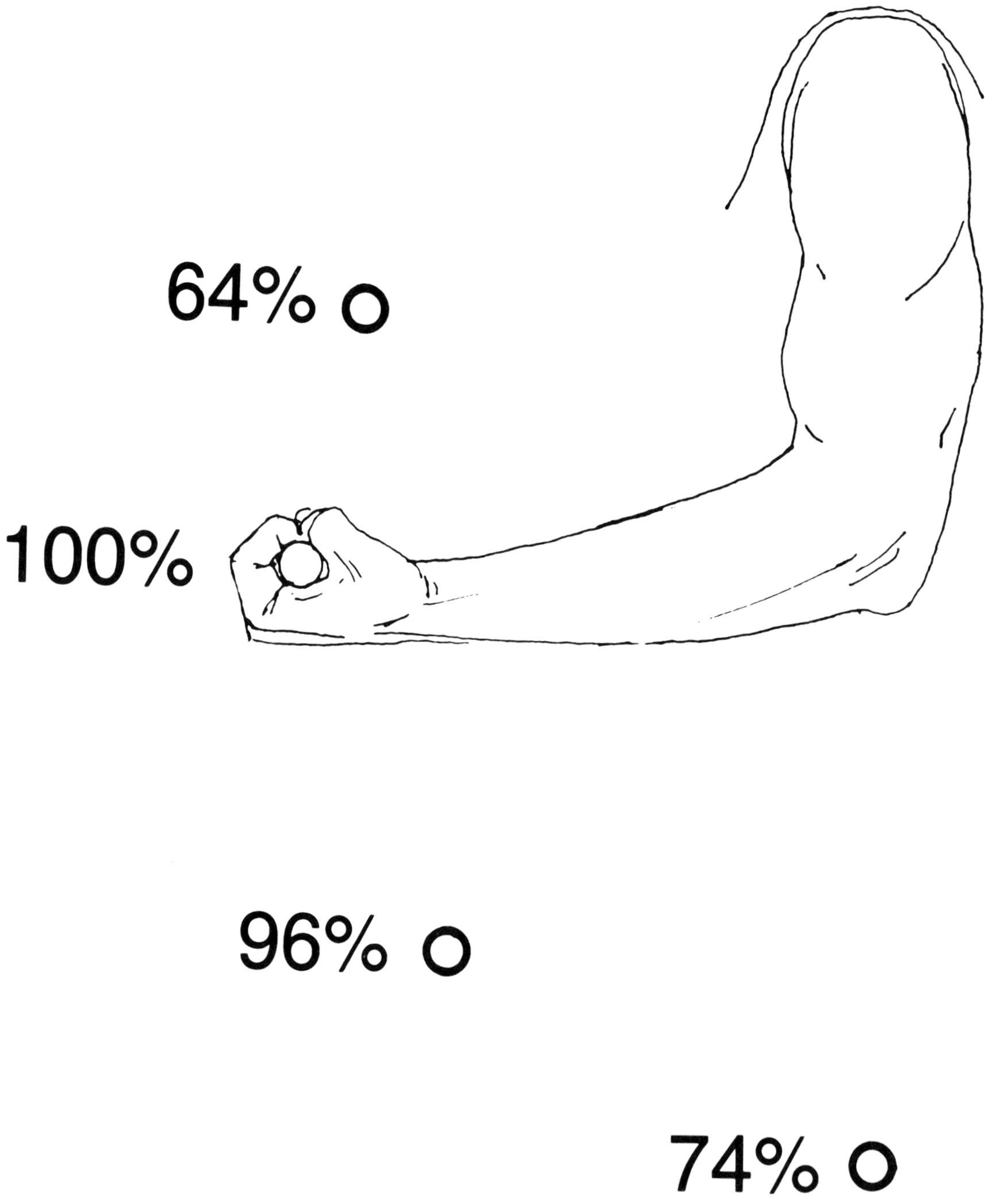

Fig. 7–10. Approximate percentage of maximal strength at different angles of pull through the elbow flexion movement. (From Jensen, C.R., and Fisher, A.G. *Scientific Basis of Athletic Conditioning,* 2nd Ed. Courtesy of Lea & Febiger, 1979.)

practically all the increased strength is accounted for by the increased muscle growth. It seems likely that the decrease in strength associated with increasing age is due to a decreased quality of muscle as well as quantity of muscle.

The strength curve relating muscle strength to age and sex shows what can be expected under normal living conditions. The curve can be altered at any point in life by using an effective strength building program. As a result of training a person can be significantly stronger at any particular age than he otherwise would have been and can retard the decline in strength that normally occurs (Fig. 7–11).

Girls increase in strength at about the same rate as boys to puberty. After puberty girls still gain strength, but at a slower rate. They typically reach maximal strength at age 21, but soon after begin to decline at about the same rate as men.

Relationship of Strength to Sex

Women are about two-thirds as strong as men and have about two-thirds as much muscle mass as men. They are about 80% as strong as men in the hip flexors and extensors, and about 55% as strong in the forearm flexors and extensors. The difference in upper and lower body strength between the sexes is probably due to the difference in typical daily activity patterns, although differences are diminishing. There is no evidence to suggest differences in muscle quality between men and women.

OVERTRAINING

It is essential that coaches and trainers exercise caution in writing training programs for entire teams without considering and monitoring the program of each individual athlete.

A basic principle of training is to *stress* or overload the physiologic system so the body will respond with increased strength or endurance. Because of this and other stresses placed on athletes, there is a risk of overtraining, which can lead to staleness and exhaustion. When planning a training program, the coach needs to consider the total stress the athlete is experiencing (work, school, social interactions, and training load) and be creative in his/her approach to allow the athlete to improve without becoming exhausted. Too much training stress can have a negative effect on the athlete leading to pain and fatigue. If the overall stress becomes too great, the athlete may experience boredom, loss of sleep, and sometimes stress between coaches and players. Some of the negative symptoms associated with staleness are:

1. increased resting and exercise heart rate
2. decreased appetite
3. decreased body weight
4. loss of sleep
5. decreased sex drive
6. generalized body aches and pains
7. decreased performance
8. personal problems
9. illness and injury
10. loss of motivation

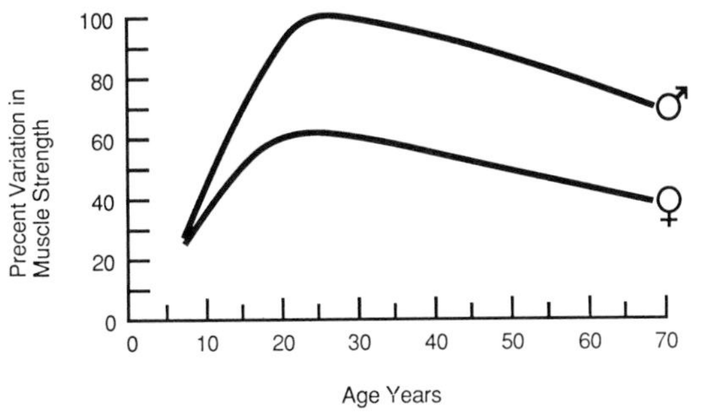

Fig. 7–11. Strength decreases with age. (From Asmussen, E.: Growth in muscle strength and power. *In* Physical Activity: Human Growth and Development. Edited by G.L. Rarick. Courtesy of Academic Press, 1973, p. 60.)

DETRAINING

Most athletes fear that muscular strength and endurance gained through training will be lost after a period of rest, especially once the competitive season is over. A few days of rest or reduction in training has actually been shown to be beneficial rather than harmful to one's state of training. In fact, periodization takes this into account with tapering techniques. Active rest periods are also recommended rather than complete inactivity. At some point in time, complete inactivity will result in deterioration of physical condition and performance.

Current research confirms the decrement in muscular strength and endurance following periods of complete inactivity. The strength losses are relatively slow during the first several months following cessation of training. Following a 12-week strength training program, a 1-year detraining period resulted in a 45% loss of the strength gains. This information is different from the losses of strength and muscle mass due to complete immobilization of a limb (such as with casting). The difference lies in the fact that although a muscle group is not being trained formally, regular daily activity is enough to retain some of the previously gained strength. The optimum stimulus for maintenance of strength during off season is probably about one workout per week.

POWER

A discussion of strength would be incomplete without relating it to *Power*, the ability to apply force rapidly. Maximal power results from the optimal combination of maximal force being applied as rapidly as possible. If two individuals lift a 200-pound weight through a 3-foot range of motion, both accomplish the same amount of work, but if the first individual takes 2 seconds to move this weight and the second could do it in 1 second, the amount of power is quite different. Likewise if two individuals were to move at the same speed, but one worked against twice the resistance as the other, he would demonstrate twice as much power. The formula for power is:

$$\text{Power} = \text{Force (strength)} \times \text{Velocity (speed)}$$

or:

$$\text{Power} = \frac{\text{Force} \times \text{Distance}}{\text{Time}} \text{ or } \frac{\text{Work}}{\text{Time}}$$

Significance of Power

Maximal power is demonstrated in athletic performances by the ability to project an object or one's body through space. Power produces momentum, which is the striking force when contact is made. Thus power has many applications in a variety of athletic events. In projecting an object, the object might be thrown, kicked or struck, and the power is determined by the combination of force and speed. For example, if a baseball batter can apply more force to the bat at a faster rate than usual, the bat will accelerate faster and will have greater velocity (and momentum) when it strikes the ball. If the batter can be strengthened to handle a heavier bat and maintain or increase swing speed, he will increase the momentum of the bat (since mass of the bat is an element of momentum). A player who is lacking in force will not be able to accelerate a heavy bat effectively.

A shot putter probably depends as much on power for success as any other athlete. If the angle of projection is constant, then the distance of the flight is related to the velocity at the moment of release. The prime objective of the shot putter is to increase initial speed of the shot. This is accomplished by applying maximal force at maximal speed over a maximal distance. The distance of force application is relatively constant for the shot putter so the amount of force applied and speed are fundamental to success.

Sprint running is dependent largely upon power because it involves a series of body projections, alternating from the two legs. The rate of these projections is dependent upon the combination of the force and speed of muscle contractions. Power plays an even more prominent role in sprinting during the acceleration phase than during the remainder of the sprint. With consideration of the prevalence of sprinting, acceleration, throwing, kicking, and impact in athletic performances, the significance of power becomes apparent.

Even though power always involves a combination of the components strength (force) and speed (time), different kinds of performances often require more emphasis on one component than on the other. Power events involving light resistance place emphasis on speed, whereas performances utilizing heavy resistances depend more on strength. Consider the continuum of throwing events and the relative importance of speed and strength:

speed				strength
baseball pitch	javelin throw	discus throw	16 lb shot	35 lb weight

So in power performances there are those which depend greatly upon speed and those that depend greatly on force. Between the two extremes there are numerous performances that require varying amounts of emphasis on each component. It is easy to see that training must be very specific and must emphasize the factor that is most important to be successful.

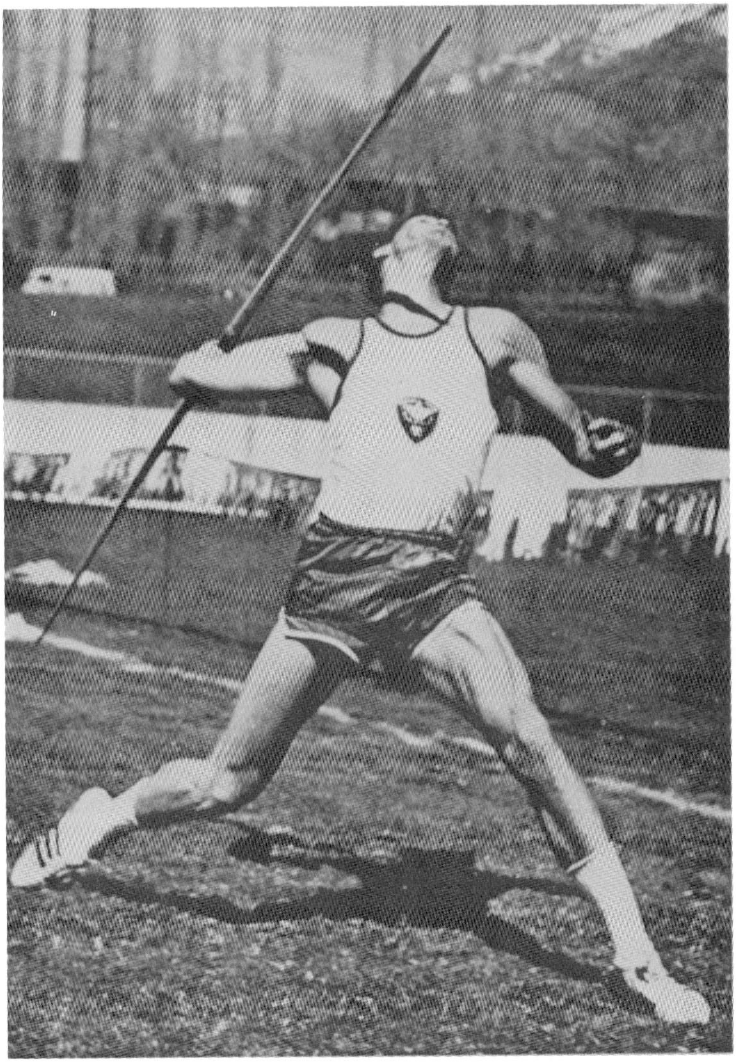

Fig. 7–12. Throwing the javelin requires power.

Increasing Power

Obviously, in order to increase power one would need to increase either the strength or speed of muscular contraction, or both. Usually the best approach for increasing power is to increase strength. Practical experience and observation support the claim that performance in many power events has been vastly improved during the past couple of decades as a result of the emphasis placed on strength training. Where two decades ago no one had thrown the shot past 60 feet, it is now a common practice, and 70 feet has been exceeded several times. Sprinting speed has increased with new records being set annually. There has been a dramatic increase in the number and type of power moves in both men's and women's gymnastics. Professional figure skating has a new image with aesthetic beauty combined with strength. Although events like speed skating and indoor track bicycle racing entail an aerobic component, there is a great deal of power involved. Realistically, an athlete cannot be expected to compete favorably in explosive events unless his training program involves effective strength-improvement procedures.

The key to improving the speed component of power is to increase the contractile speed of the muscles involved. Interestingly enough, this is accomplished best by increasing the strength of the muscle. Other ways to increase the speed component of power is to use warm-up, improve coordination of muscles, and improve efficiency of movement.

Warm-up. Hill found that speed of contraction can be increased approximately 20% by raising body temperature 2°C, and speed of contraction is diminished significantly by reduction in temperature of 10°C. The truth of this claim lacks sufficient evidence, but it is clearly established that increased body temperature does improve rate of contraction to some degree. Apparently, such increases are due to decreased viscosity in the muscles and the increased speed of chemical reactions (Q-10 effect).

Coordination. Improved coordination of muscles (skill) can increase speed of movement because as the several mover muscles become better coordinated, they can cooperatively overcome external resistance with greater speed. Increasing one's skill level also decreases the relative effort of the event, everything else remaining constant. This is especially true for athletes training in different sports in the off season. Athletes, for example, who train in the off season by swimming or aerobic dance are intially uncoordinated, and even short periods of exertion are difficult. As skill and coordination improves, the effort required decreases even though strength or speed has not changed. Coordination is enhanced through practice.

Muscle Efficiency. The efficiency of muscle contraction can be increased by training, and this may result in increased contractile speed. If fatty tissue within a muscle is eliminated and viscosity is reduced, the result is greater efficiency and faster contraction. Increased flexibility in antagonistic muscles will cause less resistance to movement resulting in greater speed.

SELECTED READINGS

1. Allen, T.E., Byrd, R.J., and Smith, D.P.: Hemodynamic consequences of circuit weight training. Res. Q. *47*(3):329–306, 1976.
2. Asmussen, E.: The neuromuscular system and exercise. In *Exercise Physiology.* N.H. Balls (Ed.). New York: Academic Press, 1968, p. 39.
3. Asmussen, E. and Mazin, B.: A central nervous component in local muscular fatigue. Europ. J. Appl. Physiol. *38*:9–15, 1978.
4. Asmussen, E. and Mazin, B.: Recuperation after muscular fatigue by "diverting activities." Europ. J. Appl. Physiol. *38*:1–7, 1978.
5. Baldwin, K.M., Winder, W.W., Terjung, R.L., et al.: Glycolytic enzymes in different types of skeletal muscle: Adaptation to exercise. Am. J. Physiol. *225*:962–966, 1973.
6. Ball, J.R., Rich, G.Q., and Wallis, E.L.: Effects of isometric training on vertical jumping. Res. Q. *35*:231, 1964.
7. Belka, D.: Comparison of dynamic, static, and combination training on dominant wrist flexor muscles. Res. Q. *39*:244–250, 1968.
8. Berger, R.: Comparative effects of three weight training programs. Res. Q. *34*:396–398, 1963.
9. Berger, R.: Comparison between static training and various dynamic training programs. Res. Q. *34*:131–135, 1963.
10. Berger, R.: Effect of varied weight training programs on strength. Res. Q. *38*:168–181, 1962.
11. Berger, R.: Optimum repetitions for the development of strength. Res. Q. *33*:334–338, 1962.
12. Berger, R.A.: Comparison of static and dynamic strength increases. Res. Q. *33*:329, 1962.
13. Berger, R.A.: Effect of varied weight training programs on strength. Res. Q. *33*:168, 1962.
14. Berger, R.A.: Leg extension at three different angles. Res. Q. *37*:560, 1966.
15. Bompa, T.: *Theory and Methodology of Training.* Kendau/Hunt, 1983.
16. Clark, D. and Stull, G.: Endurance training as a determinant of strength and fatigability. Res. Q. *41*:19–26, 1970.
17. Clark, H. (ed.): *Development of Muscular Strength and Endurance.* Phys Fit Res Digest. Series 4, No. 1, Jan., 1974.
18. Coleman, A.E.: Effect of unilateral isometric and isotonic contractions on the strength of the contralateral limb. Res. Q. *40*:490, 1969.
19. Councilman, J.E.: The importance of speed in exercise. Athletic Journal, May 1976, pp. 72–75.
20. DeLateur, B., Lehmann, J., and Fordyce, W.: A test of the DeLorme axiom. Arch. Phys. Med. Rehab. *49*:245–248, 1968.
21. DeLateur, B., et al.: Comparison of effectiveness of isokinetic and isotonic exercise in quadriceps strengthening. Arch. Phys. Med. Rehabil., Feb. 1972, pp. 60–64.
22. DeLorme, T., and Wilkins, A.L.: Progressive Resistance Exercise. New York: Appleton-Century-Crofts, 1951.
23. Duchateau, J., and Hainaut, K.: Isometric or dynamic training, differential effects of mechanical properties of a human muscle. J. Appl. Physiol. Respirat. Environ. Exercise Physiol. *56*(2), 296–301, 1984.
24. Fitts, R.H., and Holloszy, J.O.: Lactate and contractile force in frog muscle during development of fatigue and recovery. Am. J. Physiol. *231*(2):430–433, 1976.
25. Fletch, S.J., and Kraemer, W.J.: Resistance training: basic principles. Physician Sports Med. *16*(3):160–171, 1988.
26. Fletch, S.J., and Kraemer, W.J.: Resistance training: physiological responses and adaptations. Physician Sports Med. *16*(4):108–124, 1988.

27. Freeman, W.H.: Peak When It Counts. Tafnews Press, 1989.
28. Fuchs, F., Reddy, V., and Briggs, F.N.: The interaction of cations with the calcium binding site of troponin. Biochim. Biophys. Acta. *221*:407–409, 1970.
29. Gardner, G.: Specificity of strength changes of the exercised and nonexercised limb following isometric training. Res. Q. *34*:98–101, 1963.
30. Gardner, H.W.: Specificity of strength changes of the exercised and non-exercised limb following isometric training. Res. Q. *34*:98, 1963.
31. Gettman, L.R., Ayres, J.J., Pollock, M.L., et al.: The effect of circuit weight training on strength, cardiorespiratory function, and body composition of adult men. Med. Sci. Sports *10*(3):171–176, 1978.
32. Gonyea, W.J., Sale, D.G., Gonyea, F.B., et al.: Exercise induced increases in muscle fiber number. Eur. J. Appl. Physiol. *55*:137–141, 1986.
33. Grose, J.E.: Depression of muscle fatigue curves by heat and cold. Res. Q. *29*:19, 1958.
34. Hakkinen, K., and Komi, P.V.: Alterations of mechanical characteristics of human skeletal muscle during strength training. Eur. J. Appl. Physiol. *50*:161–172, 1983.
35. Hettinger, T.: Physiology of Strength. Springfield, Charles C Thomas, 1961.
36. Hettinger, T., and Muller, E.A.: Muskelleistung and Muskeltraining. Arbeitsphysiologie *15*:111, 1953.
37. Hettinger, T., and Muller, E.A.: Die Trainierbarkeit der Muskulatur. Arbeitsphysiologie *16*:90, 1955.
38. Hettinger, T., and Muller, E.: Muskelleistung und Muskeltraining. Arbeitsphysiol. *15*:11–126, 1953.
39. Hellebrandt, F.A.: Cross education: Ipsilateral and contralateral effects of unimanual training. J. Appl. Physiol. *4*:136, 1951.
40. Hellebrandt, F.A., Houtz, S.J., and Kirkorian, A.M.: Influence of bimanual exercise on unilateral work capacity. J. Appl. Physiol. *2*:446, 1950.
41. Hellebrandt, F.A., Parrish, A.M., and Houtz, S.J.: Cross education: The influence of unilateral exercise on the contralateral limb. Arch. Phys. Med. *78*:76, 1947.
42. Hickson, R.C.: Interference of strength development by simultaneously training for strength and endurance. Eur. J. Appl. Physiol. *45*:255–262, 1980.
43. Hill, A.V.: The mechanics of voluntary muscle. Lancet *261*:947, 1951.
44. Jensen, C.R.: The significance of strength in athletic performance. Coach and Athlete, December 1965, p. 22.
45. Johnson, B.L.: Eccentric vs concentric muscle training for strength development. Med. Sci. Sports *4*(2):111–115, 1972.
46. Johnson, B.L., et al.: A comparison of concentric and eccentric muscle training. Med. Sci. Sports *8*:35–38, 1976.
47. Jokl, E.: Physiology of Exercise. Springfield, Ill.: Charles C Thomas, 1964.
48. Kanehisa, H., and Miyashita, M.: Specificity of velocity in strength training. Eur. J. Appl. Physiol. *52*:104–106, 1983.
49. Karlsson, J., and Saltin, B.: Lactate, ATP, and CP in working muscle during exhaustive exercise in man. J. Appl. Physiol. *29*(5):598–602, 1970.
50. Karlsson, J., and Saltin, B.: Oxygen deficit and muscle metabolites in intermittent exercise. Acta. Physiol. Scand. *32*:115–122, 1982.
51. Klein, K.K.: Muscular strength in the knee. The Physician and Sports Medicine, December 1974, p. 29.
52. Komi, P.V., and Tesch, P.: Emg frequency spectrum, muscle structure and fatigue during dynamic contractions in man. Europ. J. Appl. Physiol. *42*:41–50, 1979.
53. Lesmes, G.R., Costill, D.L. Coyle, E.F., et al.: Muscle strength and power changes during maximal isokinetic training. Med. Sci. Sports *10*(4):266–269, 1976.
54. Lindh, M.: Increase of muscle strength from isometric quadriceps exercises at different knee angles. Scand. J. Rehab. Med. *11*:33–36, 1979.
55. Linford, A.G., and Rarick, L.: The effect of knee angle on the measurement of leg strength of college males. Res. Q. *39*:582, 1968.
56. McGlynn, G.H.: A re-evaluation of isometric strength training. J. Sports Med., December 1972, pp. 258, 260.
57. Moffroid, M., et al.: A study of isokinetic exercise. Phys. Ther. *49*:735, 1966.
58. Moffroid, M.T., and Whipple, R.H.: Specificity of speed and exercise. J. Am. Phys. Ther. Assoc. *50*:1699–1704, 1970.
59. Nakamura, Y., and Schwartz, S.: The influence of hydrogen ion concentration on calcium binding and release by skeletal muscle sarcoplasmic reticulum. J. Gen. Physiol. *59*:22–32, 1972.
60. Pauletto, B.: Sets and repetitions. NSCA Journal *7*(6):67–69, 1985.
61. Pauletto, B.: Intensity. NSCA Journal *8*(1):33–37, 1986.
62. Pauletto, B: Rest and recuperation. NSCA Journal *8*(3):52–53, 1986.
63. Pauletto, B.: Choice and order of exercises. NSCA Journal *8*(2):71–73, 1986.
64. Pauletto, B.: Periodization. NSCA Journal *8*(4):30–31, 1986.
65. Pipes, T.B., and Wilmore, J.: Isokinetic versus isotonic strength training in adult men. Athletic Journal, June 1976, pp. 26–29.
66. Rasch, P.J.: The present status of negative (eccentric) exercise. Am. Correct. Ther. J., May-June 1974, p. 77.
67. Rasch, P.J., and Morehouse, L.E.: Effect of static and dynamic exercises on muscular strength and hypertrophy. J. Appl. Physiol. *11*:29, 1957.
68. Rich, G.Q., Ball, J.R., and Wallis, E.L.: Effects of isometric training on strength and transfer of effect to untrained antagonists. J. Sports Med. Phys. Fitness *4*:217, 1964.
69. Royce, J.: Isometric fatigue curves in human muscle with normal and occluded circulation. Res. Q. *29*:204, 1958.
70. Shepherd, G.R.: A comparison of the effects of isotonic, isokinetic and negative resistance strength training programs. Doctoral dissertation. Provo: Brigham Young University, 1975.
71. Sorenson, M.B.: The Effects of Conventional and High-repetition Weight-training Programs on Strength and Cardiovascular Endurance. Unpublished doctoral dissertation. Provo: Brigham Young University, 1974.
72. Stephans, J., and Taylor, A.: Fatigue of maintained voluntary muscle contraction in man. J. Physiol. (London) *220*:1–18, 1972.
73. Stone, M.H., O'Bryant, H., and Garhammer, J.: A hypothetical model for strength training. J. Sports Med. *21*:342–351, 1981.
74. Stull, G., and Clark, D.: High-resistance, low repe-

tition training as a determiner of strength and fatigability. Res. Q. *41*:189–193, 1970.
75. Tesch, P., Sjodon, B., Thorstensson, A., et al.: Muscle fatigue and its relation to lactate accumulation and LDH activity in man. Acta. Physiol. Scand. *103*:413–420, 1978.
76. Thistle, H.G., et al.: Isokinetic contraction: A new concept of resistive exercise. Arch. Phys. Med. Rehabil., *48*:279, 1966.
77. Trivedi, B., and Danforth, W.H.: Effect of pH on the kinetics of frog muscle phosphofructokinase. J. Biol. Chem. *241*:4110–4112, 1966.
78. Van Oteghen, S.L.: Two speeds of isokinetic exercise as related to the vertical jump performance of women. Res. Q. *46*:78–84, 1975.
79. Wilmore, J.H., Parr, R.B., Girandola, R.N., et al.: Physiological alterations consequent to circuit training. Med. Sci. Sports *10*(2):79–84, 1978.
80. Whithers, R.: Effect of varied weight training loads on the strength university freshman. Res. Q. *41*:110–114, 1970.

8

Endurance and the Energy Systems

Three sources of energy for muscular activity have been mentioned and discussed in previous chapters. The first of these is the ATP and PC found in the cell. This is called the alactacid system and can support intense work only for 10 to 15 seconds before it is used up. The second major source of energy is that produced by the glycolytic pathway. This is often referred to as the lactacid system, because lactic acid is produced as a by-product when it is used for energy production. Energy from this source can support intense work only for 45 to 60 seconds. The third source of energy comes from the oxidative pathways in the cell and yields water and carbon dioxide as normal by-products. Of course, this system can support low levels of work almost indefinitely, and moderate levels for long periods. This is the most efficient of the energy systems, and is able to produce ATP from food products at an efficiency of about 50%.

Each of these systems can be trained to become more effective in the production of energy, and should be trained either alone or together for all athletic events. The purpose of this chapter is to discuss the techniques of training these energy systems and the principles involved in using these techniques.

SPECIFIC TRAINING GUIDELINES

Although few athletic events use a single system, it might be helpful to discuss first how each system can be trained with minimal involvement of other systems.

Alactacid System (ATP-CP)

The alactacid system can be improved best by short (10 seconds or so) bouts of high-intensity work, followed by rest periods of at least the same duration or preferably longer. High-intensity work bouts of 10 seconds, followed by 10-second rest periods raised blood lactate only from 10 mg/1 mmole/l of blood to a little over 2 mmole/l after 30 minutes of work. Fifteen-sec work bouts followed by 30 seconds of rest yielded an increase in lactate of less than 2 mmole/l of blood. Athletes trained with short, high-intensity sprint training increase their power potential dramatically as measured by a test such as the Margaria-Kalamen power test. This would indicate that specific training of this system is accomplished easily. This increase in power is a result of increased levels of ATP-CP in the muscle. This increase has been reported at 25% to 40%.

Lactacid System

The best way to train the lactacid system is to use longer bouts (45 to 60 sec) of high-intensity work, followed by recovery periods at least as long as the work period or longer. Four or five such work bouts increase the lactic acid levels to maximal values (20 mmoles/liter) and are strenuous for the subject. There is no doubt that training of this type increases the athlete's ability to develop high blood lactate levels. The enzymes of glycolysis also are increased significantly.

Oxidative or Aerobic System

The best way to train the oxidative system *only* would be to work at moderate levels of intensity for long periods of time.

The following "rules" have been proven through research to yield changes in aerobic conditioning (as measured by VO_2max changes):

1. *Type.* Choose activities involving large muscle groups of the body in a rhythmic, continuous way. Jogging, walking, rope jumping, swimming, and bicycling are excellent activities which meet these criteria.

2. *Intensity.* The intensity should be hard enough to cause the heart rate (HR) to increase between 65 and 90% of maximum. This is the point at which stroke volume is maximal and yields a volume overload on the myocardium. Karvonen found the minimal level of intensity to be 60% of the difference between resting HR and maximal HR, added to the resting HR. Within limits, the higher the intensity, the better is the effect. Of course, as stress levels increase, the involvement of the anaerobic systems will also increase.

3. *Duration.* The workout must be from 15 to 60 minutes duration at the proper intensity. Most errors in aerobic conditioning involve the violation of the duration principle. Short exercise bouts (4 or 5 min.) followed by rest periods long enough to allow the heart rate to decrease below the minimal training intensity are not as effective for training the aerobic system as is continuous exercise at the proper duration.

4. *Frequency.* Workouts should be scheduled on a daily basis, if possible, for maximal effect. However, a frequency of three times a week or every other day will be effective.

It should be emphasized that aerobic conditioning can be accomplished using interval training techniques (see section on interval training in this chapter for more information).

These aforementioned increase the $\dot{V}O_2$ max, cardiac output, and stroke volume of the heart, and are associated with increased running speed, decreased submaximal and resting heart rates, and the number of mitochondria and the concentration of oxidative enzymes in the mitochondria of the muscle involved in the exercise.

SELECTION OF THE ENERGY SYSTEM

Most athletic events involve two, and sometimes all, energy systems. However, there is always a predominant system which must receive the most emphasis. How can you tell which system requires the most emphasis? Table 8–1 illustrates the relationship between different track events and the primary energy systems involved. From this table, it is apparent that an athlete who is training to run the mile should devote 20% of his program to speed (alactacid), 55% to lactacid programs, and 25% to aerobic work. Notice that the time of each performance also is included. This allows the coach or athlete to use this information for other events. For example, a swimming event lasting 4 to 5 minutes would require approximately the same training emphasis as the mile run, which also lasts 4 to 5 minutes. Of course, the training stimulus would vary depending on the activity involved. *The point is that the energy source to be emphasized is time-dependent.* This relationship is more graphically shown in Figure 8–1, which shows the total contribution of anaerobic energy (both alactacid and lactacid) and aerobic energy as related to time of the activity.

Using the information in Table 8–1, Mathews and Fox have developed a table showing their idea of the energy requirements of various activities (Table 8–2). It is difficult to assess the contribution of the various energy systems in a sport such as football, however, because of several complicating factors. For instance, the energy needs for a lineman may differ significantly from those of a split end. It also is difficult to assess the contribution of the aerobic system in games that last for several hours. An increased emphasis on aerobic conditioning may be extremely valuable during the last quarter of a contest, during which the high aerobic capacity would result in a more rapid payoff of oxygen debt and allow the player to perform at his early game level of skill.

Table 8–1. Percentage of Training Time Spent in Developing the Energy Sources for Various Track Events

Event	*Performance Time*	*(alactacid) Speed %*	*Aerobic Capacity %*	*Anaerobic Capacity %*
Marathon	135:00 to 180:00	5	90	5
6 mile	30:00 to 50:00	5	80	15
3 mile	15:00 to 25:00	10	70	20
2 mile	10:00 to 16:00	20	40	40
1 mile	4:00 to 6:00	20	25	55
880 yards	2:00 to 3:00	30	5	65
440 yards	1:00 to 1:30	80	3	15
220 yards	0:22 to 0:35	95	3	2
110 yards	0:10 to 0:15	95	2	3

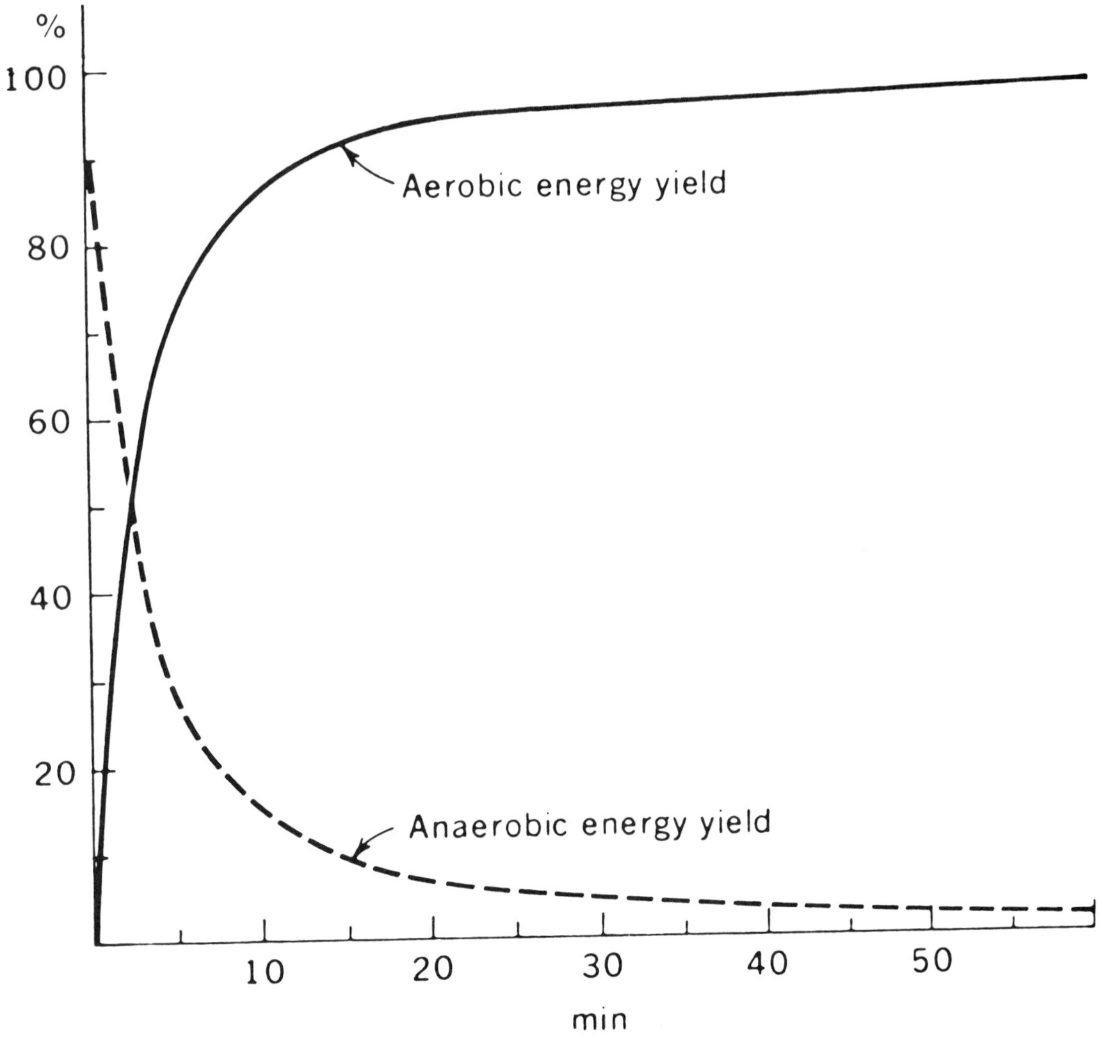

Fig. 8–1. Relative contribution in percentage of total energy yield from aerobic and anaerobic processes, respectively, during maximal efforts of up to 60 min. duration for an individual with high maximal power for both processes. Note that a 2-mi. maximal effort hits the 50% mark, meaning that both processes are equally important for success. (From Astrand, P.O., and Rodahl, K. *Textbook of Work Physiology: Physiological Basis of Exercises,* 2nd Ed. Courtesy of McGraw Hill, 1986.)

Table 8–2. Various Sports and Their Predominant Energy System (S)

	% Emphasis According to Energy Systems		
Sports or Sport Activity	*ATP-PC and LA*	*LA-O_2*	*O_2*
1. Baseball	80	20	—
2. Basketball	85	15	—
3. Fencing	90	10	—
4. Field Hockey	60	20	20
5. Football	90	10	—
6. Golf	95	5	—
7. Gymnastics	90	10	—
8. Ice Hockey			
a. forewards, defense	80	20	—
b. goalie	95	5	—
9. Lacrosse			
a. goalie, defense, attack men	80	20	—
b. midfielders, man-down	60	20	20
10. Rowing	20	30	50
11. Skiing			
a. slalom, jumping, downhill	80	20	—
b. cross-country	—	5	95
c. pleasure skiing	34	33	33
12. Soccer			
a. goalie, wings, strikers	80	20	—
b. halfbacks, or link men	60	20	20
13. Swimming and diving			
a. 50 yds., diving	98	2	—
b. 100 yds.	80	15	5
c. 200 yds.	30	65	5
d. 400, 500 yds.	20	40	40
e. 1500, 1650 yds.	10	20	70
14. Tennis	70	20	10
15. Track and field			
a. 100, 220 yds.	98	2	—
b. field events	90	10	—
c. 440 yds.	80	15	5
d. 880 yds.	30	65	5
e. 1 mile	20	55	25
f. 2 miles	20	40	40
g. 3 miles	10	20	70
h. 6 miles	5	15	80
i. marathon	—	5	95
16. Volleyball	90	10	—
17. Wrestling	90	10	—

Modified from Mathews, K.D., and Fox, E.L.: *The Physiological Basis of Physical Education and Athletics.* Philadelphia: W.B. Saunders Co., 1976.

TRAINING PROGRAMS

There is no question that the best approach to training athletes in almost any activity involves some type of *interval training* program. Interval training allows the athlete to work at the proper intensities to train any energy system, and yet do enough total work to receive a proper training effect without undue fatigue. Consider an example of an offensive lineman running a single 60 second 440 yard run. Compare this to the same lineman running a series of 6 to 10 second intervals at maximum speed, with a short rest between each interval. Although the amount of work is similar in each case, the amount of fatigue would be much less following the interval training and the energy system involvement would be quite different. In the intermittent sprints, the contribution of the ATP-CP system is greater because the time is so short that most of the energy needs can be met by the ATP-PC stores, and they can be restored during the rest periods. In the 440, the lactic acid (LA) system is maximally utilized, because the ATP-CP stores are used in the first 10 seconds or so and the body must rely more on energy from the glycolytic pathway to complete the run. Although there are events where interval training may not be the best method of training, it is so useful in so many events, that its use will be discussed in some detail in this section.

Application of overload to interval training programs is accomplished by manipulating 4 important variables:

1. The intensity and duration of the work interval.
2. The number of repetitions and sets in each workout.
3. The duration and activity of the relief interval.
4. The frequency of weekly training sessions.

The Intensity and Duration of the Work Interval

It is this variable that allows the coach or athlete to train the proper energy system. For training the ATP-PC system, the work interval would be from 10 to 20 seconds at high intensities; for the LA system, from 20 seconds to about 1:30 seconds at moderate intensities; for aerobic training, from 1:30 to as long as desired at lower intensities. For many sports, distance is used because of convenience. For instance, instead of swimming for some specific time, a sprint swimmer would be wiser to swim a certain number of lengths of the pool that relates to the desired time for the specific energy system being trained, so that he/she ends up at one end or the other of the pool at the end of the work interval. The same rule may apply to track. It would be best to use some natural distance (that takes the proper time for the energy system being trained) on the track such as 220, 440, etc., rather than just a time.

The most difficult problem related to this variable is determining the proper intensity of exercise. There are several alternatives that can be used:

1. Heart rate. The heart rate can be counted for 6 seconds (then multiply by 10 for beats per minute) immediately after the interval to determine a rough idea of the heart rate response during the training interval. For short high intensity intervals, the heart rate will be close to maximum (and maximum heart rate can be estimated by subtracting age from 220 or by counting the heart rate for 15 seconds immediately following an all-out 400 meter run). For moderate intervals, heart rate will be between 90 to 95% maximum (about 190 for young athletes). The heart rate for aerobic intervals will depend on the length of the interval. However, they will of necessity be lower (usually between 85 to 90%), especially if the interval is 5 to 10 minutes or longer.

2. Subjective feeling of athlete. If an interval program is set up that is too demanding, the athlete will be unable to accomplish it. If it demands too little, more repetitions than were assigned can be accomplished. Based on this response, the coach can alter the program to fit the athlete's needs.

3. Best-time adjustment. The best program for proper interval times for runners was published in the book *Computerized Running Training Programs,* by Gardner and Purdy. This book contained computerized training tables for various levels of performance. The first step was to "score" an athlete in his event and enter the "pacing" tables based on that score. The pacing tables showed various combinations of repetitions and times, as well as the recommended rest interval based on the person's ability to perform. The times were used to pace the athlete so that he could complete the amount of work desired, rather than as a means of increasing the speed of each interval. A similar, though not as scientific, procedure can be used by adding time to the athlete's best time for various distances (see Table 8–3).

The Number of Repetitions and Number of Sets

The number of repetitions depends on the length of the work interval; the shorter the interval, the more of them that must be done. For running training, the total mileage should be about 1.5 to 2.0 miles (about 1/4th of this for swimming). Of course, this can be divided up into *sets,* emphasizing different energy systems. However, the total workout cannot be too difficult or the athlete could get fatigued to the point where recovery could not occur before the next workout and overtraining would result. *Sets* are a group of work and relief intervals, used to allow additional rest between groups of work and relief intervals.

Table 8–3. Guidelines for Determining a Sufficient Work Rate for Running and Swimming ITP's

Training Distance (yards)		
Run	*Swim*	*Work Rate*
55	15	1½ seconds slower than best times from moving starts
110	25	3 seconds slower than best times from moving starts
220	55	5 seconds slower than best times from moving starts
440	110	1 to 4 seconds faster than average 440 (run) or 110 (swim) than best times in mile (run) or 440 (swim)
660–1320	165–330	3 to 4 seconds slower than average 440 (run) or 110 (swim) than best times in mile (run) or 440 (swim)

Fox & Mathews, '74—Int. Training

This added rest allows higher intensity to occur in the work intervals and better overall training results.

For many athletic events, training of energy systems can be done along with teaching certain skills. For example, basketball coaches use fast-break drills to train the ATP-PC system as well as teach ball handling skills. Receivers in football run patterns during practice to train energy systems and learn receiving skills. This approach makes sense in terms of the limited time available to train athletes and teach proper skills.

The Relief Interval

The time of the relief interval between each work interval is determined by how long it takes for the heart rate to return to about 150 beats per minute (partial recovery). Between sets, the time is increased until the heart rate is about 120 beats per minute (use 1 beat less per year for older athletes). For short, high intensity work intervals, the relief interval may be 2 or 3 times as long as the work interval. For longer, more moderate intensity work intervals, the relief interval may be equal to or less than the work interval. After checking heart rate during relief intervals, the time of the interval can be determined and heart rate checks would no longer be necessary except on an occasional basis.

The type of activity during the relief interval depends on the energy system being trained. Use rest (walking, light movement) for relief when training the ATP-PC system to allow the ATP-PC stores to be re-established. For LA, use mild work (rapid walking or jogging) to speed up the removal of lactate. Rest relief for aerobic conditioning would probably be best so that LA is prevented from forming.

Frequency

Typically, athletes train on a daily basis (5 to 7 days/week). However, non athletes can get a good training effect with only 3 to 4 days/week. Frequency might be modified somewhat during the competitive season to avoid staleness.

For more detailed information on interval training, see the excellent book by Fox and Mathews (1974) Interval Training, W.B. Saunders.

Running Programs Using Interval Training Principles

It is easy to use time-energy relationships to train runners. Table 8–4 lists various types of training programs involving speed training, aerobic training, and anaerobic training. A coach or an athlete can refer to Table 8–1 for the type of program needed in training for his event, then to Table 8–4 for a description of the training program to be used. For example, a 2-miler should use a training program with 20% of the emphasis on speed, 40% on aerobic capacity, and 40% on the lactacid system. He would then attempt to match these percentages to a training program listed in Table 8–4. Speed play, or fartlek training, is the type of training most nearly matched to the training requirements of a 2-miler, but repetition running could be used with good results.

The different types of training listed in Table 8–4 are described below:

Repetitions of sprints involve the repetition of short sprints as a means of preparation for competitive running. Since sprinting means running at absolute maximal speed, there is

Table 8–4. Endurance Development Programs Specifying Type of Training

Types of Training	*Speed* %	*Aerobic Endurance* %	*Anaerobic Endurance* %
Repetitions of sprints	90	4	6
Continuous slow running	2	93	5
Continuous fast running	2	90	8
Slow interval	10	60	30
Fast interval	30	20	50
Repetition running	10	40	50
Speed play (fartlek)	20	40	40
Interval sprinting	20	70	10
Acceleration sprinting	90	5	5
Hollow sprints	85	5	10

not an "easy sprint." The effect of sprinting as a means of training is the development of speed and muscular strength.

Continuous slow running refers to running long distances at relatively slow speeds. The distances covered in this type of training should be related to the racing event. For example, a miler might run five times his racing distance or more. The heart rate should be between 80 and 90% maximum during this type of training, and the speed depends upon the ability of the athlete.

Continuous fast running differs from continuous slow running in terms of speed. Because the pace is faster, fatigue is encountered sooner. This training develops aerobic endurance. It represents a form of effort that seeks gradually to condition the organism to tolerate the stress encountered in running at faster and faster speeds.

Slow interval develops aerobic endurance. The speed is faster than in continuous fast-running training, thus adapting the athlete to running at a more intense effort. In this type of formal fast-slow running, the heart beats at the rate of approximately 180 beats per minute or more during the heavy work phase.

Fast interval develops anaerobic endurance or speed endurance. It is used after a background of aerobic or general endurance has been established. The heart should beat at maximal or near-maximal rate during the work phase. It develops the ability of the runner to withstand fatigue in the absence of an adequate oxygen supply.

Repetition running differs from interval training in terms of the length of the fast run and the degree of recovery following each fast effort. It involves repetitions of comparatively longer distances with relatively complete recovery (usually by walking) after each effort. Repetition running is usually concerned with repetitions of distances such as 880 yards to 2 miles with relatively complete recovery between, during which time the heart rate falls below 120 beats/minute. Conversely, interval training includes repetitions of shorter distances (ordinarily 110 to 440 yards) with less than complete recovery after each by jogging a distance equal to the fast run in a time period two to three times as long as required to complete the fast run.

Speed play is a form of training featuring informal fast-slow running, as opposed to the formal fast-slow running in interval training. It involves running preferably, but not necessarily, over natural surfaces such as golf courses, grass, or trails through woods, with emphasis on fast running. Fast and slow interval running, repetition running, sprinting, walking, and continuous fast-running training are informally combined in speed play. This type of training is also known as fartlek training.

Interval sprinting is a method of training whereby an athlete alternately sprints about 50 yards and jogs 10 yards for distances up to 3 miles. After the first few sprints, fatigue tends to inhibit the athlete from running at his absolute top speed. Similarly, fatigue causes the athlete to slow his recovery jogging to a slow rate.

Acceleration sprinting is the gradual acceleration from jogging to striding to sprinting. For example, an athlete may jog 25 yards, stride 50 yards, and sprint 50 yards, followed by 50 yards of walking, then repeat the procedure several times. This type of training emphasizes both speed and endurance, provided enough repetitions are performed to cause endurance overload.

Hollow sprints are two sprints joined by a "hollow" period of recovery jogging. Examples include sprint 50, jog 50, sprint 50, and walk 50 yards for recovery prior to the next repetition; sprint 110, jog 110, sprint 110, and walk 110 yards before the next repetition; sprint 220, jog 220, and walk 220 yards before repeating.

Many of the programs mentioned here are a type of *interval training* since any interval-training program consists of a series of work bouts with a short rest interval between bouts. Astrand and Rodahl reported that a work load that could be tolerated continuously for only 9 minutes could be carried on for an hour when done intermittently. This means that much more total work can be accomplished before fatigue when interval training is used than when continuous training is used.

In order for an interval-training program to continue to be effective over a period of time, the intensity must be increased as endurance is gained so that overload may continue to be applied. In other words, as an athlete becomes better conditioned, he must do more work during each of the training periods to cause additional endurance gains.

It should be emphasized that aerobic conditioning can be accomplished using interval training procedures which have been selected primarily to train other systems (alactacid; lactacid). For example, you desire to develop the aerobic capacity of a group of basketball players while emphasizing the anaerobic energy sources, and at the same time have them practice the skills involved in basketball. You can do this easily by having the players perform a series of high-intensity drills (such as fast-break drills), and still keep their heart rates between 120 and 150 beats per minute during the rest period by having them jog back to their starting positions on the basketball floor. You must force the intensity of the drill during the fast-break portion and never allow the heart rate to return to normal during the recovery portion, for a total period of 15 to 20 minutes. You can go from drill to drill, but you must not stop the activity and allow the heart rate to drop until the total time has elapsed. Many successful coaches use this technique without realizing why it works.

SPECIFICITY OF TRAINING

Someone has suggested that if an athletic training book were written which was only one page long, it should have as its central theme *specificity of training*. It is important to realize that the body responds to any training program specifically. The long-distance runner needs to run rather than to swim, the tennis player will get little help from shooting baskets. Although these examples are fairly obvious, there are still many unanswered questions concerning specificity of training. For instance, the interpretation of literature dealing with weight training has been difficult because of the specific effects of certain programs on subjects. Researchers compare isometric to isotonic programs using a cable tensiometer (static tension) as the criterion measure. It is now known that subjects who train isometrically will show the greatest gains if tested with static devices and those who train isotonically show better gains if tested using the isotonic techniques. This means that a study comparing two different training programs often finds in favor of the program that used a testing method similar to the training method.

Specificity of training also has been demonstrated in cardiovascular endurance programs. When two groups of men were trained on different apparatus (treadmill vs. bicycle ergometer), the improvement in $\dot{V}O_2$ max for the bicycling group was significantly greater when tested on a bicycle ergometer than when tested on a treadmill. This same principle was demonstrated graphically with identical twins who had both been outstanding swimmers. They were tested some time after one of the twins had stopped competitive training (but had remained active). The $\dot{V}O_2$ max of the highly trained twin was much higher when tested in the swimming flume. However, there was no significant difference between the two when tested on a treadmill.

Subjects who train specific body areas (arms vs. legs) always show greater effects in the trained limbs than in the untrained limbs.

These experiments show that specificity of training applies to specific muscle groups also.

When two groups of subjects were trained using either a fast sprint interval or a slower endurance interval, the changes were related to the type of training performed. Both groups made significant $\dot{V}O_2$ max improvements, but the capacity of the ATP-CP systems was much greater in the sprint group, whereas in the endurance group the amount of lactic acid produced during a submaximal exercise decreased. These data are convincing evidence that specificity of training also applies when training the energy systems of the body.

It is clear that the body adapts to the stresses placed upon it in a rather specific manner, and in order to maximize the training effect, one must identify the specific energy systems and movements of the sport or activity and develop training programs for them.

OTHER FACTORS

The following factors relate to endurance and influence it in different ways.

Pace

The most economical pace is an even rate over the entire distance. In walking, running, swimming, and other locomotive activities, stopping, starting, accelerating, and decelerating are costly in terms of energy. Coaches sometimes insist that runners "keep contact" with the pack. However, it would be better for the runner to maintain a fairly even pace to avoid excessive lactate production until near the end of the race; then the runner can increase pace to finish with his or her best effort. The idea of an even pace also has strong application to long-duration games, such as basketball, soccer, tennis, or handball. Playing in "bursts" requires much additional energy and should be avoided when endurance is of prime concern.

Skill

During performance a certain amount of energy is wasted in unnecessary and uncoordinated movements. A skilled individual wastes less energy than the unskilled. For example, an unskilled swimmer may use more than five times as much energy as a skilled person to swim the same distance. Similar comparisons could be made between skilled and unskilled performers in other activities. Repeated practice improves skill and efficiency, and thus influences endurance favorably.

Age

Endurance increases with age to a certain point, after which endurance decreases as age increases. Among trained individuals, maximal endurance usually occurs slightly later than maximal strength; the early 20s among women, and the middle to late 20s among men. Morehouse and Miller state that the ability of boys to perform endurance activities increases steadily to about the age of 20. (With training, endurance will increase beyond this age.) They make these observations about the endurance of children: "The physiological systems of younger children are apparently not as well developed to meet the demands of strenuous exercise as they become when puberty is reached. Children under twelve years of age possess a highly active sympathetic nervous system that predisposes to a high heart rate and an easily depleted capacity to utilize oxygen." They further state that children have a small stroke volume of the heart and consequently a small capacity for increased circulation of blood. These limitations on endurance gradually diminish as the person matures into young adulthood, and endurance reaches its peak potential soon after full physical maturation is achieved.

After maximal endurance is reached, it holds fairly constant for 3 to 5 years, then begins to decline gradually because of several changes that occur in the circulatory and respiratory systems with increased age. Men in their 70s or 80s have lost about one half of their capacity for transforming energy aerobically. The ability to supply blood to active tissues has decreased, and skeletal muscles are weak. Nevertheless, when working within the limits of their ability, many men well advanced in years can carry on work with a lower heart rate and less evidence of fatigue than that exhibited by certain younger men. It should be noted that the loss of endurance at any stage in life can be reduced significantly as a result of training.

Sex

Studies show that up to the beginning of puberty, girls are about equal to boys in endurance. Women reach maximal endurance potential at about the age of 20, whereas men continue to increase until at least the mid 20s.

There is only a slight difference in endurance in moderate exercise, between adult men and women, but the endurance of women in strenuous activities is considerably less than that of men. Limiting factors of endurance among women for vigorous activity are (1) a more rapid heart rate; (2) a small heart with a resultant smaller capacity to deliver blood; (3) smaller chest cavity, resulting in a lower lung capacity; and (4) the blood of women is limited in its oxygen-carrying capacity owing to fewer red blood cells and less hemoglobin (see Chapter 14 for more details).

Body Type

Physique studies by Cureton show that only swimmers with high mesomorphic (a naturally muscular build) characteristics have held world records. A few slightly built ecto-mesomorphic swimmers have achieved high success at the long distances. Cureton also learned that champion runners have slight frames with long and well-muscled legs. Distance runners are typically more slight and less heavily muscled than sprinters.

Morehouse and Miller claim that people of moderate build have the greatest ability to sustain prolonged muscular effort. Sills and Everett, in a study of the relationship between extreme body types and performance, found that mesomorphs were only slightly better than ectomorphs in endurance tests, and endomorphs were far inferior to the other two body types. Bookwalter's evidence generally supports Sills' findings.

In summary, it can be said that most persons who find success in endurance activities have a high degree of mesomorphy, and are also inclined toward ectomorphy. Individuals of heavier body types (more endomorphy) are inclined to be more successful in activities requiring endurance, such as swimming, rather than in those involving running. This is because in swimming the body weight is not carried by the muscles.

Overweight

Fat lacks the ability to contract; therefore, it does not contribute to performance. In fact, it hinders performance since it adds dead weight and thereby increases resistance against movement. Fatty tissue also places an overload on the circulatory system, because it is estimated that 1 pound of fat increases the vascular system by 1 mile (mostly in the form of capillaries).

Temperature

Grose found that endurance is adversely affected by immersion of the arm for 8 minutes in water at 120°F. Conversely, the effects of cold have proven to be advantageous, until a muscle temperature of 80°F is reached. According to Clark and associates, 80°F appears to be the optimal muscle temperature for endurance, and muscle temperatures below this level produce adverse effects on endurance.

Hyperventilation

Hyperventilation may occur in an athlete either unintentionally or intentionally. It is brought on intentionally by forced deep breathing which results in a greatly increased exchange of air to the lungs. Hyperventilation results in an appreciable decrease in CO_2 in the circulorespiratory system, but it does not increase the amount of O_2 in the blood, as commonly believed. The amount of oxygen transferred to the blood is not usually limited by the amount entering the lungs, but rather by the available area of contact between the alveoli and the capillary bed and by the carrying capacity of the blood. If the blood is already fully saturated, the excess oxygen in the lungs will be expelled only in normal expiration, because oxygen cannot be stored.

DeVries found that hyperventilation can approximately double breath-holding time. Consequently, it would definitely improve performance where breath holding is important, such as underwater swimming, or crawl-stroke sprinting. However, since hyperventilation depletes blood CO_2 levels, a person may pass out from lack of oxygen to brain cells before feeling a need to breathe. This is a significant problem and causes several deaths each year.

Vital Capacity

Vital capacity, the total amount of air that can be forcibly expired after a complete inspiration, has been used frequently as a measure of adequacy of the respiratory system. Although it measures the approximate capacity of the lungs, recent information indicates it is of little use in predicting ability to perform tasks of endurance. Obviously, other factors are more significant. For example, any limitation of the oxygen delivery system to the cells will reduce the effectiveness of the delivery, regardless of vital capacity.

Probably a large vital capacity is important in intense exercise when there may be a lack of oxygen in the alveoli, but it is of little value when the exercise is less demanding. The main advantage of a large vital capacity is the ability to take in more air per unit of time with fewer, but deeper, inspirations, thus prolonging the onset of fatigue in the respiratory muscles.

SELECTED READINGS

1. American College of Sports Medicine: *Guidelines for Graded Exercise Testing and Exercise Prescription.* 3rd Ed. Philadelphia: Lea & Febiger, 1986.
2. Astrand, I.: Aerobic work capacity in men and women with special reference to age. Acta Physiol. Scand., *49*(Suppl. 169) 1960.
3. Astrand, I., Astrand, P.-O., Christensen, E.N., and Hedman, R.: Intermittent muscular work. Acta Physiol. Scand., *48*:448, 1960.
4. Astrand, P.-O.: *Experimental Studies of Physical Working Capacity in Relation to Sex and Age.* Copenhagen: Ejnar Munksgaard, 1952.
5. Astrand, P.-O., Hallback, J., Hedman, R., and Saltin, B.: Blood lactates after prolonged severe exercise. J. Appl. Physiol., *18*:619, 1963.
6. Astrand, P.-O., and Rodahl, K.: *Textbook of Work Physiology.* 3rd Ed. New York: McGraw-Hill Book Co., 1986.
7. Bowles, C.J., and Sigerseth, P.O.: Telemetered heart rate responses to pace patterns in the one mile run. Res. Q., *39*:36, 1968.
8. Carlsten, A., and Grimby, G.: *The Circulatory Response to Muscular Exercise in Man.* Springfield, Charles C Thomas, 1966.
9. Christensen, E.H., Hedman, R., and Saltin, B.: Intermittent and continuous running. Acta Physiol. Scand., *50*:269, 1960.
10. Costill, D.L.: *Inside running: Basics of sports physiology.* Indianapolis, IN: Benchmark Press, Inc., 1986.
11. Cureton, T.K.: *Physical Fitness of Champion Athletes.* Urbana, Ill.: University of Illinois Press, 1951.
12. DeVries, H.A.: *Physiology of Exercise for Physical Education and Athletics,* 4th ed. Dubuque: Wm. C. Brown Co., 1986.
13. Fox, E.: Differences in metabolic alterations with sprint versus endurance interval training programs. In *Metabolic Adaptations to Prolonged Physical Exercise.* H. Howard and J. Poortmans (Eds.). Basel: Birkhauser Verlag, 1975, pp. 119–126.
14. Fox, E., McKenzie, D., and Cohen, K.: Specificity of training: Metabolic and circulatory responses. Med. Sci. Sports, *7*:83, 1975.
15. Fox, E.L., Bowers, R.W., and Foss, M.L.: *The Physiological Basis of Physical Education and Athletics.* 4th Ed. Philadelphia: Saunders College Pub., 1988.
16. Fox, E.L., Robinson, S., and Wiegman, D.L.: Metabolic energy sources during continuous and interval running. J. Appl. Physiol., *27*:174, 1969.
17. Gaesser, G.A., and Rich, R.G.: Effects of High- and Low-Intensity Exercise Training on Aerobic Capacity and Blood Lipids. Med. Sci. Sports Exerc., *16*:269, 1984.
18. Gardner, J.B., and Purdy, J.G.: *Computerized Running Training Programs.* Los Altos: Tafnews Press, 1970.
19. Gollnick, P., et al.: Effect of training on enzyme activity and fiber composition of human skeletal muscle. J. Appl. Physiol., *34*:107–111, 1973.
20. Grose, J.E.: Depression of muscle fatigue curves by heat and cold. Res. Q., *29*:19, 1958.
21. Hodgkins, I.: Influence of unilateral endurance training on contralateral limbs. J. Appl. Physiol., *6*:991, 1961.
22. Holmer, I., and Åstrand, P.-O.: Swimming training and maximal oxygen uptake. J. Appl. Physiol., *33*:510–513, 1972.
23. Karlson, J., Nordesjö, L., Jorfeldt, L., and Saltin, B.: Muscle lactate, ATP, and CP levels during exercise after physical training in men. J. Appl. Physiol., *33*:199–203, 1972.
24. Karvonen, M.J.: Effects of vigorous exercise on the heart. In *Work and the Heart.* F.F. Rosenbaum and E.L. Belnap (Eds.). New York: Paul B. Hoeber, Inc., 1959.
25. Knuttgen, H.G.: Oxygen debt, lactate, pyruvate and excess lactate after muscular work. J. Appl. Physiol., *17*:639, 1962.
26. Lortie, G., Simoneau, J.A., Hamel, P., et al.: Responses of Maximal Aerobic Power and Capacity to Aerobic Training. Int. J. Sports Med., *5*:232, 1984.
27. McCafferty, W.B., and Horvath, S.M.: Specificity of exercise and specificity of training: A subcellular review. Res. Q., *48*:358–371, 1977.
28. Milesis, C.A., et al.: Effects of different deviations of physical training on cardio-respiratory function, body composition, and serum liquids. Res. Q., *47*:716–725, 1976.
29. Morehouse, L.E., and Miller, A.T.: *Physiology of Exercise,* 7th ed. St Louis: C.V. Mosby Co., 1976.
30. Pechar, G., et al.: Specificity of cardio-respiratory adaptation to bicycle and treadmill training. J. Appl. Physiol., *36*:753–756, 1974.

31. Pipes, T.V., and Wilmore, J.H.: Isokinetic vs. isotonic strength training in adult men. Med. Sci. Sports, 7:262–274, 1975.
32. Pollock, M.L., Wilmore, J.H., and Fox, S.M.: *Exercise in Health and Disease: Evaluation and Prescription for Health and Rehabilitation.* Philadelphia: W.B. Saunders Co., 1984.
33. Ricci, B.: *Physiological Basis of Human Performance.* Philadelphia, Lea & Febiger, 1967.
34. Saltin, B.: Aerobic work capacity and circulation at exercise in man. Acta Physiol. Scand., *62*(Suppl. 230), 1964.
35. Saltin, B., and Astrand, P.-O.: Maximal oxygen uptake in athletes. J. Appl. Physiol., *23*:353, 1967.
36. Sills, F.D., and Everett, P.W.: The relationship of extreme somatotypes to performances in motor and strength tests. Res. Q., *24*:223, 1953.

9

Applying the Principles of Conditioning

The various factors of performance have been discussed in some detail in the preceding chapters. However, it is sometimes difficult to apply this information to "real" situations. The purpose of this chapter is to show how the information you have learned is used. It should be fairly obvious by now that each athletic event requires a different training emphasis. Hopefully the guidelines below will help the reader use the specific information contained in previous chapters to place the proper emphasis for the event or activity of interest to him.

RULES FOR WRITING PROGRAMS

Writing training programs for athletes (or non-athletes for that matter) should involve the following simple rules:

1. *Determine the primary (and secondary) energy system(s)* used for the activity under consideration and set up an interval training program to develop these systems. For team sports, it might be necessary to analyze the energy system for each position involved if they are different. For instance, running backs may need quite a different program from offensive and defensive linemen. There will also be major differences among the various track and field athletes because of their different requirements for energy.

2. *Evaluate the strength needs for the activity.* Decide which muscle groups must be strengthened for the activity or position and organize a strength program to work on these specific muscle groups. Be sure not to ignore stabilizer and other ancillary muscles.

3. *Look at the activity in terms of flexibility.* Organize a basic flexibility program, emphasizing the joints most used for that activity. Flexibility is critical to developing skill and avoiding injury in all activities and sports.

4. *For activities and sports that have a high skill component, find or invent drills* that teach skill and develop strength and/or energy systems at the same time. These drills can decrease the total training time to make your program more efficient.

5. *Remember specificity.* The best programs are specifically structured for the athlete to meet his needs and level of training.

EXAMPLE PROGRAMS

There are so many different activities and sports events, it would be impossible to include them all in a book of this type. In addition, it is much better for you to understand the principles, and use them to develop your own programs. However, examples of how to approach the analysis of activities may be helpful. The first two examples will look at each end of the running spectrum and show you the analysis process for individuals who are pure sprinters, and those who are long-distance runners. The game of volleyball will also be analyzed as the team-sport example.

Pure Sprinters (100 and 200 Meters)

1. *Energy system.* Almost entirely ATP-PC, but can use aerobic base to enhance recovery

and to support training program. Regular training program would include intervals just longer and just shorter than the competition distance. Could include:

A. Repeat 100's or 200's, fairly long recovery to allow ATP-PC stores to be refilled.

B. Work up or work down intervals such as 1–300, 2–200, 3–100, and 4–50 meters series or just the reverse. Longer intervals would be run at slower than race pace. Shorter intervals at faster than race pace.

2. *Strength.* Great need for overall body strength, but emphasis on lower body and hips.

Strength training is especially helpful because it can help convert type IIA fibers into type IIB, which have a greater capacity for ATP-PC generation. It also thickens the muscle fiber which adds cross-bridges and increases the potential for power.

3. *Flexibility.* Emphasize hip flexion and extension; shoulder extension and flexion.

4. *Drills.* Must work on starts. These could be practiced with shorter distances to increase the number of starts practiced.

5. *Specificity.* Some coaches have sprinters train on a mild grade to develop running power (called strength-endurance). Use a mild grade ($<7\%$) and have sprinter run 75 to 150 meters up the hill and walk back.

As can be seen, the main elements of sprint training are regularly repeated short sprints separated by brief recovery periods, strength training, and development of skill in starting.

Long Distance Runners (10K through Marathon)

1. *Energy system.* Almost completely oxidative or aerobic. The major goal with this athlete is to build a strong aerobic base with enough speed work to allow a "kick" at the end of the race.

A. Aerobic base. The aerobic base is best reached by a massive total mileage. Many long distance runners run from 120 to 140 miles per week at some moderate rate (6 minute mile pace for world class men runners; 7 minute mile pace for world class women runners). Since the injury potential is increased with this much distance, some coaches have athletes train in the pool using flotation devices for an hour twice a week. This helps build and maintain the aerobic base with less chance of injury.

B. Intervals. There is some discussion whether training for a marathon should consist of running long distances (sometimes called "overdistance" training or "long, slow distance training" (LSD), without interval training or whether intervals should be included. Most coaches agree now that intervals should be included. It is unlikely that maximum oxygen uptake can be reached without working at a point nearer aerobic capacity. However, any attempt to do this for a long period is terminated by fatigue due to lactic acid accumulation. Intervals allow for high intensity workouts with time for lactate removal. In fact, some training needs to be done at a pace faster than race pace for success in long distance running. Some coaches believe that marathoners should train in much the same way as elite 10 K racers. This involves repeat miles and half miles. One elite racer does 6 repeat miles per workout at a 4:25 pace.

It should be pointed out that speed work alone is not enough since there is little stress on the systems that are involved with fuel mobilization and utilization (glucose from the liver, fat from the fat cells). Long distance running is probably the best way of stressing these control mechanisms. It is also the best way to increase the aerobic base and the percent of VO_2max that can be utilized without significant lactate production. Be sure to vary the program using periodization principles to avoid burnout and fatigue (see Chap. 7).

2. *Strength.* It would be a disadvantage to carry a large upper body muscle mass for long distances, so strength programs for runners are necessarily different from those used for power athletes. Long distance runners should strength train, but the repetitions should be increased to a higher level to avoid hypertrophy. Leg strength should be increased and many runners now work on their arms to help avoid fatigue associated with holding them in position for several hours.

3. *Flexibility.* Runners tend to lose flexibility in the lower body and must work on this aspect of training regularly. Hurdle stretches, hip flexion, and heel stretches are important for a long distance runner.

4. Drills. Not very applicable

5. Specificity. Another technique often used by endurance athletes is to run fairly long hills (8 to 10 miles) to develop running "strength" as well as endurance. This technique is good because many races include a significant up and down slope. Training on hills allows specific changes to take place to allow better hill running.

Volleyball

1. Energy systems. Without much hesitation, most people would respond "ATP-PC" if asked which energy system was most used in volleyball. Although the ATP-PC system is important and is used often during the power moves (spiking, blocking, etc.) of a match, there is also a high aerobic requirement. A recent study of volleyball players before, during, and after a tournament showed that slow twitch, rather than fast twitch, fibers became glycogen depleted. This indicates that the non-power activities of the game (awaiting service, positioning for defense, etc.) depend primarily upon aerobic fibers. When one considers the fact that some Olympic level matches last up to 3 hours, and that some tournaments last all day, it becomes apparent that endurance is a major factor in the training program. The following ideas may be helpful in analyzing this activity:

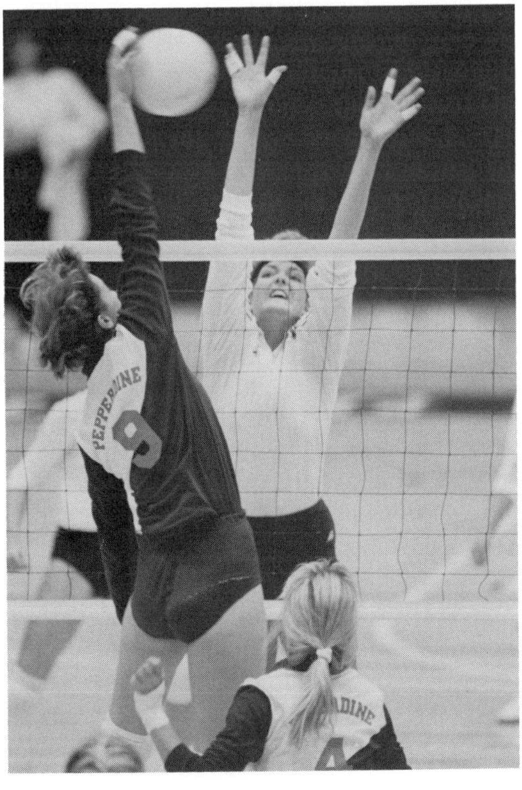

Fig. 9–1.

A. Training ATP-PC. The traditional approach to training the ATP-PC system is little different from that used by sprinters or other power athletes. The program would include short intervals (called wind sprints) of up to 440 yards, with shorter intervals (20, 40, etc.) predominating. Most volleyball programs use many different jump-training techniques including plyometrics. Some coaches have rigged rubber bands to act as resistance to jumping; others have athletes jump back and forth across a mesh of rubber bands between chairs; some have athletes simply do a series of maximum jumps. The US Olympic team worked up to 45 minutes of maximum jumps a day, and in the process increased total vertical jump in these already well-trained athletes by about 4 inches.

A less traditional approach to training is to "practice hard." This approach will be discussed under "drills" below.

B. Training for endurance. Volleyball players should probably use traditional programs for aerobic conditioning during the off season, but emphasize playing time during season to develop endurance. The "endurance" needed for volleyball is quite different from that needed for long distance running. This difference shows up in the measures of $\dot{V}O_2$max where long distance runners are above 80 ml/kg/minute and volleyballers are between 50 and 60 ml/kg/minute. Aerobic capacity as measured by $\dot{V}O_2$max and the endurance necessary to stay in a "ready" position for an entire match or tournament may be quite different. This is why actual playing time may be so important for training endurance. More about this under "specificity."

2. Strength. Volleyball players need an all-around strength program with emphasis on the lower body (jumping muscles) and the arms (hitting muscles). Squats, hip extension, and leg extension exercises are always used. Wall pulley exercises could be used for arm motion. Some coaches used surgical tubing to provide resistance for the hitting motion.

3. Flexibility. Although important for any activity, little work is done on flexibility in volleyball. Athletes tend to "loosen up" and "stretch" prior to games and practice but on an unorganized basis. An all-around flexibility program would be helpful for a sport of this type.

4 and 5. Drills and Specificity. Volleyball lends itself to practice drills. Traditionally, coaches have stood on tables and hit balls to receivers and tossed balls to each side as players practiced receiving skills. Hitting drills have consisted of hitters passing to the setter, then moving in for the kill. Some motor learning experts feel that these drills should all be done in a game situation to make the skills more "game like." In this situation, the coach can emphasize certain aspects of the game, while practicing the other game skills. This approach makes good sense in terms of specificity. It can also make good sense in terms of conditioning, especially for less skilled players. Players at the high school and college level often have too little time to do everything separately and often lack the skills (especially in high school) to play well. By using some creativity, a coach could work out ways to condition as well as teach skills. For example:

A. Play regular games, but focus on blocking, hitting, or some other specific part of the game. Stop the game briefly to help with technique, then continue play.

B. Different sided games. Have the team play 2-, 3-, or 4-sided games to increase the work involved with play. Work on specific skills during these games, but work hard.

C. Throw in the ball. A game could be played at a much higher level of intensity if a new ball were tossed in whenever a fault occurred and the game continued without waiting for a new serve.

For relatively unskilled players, focus on playing skills in actual playing situations. These players need more time for skill development, so conditioning should occur during skill-type situations. For more highly skilled players, broaden the program to include specific energy system training and weight training. However, playing hard is a good way to develop fitness for playing (specifically) as well as skills and can be used as a primary mode of developing both.

General Notes

Most coaches divide the year into at least three different phases; off-season, pre-season, and in-season. The training program during these phases also differs to some extent. Off-season training is at a much lower key, and may emphasize endurance as a basis for other programs during the pre- and in-season training phases. Pre-season programs should try to maximize training for the predominant energy systems involved. In-season training for most sports must emphasize skill, using techniques to maintain energy system production and strength without overtraining. The comments on periodization are appropriate when considering the differences for these phases.

APPLYING THE PRINCIPLES OF CONDITIONING TO ADULT FITNESS PROGRAMS

Because of the interest in adult fitness and the known beneficial effects of exercise in terms of health, it is important for physical educators and coaches to know how to apply the principles of conditioning for developing a fitness program for adults. Adults who are interested in competing in various athletic or sports events can use the principles discussed for training athletes. However, a different approach should be used for those who are interested in fitness only with the goal of feeling better and improving their chances of living a longer, more healthful life. The major energy system to be trained for health is the aerobic system. Strength and flexibility programs should be added for a well-rounded program, but these programs would typically take much less time than the aerobic portion. The following general guidelines can be used for adults:

Aerobic Program

Medical Clearance. Since some adults have known or unknown medical problems, the American College of Sports Medicine has suggested the following guidelines:

1. Apparently healthy individual under age 45 can usually begin exercise programs without the need for exercise testing. At or above

45, it is desirable for these individuals to have a maximal exercise test before beginning exercise programs.

2. Individuals with any or all of the following risk factors: (a) a history of high blood pressure (above 145/95), (b) an elevated total cholesterol/high density lipoprotein cholesterol ratio (above 5), (c) smokers, (d) an abnormal resting ECG, (e) a family history of heart disease prior to age 50, or (f) diabetes should probably have an exercise test prior to beginning a vigorous exercise program, especially if they are above 35 years of age.

3. Individuals who have any symptoms of heart disease (chest pain, shortness of breath, irregular beats, etc.) should have an exercise test before starting an exercise program at any age.

In addition to these guidelines, individuals who have questions about their health should see their physician before beginning any major change in physical activity.

Developing a Program

Four basic principles apply to all programs involving cardiovascular endurance for adults: (1) type of activity, (2) intensity of activity, (3) duration of activity, and (4) frequency of activity.

Type of Activity. Any activity that uses the large muscle groups of the body (primarily the large muscles of the hips and legs) and is rhythmic and continuous in nature will cause the desired changes in cardiovascular fitness to occur. Good examples of these activities are walking, jogging, bicycling, swimming, cross-country skiing, and rope jumping. These activities are termed "aerobic" because of the predominant use of the oxidative system as the major metabolic pathway. With regular training, these activities lead to the adaptations described later in this chapter. Activities using other than continuous rhythmic movements which are aerobic in nature will be less effective in stimulating the cardiovascular and metabolic adaptations expected with chronic exercise. Strength or muscular endurance exercises or noncontinuous exercises of low intensity (golf, bowling) are less effective.

Certain competitive activities such as handball, racquetball, and tennis are appropriate if played with enough vigor to keep the heart rate in the training zone for the entire workout. However, it is difficult to use these activities properly until proficiency in applying the principles of exercise training has been gained. It is recommended that some type of aerobic activity complement participation in competitive activities. For instance, a person could walk or jog on Monday, Wednesday, and Friday, and play handball on Tuesday, Thursday, and Saturday.

The decision concerning the activities to use depends on the availability of facilities (such as a pool or track), and on special health problems (such as arthritic knees or sore ankles). Activities should be rewarding, pleasant, and fun as long as they meet the requirements stated. Remember, the activity must allow a large return of blood to the heart to be effective.

Warm-up and Cool Down. Regardless of the activity chosen for a cardiovascular endurance program, the activity must always include warm-up and cool-down periods. Warming up helps open the blood vessels in the muscles and helps stretch the tendons and ligaments so that injury will not occur so easily. The heart increases its rate gradually, the lungs begin to move the air in and out, and the whole metabolic system prepares itself for the workout ahead.

An interesting study that rather conclusively proves the need of warm-up for adults was conducted. Forty-four normal men (ages 21 to 52 years) were tested on two different occasions with and without a warm-up. In the second test (without a warm-up) 31 (70%) of the men developed abnormal changes on the ECG during the exercises.

Cooling down is even more important than warming up. During aerobic exercise, the large muscles of the legs provide a real boost to the circulating blood to help it get back to the heart. This is done by the action of the muscles on the large veins of the leg. Each time the leg muscles contract, blood is forced up the veins toward the heart. As the muscles relax, blood fills the veins but is not allowed to go backward because of the valves in the vein.

Once the activity is stopped, the recovery period allows for the cardiovascular system and metabolism to return to normal. The time

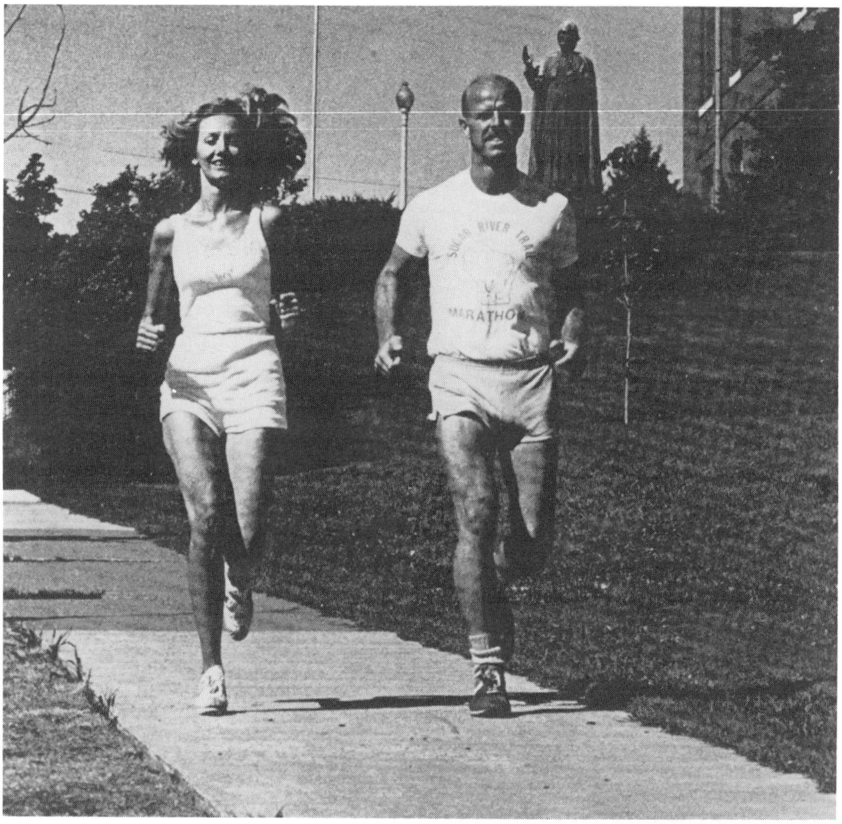

Fig. 9–2. Fisher, A.G., and Allsen, P.E. *Jogging,* 2nd. Copyright 1987, William C. Brown Publishers, Dubuque, Iowa. Reprinted by permission.

needed for complete recovery is dependent on the type and intensity of the exercise. However, from 10 to 20 minutes is usually enough time for cool down to occur. Complete recovery may take several hours. If activity is stopped without appropriate recovery and cool down, the systems of the body may be stressed and complete recovery may be delayed. The recovery period following exercise should include low intensity activity, such as walking, so the muscle pump remains operative and continues to circulate blood from the muscles to remove metabolic wastes and dissipate heat. Following an active period of recovery, there should be a period of passive rest, which includes stretching. Generally, following aerobic exercise, the recovery period should allow the heart to return to at least 100 bpm.

Intensity of Activity. Exercise intensity refers to the vigorousness of exercise. Much research has been done to determine how much exercise is needed to cause cardiovascular changes to occur. Researchers have found that changes in cardiovascular fitness are directly related to the intensity of the training load; therefore, intensity is one of the major factors influencing response to training. Of course, the more intense the exercise, the better will be the training effect. Athletes often train at or near maximal intensity for long periods of time. Athletes also can run 4-min miles and perform other feats which cannot be accomplished by the average person. The average person can get a fine training effect at a much lower intensity of performance than the athlete and should train at this lower intensity for safety and comfort. The question, then, is how intense should activity be for the average person?

Most exercise physiologists agree that the physiological and biochemical changes associated with training occur at about 70% of the individual's maximal aerobic capacity, whereas intensities of less than 60% are not nearly as efficient. These same experts also have warned adults against exceeding 90% of their maximal aerobic capacity, even during peak exercise effort. They recommend that most adults work at an intensity somewhere between 60% and 80% of their maximal aerobic capacity for safe, effective training. These levels can be estimated by using heart rate as a guide. Research has shown the heart rate, expressed as *percent of maximal heart rate,* bears a significant relationship to *percent of maximal aerobic capacity.* This relationship is shown in Figure 9–3. Note that 60% maximal aerobic capacity is related to about 70% maximal heart rate, and that 80% maximal aerobic capacity is related to about 85% maximal heart rate. This means that the proper intensity for training is between 70% and 85% of the maximal heart rate.

Maximal heart rate can be predicted using the formula

$$220 - \text{Age} = \text{Maximal heart rate}$$

Of course, the predicted value may vary somewhat among adults. However, with this information, the approximate training heart-rate range for a person of any age can be

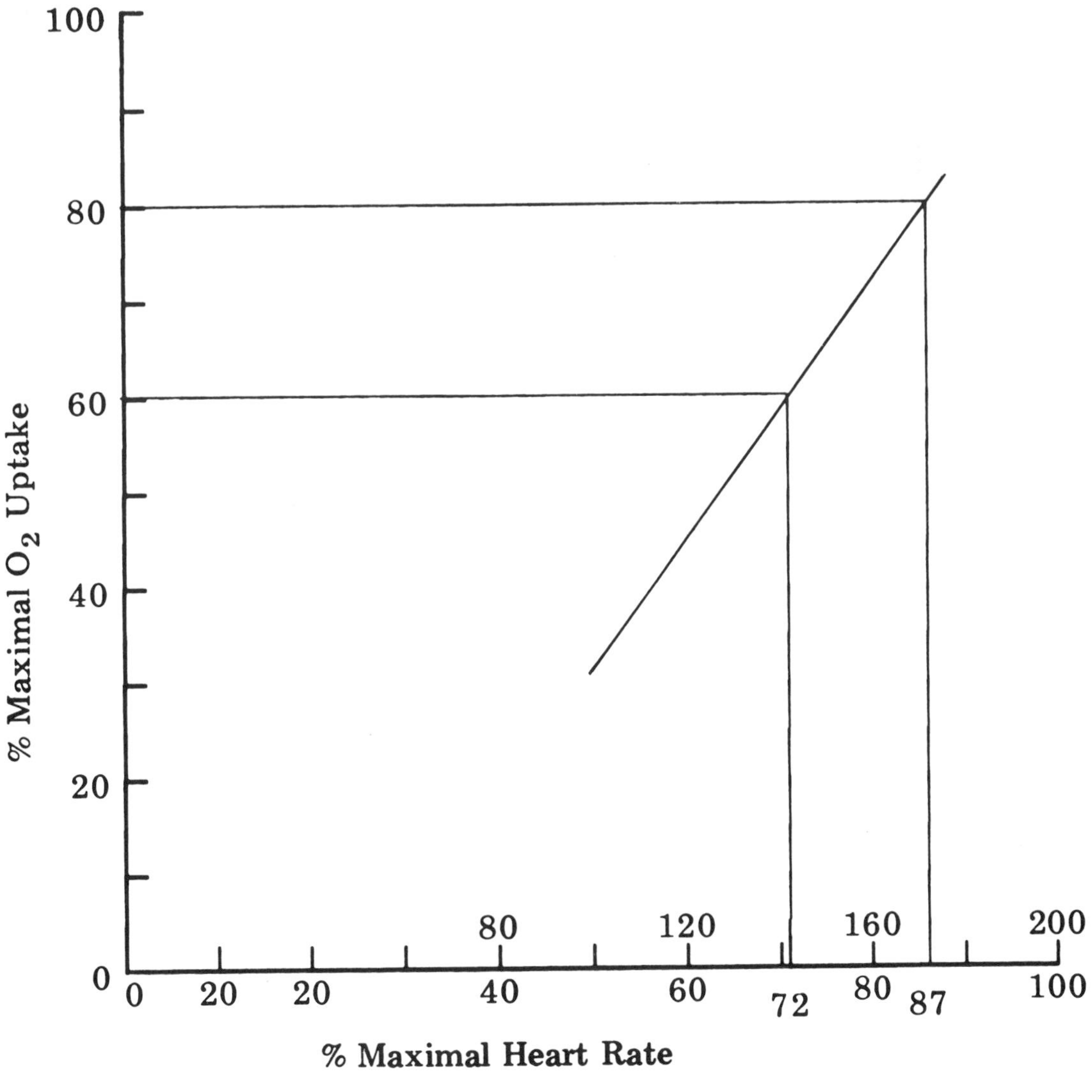

Fig. 9–3. Relationship between percentage of maximal oxygen uptake and percentage of maximal heart rate. (From Fisher, A.G. *Your Heart Rate—Key to Real Fitness.* Courtesy of Brigham Young University Press, 1976.)

computed by multiplying the predicted maximal heart rate by the recommended heart-rate percentage for effective training (between 70% and 85%). This is called the *training zone*. Using the training zone will allow almost anyone to regulate the intensity of his or her own exercise program effectively and safely, and will result in a fine aerobic training effect (Table 9–1).

For example, the training zone for a 40-year-old man was computed by multiplying his maximal heart rate (180 beats/minute) by 70% and 85%. His training heart rate is between 126 beats/minute (70%) and 153 beats/minute (85%).

How to Monitor Heart Rate. Heart rate must be monitored during exercise for the best results and should be counted during the first 10 sec following exercise. Several locations can be used to monitor this pulse; the carotid artery on each side of the voice box, the radial artery at the base of the thumb on either arm, or to the temple in front of the ear. A problem exists in counting the pulse at the carotid artery. Because of the carotid sinus reflex, palpation of this artery sometimes causes the pulse to slow and may yield an inaccurate count. Either of the other two areas may be used successfully, and with a little practice will give an accurate indication of intensity.

One of the most difficult things to learn is how to count the pulse during exercise. Research has shown that pulse rate immediately after exercise will be similar to that during exercise.

A person using jogging as his type of exercise would slow down to a walk, and immediately count his pulse for 10 sec. Table 9–2 shows training heart rate expressed in 10-sec counts. For example, a 40-year-old man would use a 21 to 22 count in 10 sec (130 beats/minute) for the low end of the exercise zone and a 26 count in 10 sec (156 beats/minute) for the high. This simplifies the counting task and is an effective way to use heart rate information during exercise.

Table 9–1. Training Heart Rates in Beats/Min. for Different Ages

Age	*70%*	*85%*
20	140	170
30	133	162
40	126	153
50	119	145
60	112	136
70	105	128

Table 9–2. Training Heart Rate Expressed in 10 Sec. Count

Age	*70%*	*85%*
20	23	28
30	22	27
40	21	26
50	20	24
60	19	23
70	18	21

The proper intensity of exercise can be determined by simple trial and error. If an exercise bout results in a heart rate that is below the training heart rate, increase the speed or intensity of the next bout; if the heart rate is above the training heart rate, decrease the intensity of the next bout.

One of the great advantages of this type of program is that it allows exercise in many varied and different conditions with minimal danger. The heart rate will accurately reflect the stress level on the body and allow an adult to exercise safely in the heat or at altitude. The speed of the activity may decrease, but the training effect will still be nearly the same and the exercise will be safe.

This principle works the other way too. As the cardiovascular system becomes more efficient, work will become easier and the tempo of the activity will necessarily increase to maintain the training heart rate. By using the training heart rate, there is an automatic compensation for this increased fitness. Training by heart rate has many advantages over training by time and distance for fitness.

Duration of Exercise. The principle of duration is easily understood and is critical to the training effect received from any activity. It is inversely related to the intensity of the activity. The more intense the activity, the shorter the duration can be. The less intense the activity, the longer the duration should be. The minimal duration is about 15 minutes. Anyone who desires a good training effect without danger should exercise in the training zone for 15 to 60 minutes daily. Exercise in the lower part of the training zone (70% to 75%) should be extended to the longer of the time period. Research seems to indicate that trained adults enjoy working at

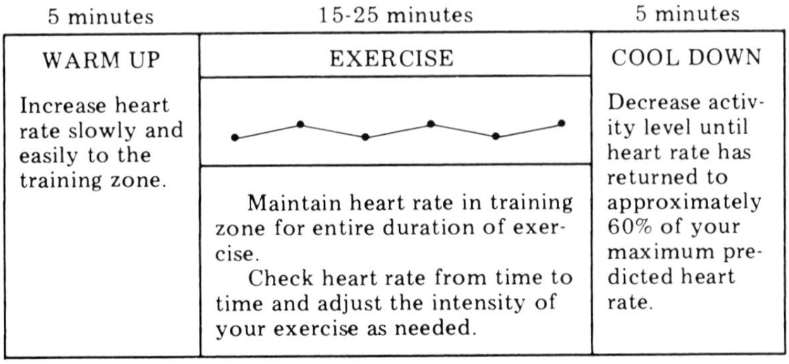

5 minutes
15-25 minutes
5 minutes
WARM UP
EXERCISE
COOL DOWN
Increase heart rate slowly and easily to the training zone.
Maintain heart rate in training zone for entire duration of exercise.
Check heart rate from time to time and adjust the intensity of your exercise as needed.
Decrease activity level until heart rate has returned to approximately 60% of your maximum predicted heart rate.

Fig. 9–4. Example of steady state exercise program. (From Fisher, A.G. *Your Heart Rate—Key to Real Fitness*. Courtesy of Brigham Young University Press, 1976.)

between 80% and 85% of their maximal heart rate. If they are forced to work at a higher level (90%), they tend to decrease their intensity to about 80% to 85%. If they are asked to work more slowly, they increase to a slightly higher level. Everyone should probably begin at the lower part of the zone and work harder as training occurs.

Figure 9–4 is a graphic representation of a typical workout. The exercise period should always begin with a warm-up and end with a cool-down period.

Interval training can be used with certain exercises such as rope jumping in which the work load is so intense that the heart rate may reach maximal if not broken by short rest periods (Fig. 9–5).

Remember that the key to any training program is to stay in the training zone for the entire duration of the exercise. It really does not matter if the heart rate varies, but it must stay in the training zone. This is crucial. The aerobic system does not train well if the proper intensity is not maintained for 15- to 20-minute workout.

Frequency of Activity. Frequency of exercise is related to the intensity of exercise as well as its duration. Research indicates that four workouts per week are better than three, and that five are even better than four. Similar training effects can be obtained from three workouts a week *by increasing the duration of each workout by 5 to 10 minutes.* These sessions should be scheduled on alternate days. Two workouts a week are not effective for training the cardiovascular system even though they will maintain a level of fitness once it has been reached.

Adults should be encouraged to begin and progress slowly. Those who have been extremely inactive should ignore the intensity

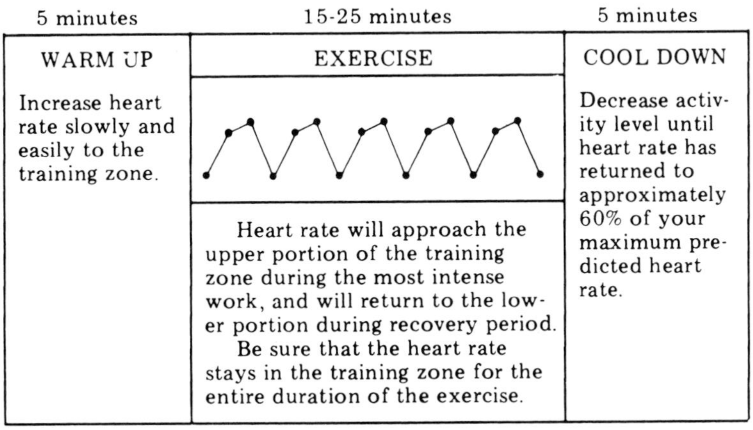

5 minutes
15-25 minutes
5 minutes
WARM UP
EXERCISE
COOL DOWN
Increase heart rate slowly and easily to the training zone.
Heart rate will approach the upper portion of the training zone during the most intense work, and will return to the lower portion during recovery period.
Be sure that the heart rate stays in the training zone for the entire duration of the exercise.
Decrease activity level until heart rate has returned to approximately 60% of your maximum predicted heart rate.

Fig. 9–5. Example of interval training exercise program. (From Fisher, A.G. *Your Heart Rate—Key to Real Fitness*. Courtesy of Brigham Young University Press, 1976.)

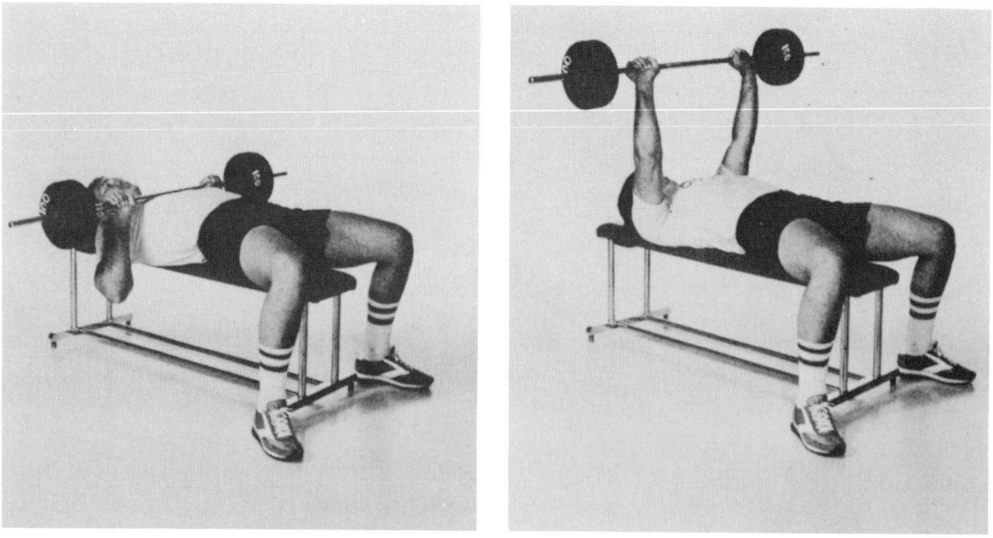

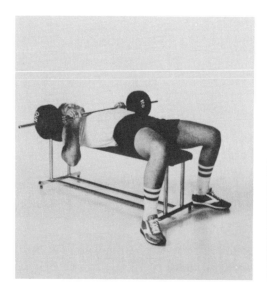

Fig. 9–6. Bench press. An excellent exercise to develop the muscles of the chest and upper arm. (From Fisher, A.G., and Conlee, R.K. *The Complete Book of Physical Fitness*. Courtesy of A.G. Fisher and R.K. Conlee, 1979.)

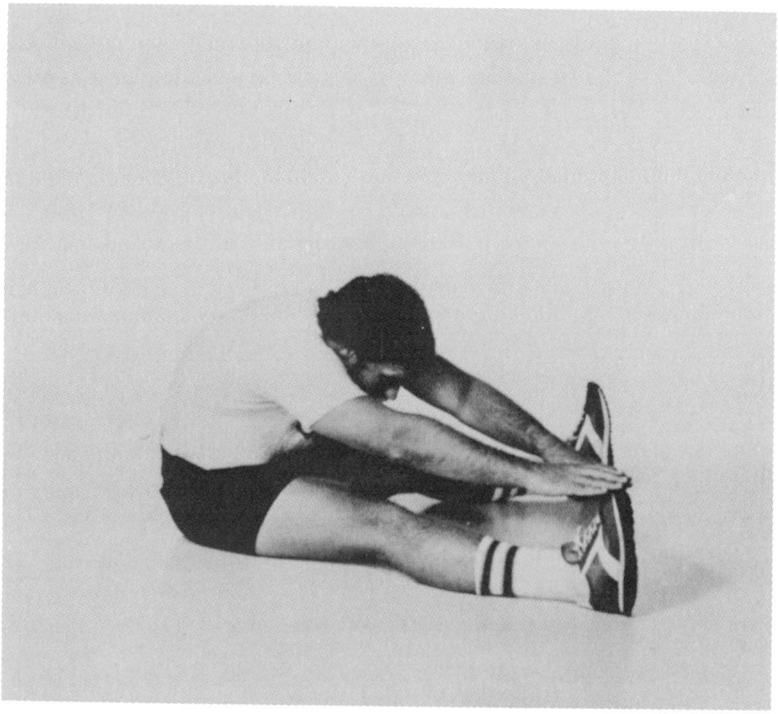

Fig. 9–7. Toe Touch (sitting). Flexibility of the lower back can help avoid lower back pain for many people. (From Fisher, A.G., and Conlee, R.K. *The Complete Book of Physical Fitness*. Courtesy of A.G. Fisher and R.K. Conlee, 1979.)

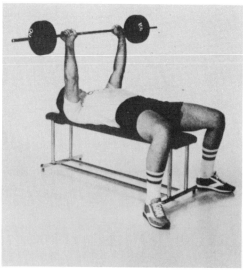

principle for the first few weeks and exercise at a low intensity for the required duration. After several weeks, the heart rate can be checked and the intensity increased to the low level of the training zone. Later, as changes in fitness occur, the heart rate will naturally move up to the higher side of the training zone, and exercise will become more effective.

Possible Physical Problems

Certain physical problems such as sore muscles, shin splints, and side ache sometimes occur as the result of exercise. These problems are not serious and can usually be taken care of at home using fairly simple remedies.

Adults who experience any abnormal heart action such as irregular, fluttering, or skipping pulse, sudden rapid heart rate, sudden slowing of the pulse during exercise, or pain or pressure in the chest, arms, or throat should *cool down and stop exercise immediately.* These conditions may or may not be dangerous, but they should be checked by a physician prior to resuming exercise.

Those who get dizzy or lightheaded, or feel sudden uncoordination or confusion, should *stop exercising immediately and lie down or put their head between their legs until the symptoms pass.* These symptoms should also be checked by a physician prior to resumption of exercise.

Strength Program

The goal of the strength program is to develop muscular strength and endurance in all of the major muscle groups of the body (Fig. 9–6). Adults often lack sufficient muscle strength to accomplish daily tasks efficiently and need to lift moderately to maintain their muscle mass. Adults should use from 8 to 15 repetitions and up to three sets of exercises for each of the major muscle groups. The danger with lifting is the extremely high blood pressure that can occur with intense effort. One study using arterial catheters recorded blood pressures in excess of 450/400 mm Hg during intense lifting. These pressures could be dangerous for adults. Following are a list of possible exercises to work the major muscle groups:

Muscle group	*Exercise*
arms	bicep curl
shoulders (back of arms)	overhead press
chest (back of arms)	bench press
stomach	abdominal curl
outside chest (arms)	lat pulldown
hips, upper legs	squat

Flexibility Program

Flexibility is an important aspect of total fitness in adults. The program can consist of any activity that stretches muscles around their joint. The most important specific flexibilities probably are neck and shoulder flexibility, back extension, and hip flexion. The most important area for flexibility is the lower back. It is believed that low back pain is associated with lack of flexibility in the lower back along with lack of strength in the abdominals. This imbalance can cause poor posture in the lower back region which can result in pain. Little is known about the minimum requirement for producing gains in flexibility, but most research recommends longer periods of holding the stretch, a short relaxation period, then a longer stretch. It is probably helpful to stretch *after* aerobic exercise when muscles are warm and full of blood (Fig. 9–7).

SELECTED READINGS

1. American College of Sports Medicine: *Guidelines for Graded Exercise Testing and Exercise Prescription.* 3rd Ed. Philadelphia: Lea & Febiger, 1986.
2. Barnard, A.J., et al.: Cardiovascular response to sudden strenuous exercise on heart rate, blood pressure and ECG. J. Appl. Physiol., *34*:833, 1973.
3. Conlee, R.K., et al.: Physiological Effects of Power Volleyball. The Phys. and Sports Medicine. Vol. 10:2, Feb. 1982.
4. Fisher, A.G.: *Your Heart Rate—Key to Real Fitness.* Provo: Brigham Young University Press, 1976.
5. Fox, S.M., Naughton, J.P., and Haskell, W.L.: Physical activity and the prevention of coronary heart disease. Ann. Clin. Res., *3*:404–432, 1971.
6. Hellerstein, H.K., et al.: Principles of exercise prescription. In *Exercise Testing and Exercise Training in Coronary Heart Disease.* J.P. Naughton and H.K. Hellerstein (Eds.). New York: Academic Press, 1973.
7. Skinner, J.S. (ed): *Exercise Testing and Exercise Prescription for Special Cases.* Philadelphia: Lea & Febiger, 1987.
8. White, J.R.: EKG changes using carotid artery for heart rate monitoring. Med. Sci. Sports, *9*:88–94, 1977.

10

Physiologic Responses and Adaptations to Exercise

The purpose of this chapter is to review the *acute* responses that occur as the body begins to exercise and then to discuss the *chronic* changes that occur as a result of training. Most of the acute responses have been mentioned in previous chapters, but they are sometimes difficult to pull out of the discussion. The chronic responses to exercise are important to an understanding of how the body is finally able to meet the increased demands placed upon it as a result of regular training.

ACUTE RESPONSE TO EXERCISE

Cardiovascular System

Heart Rate. The heart rate increases linearly from about 60 beats per minute to a maximum of about 200 beats per minute (220 − age = predicted maximum heart rate) (Fig. 10–1). The resting heart rate is influenced by age, body position, fitness level, and environmental factors such as altitude, heat, and cold.

The lowest resting heart rate is found when a person rests, in a supine position. This rate increases as a person stands up, and will increase even more as exercise begins. At submaximal exercise, the heart rate levels off and then drifts slowly upward (cardiac drift). A further increase in work load will cause a progressive increase in heart rate until maximum heart rate is reached.

Stroke Volume. Stroke volume (the amount of blood pumped out of the heart each beat) increases during the first 25 to 40% of an increasing work bout to maximum and then levels off (Fig. 10–2). It then remains stable until near-maximum levels where it may decrease slightly due to decreased ventricular filling time. The response just described is from studies of supine cycling and newer ev-

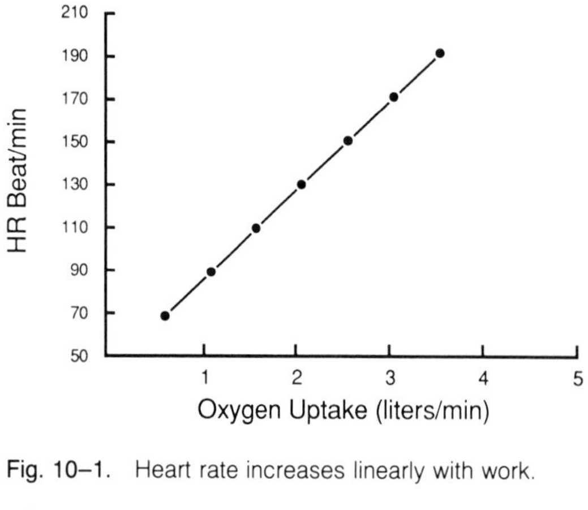

Fig. 10–1. Heart rate increases linearly with work.

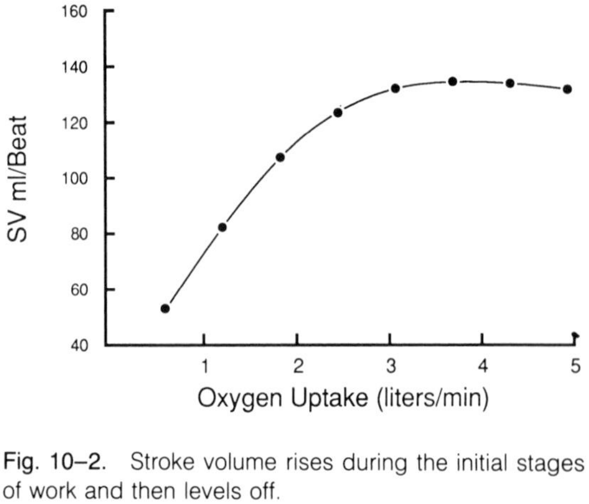

Fig. 10–2. Stroke volume rises during the initial stages of work and then levels off.

idence suggests that SV may increase more linearly than previously thought. SV can increase from about 30 to 50% above resting values during supine exercise, to almost doubling in upright work. Typically, stroke volume ranges from 50 to 110 ml/beat at rest to 100 to 200 ml/beat during maximum work.

Cardiac Output. Cardiac output ($\dot{Q}$) is defined as the amount of blood pumped out of either ventricle per minute. The formula for calculating $\dot{Q}$ is:

$$\dot{Q} = HR \times SV$$

At rest, $\dot{Q}$ is about 5 liters/minute. This value increases linearly with exercise to a level between 20 and 40 liters/min., depending on the size of the ventricle and the resulting stroke volume (Fig. 10–3). In early exercise, the increase is related to increases in both HR and SV. Later increases are due to increases in HR only (assuming that SV plateaus).

Arteriovenous Oxygen Difference (a-$\bar{v}O_2$ diff). As blood flows through the body, some of the oxygen is extracted and used by the mitochondria. The difference between the amount of oxygen leaving the heart and the amount returning to the heart is called a-$\bar{v}O_2$ diff. At rest, this difference is about 5 ml/dl. During maximum exercise, more oxygen is used and the difference between the blood carried away from the heart and that returning to the heart increases to about 15 ml/dl. The blood draining from working muscle tissue may be almost completely depleted of oxygen. However, the mixed venous blood would still have around 5 ml/dl because it is a mixture of blood from the working muscles and less active parts of the body combined. The arteriovenous oxygen difference is an important adjustment mechanism that allows a much greater increase in metabolic rate than would be possible if the muscles depended on increased blood flow alone for an increase in oxygen consumption (Fig. 10–4).

It should be mentioned that the a-$\bar{v}O_2$ diff in the heart is fairly large even at rest (about 15 ml/dl). During work, the increased oxygen demand of this organ is met almost entirely by increased flow. This is one reason why blockage of coronary arteries is such a troublesome matter.

Blood Flow. Since the vascular system is much too large for the amount of blood in it, the blood must be shunted to the system or systems which need it the most. The sympathetic nervous system sends vasoconstrictor and vasodilator fibers to the smooth muscles of the arterioles. As work begins, the blood is shifted from the gut and other nonessential areas to the muscle beds. At the same time, the heart is stimulated by the accelerator nerve and the vagus nerve is inhibited to increase the total flow of blood. The precapillary sphincters are then locally dilated in the areas needing blood, and the blood flow serves the tissues which have the need. As heat builds up, some of the blood is shifted to the skin to help maintain internal temperatures within acceptable limits. This limits the amount of blood available to muscles and can have a negative effect on performance.

Blood. During moderate to intense work, there is a decrease in total blood volume as a

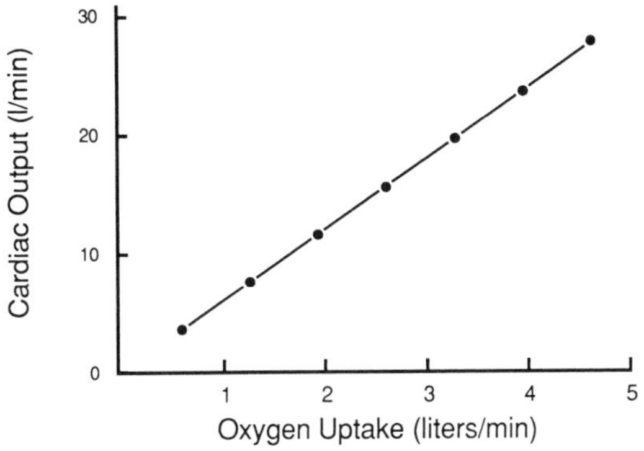

Fig. 10–3. Changes in cardiac output associated with increased work.

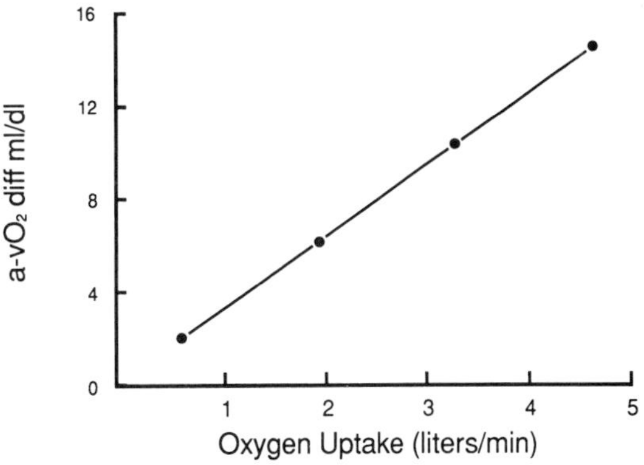

Fig. 10–4. The a-$\bar{v}O_{2diff}$ at various levels of work.

result of water loss from increased hydrostatic pressure and sweat. This decrease in total fluid volume has a negative effect on the heart (lowers cardiac output) but the hemoconcentration increases the carrying capacity (more RBC's per liter of blood) in terms of oxygen. However, there is also an increase in temperature and a decrease in pH, both of which tend to decrease the oxygen-carrying capacity of the RBC through the Bohr effect. Interestingly, there is really very little change from all this in the body's ability to carry oxygen to the cells.

Blood Pressure. At rest, systolic pressure is about 120 mm Hg and the diastolic pressure is about 80 mm Hg. These numbers indicate that the heart is pushing blood into the vessels with a force of about 120 mm Hg and that the pressure between beats is about 80 mm Hg (120/80). The systolic pressure rises with increased work to a level above 150 mm Hg, whereas the diastolic pressure usually remains about the same or decreases slightly to allow easy flow into the aorta (Fig. 10–5).

The systolic pressure in the pulmonary system also increases during work from about 20 to 35 mm Hg. The diastolic pressure is fairly constant and stays somewhere between 0 to 5 mm Hg in either case.

Respiratory Response

Since the exchange of respiratory gases occurs in the lungs, it is important that the amount of air ($\dot{V}_E$) moved by the lungs is sensitive to increased oxidative need. Resting $\dot{V}_E$ is about 5 to 7.5 liters/minute, consisting of a tidal volume (V_T) of about 0.5 liters/breath, and a frequency (f), of about 10 to 15 times/minute.

$\dot{V}_E$ increases linearly with increased activity, in the ratio of about 20 to 25 liters of air per liter of oxygen used at lower levels of work and 30 to 35 liters of air per liter of oxygen at higher levels. The increased air to oxygen ratio is caused by hyperventilation that occurs above the lactate threshold (Fig. 10–6).

Maximum $\dot{V}_E$ is between 75 and 200 liters/minute in most people, depending on their vital capacity, since only about 50 to 60% of VC is used during maximum work. The frequency of breathing increases to somewhere between 40 and 60 breaths per minute. Since VC is related to body size and age, a large young subject will have a larger maximum $\dot{V}_E$ than a smaller, older subject. $\dot{V}_E$ cannot be used as an indicator of fitness.

Metabolic Response

Oxygen consumption, or $\dot{V}O_2$, reflects the metabolic activity of the body and increases linearly with work (Fig. 10–7). Expressed in liters per minute, it is related somewhat to metabolic mass or body size. When expressed in ml/kg/min. it indicates potential for aerobic activity.

Resting $\dot{V}O_2$ is about .25 liters/minute or 3.5 ml/kg/min. (1 MET). Walking requires about 1 l/min. or 10 ml/kg/min. (depending on body size), and jogging doubles these values. There is a wide variation in $\dot{V}O_2$max because of the difference in size and the difference in fitness levels. A highly trained male athlete may have a $\dot{V}O_2$max between 4 and 5

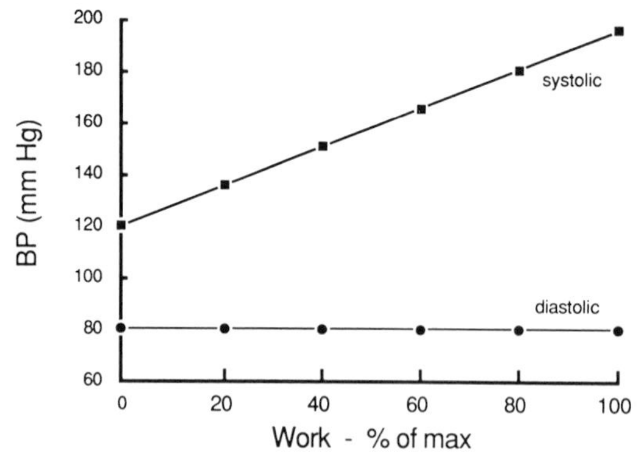

Fig. 10–5. Response of blood pressure during exercise.

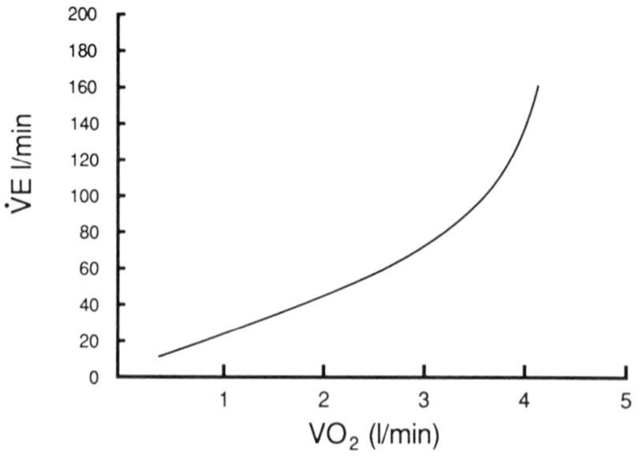

Fig. 10–6. $\dot{V}_E$ increases with work during the initial levels and then increases out of proportion to need (hyperventilation).

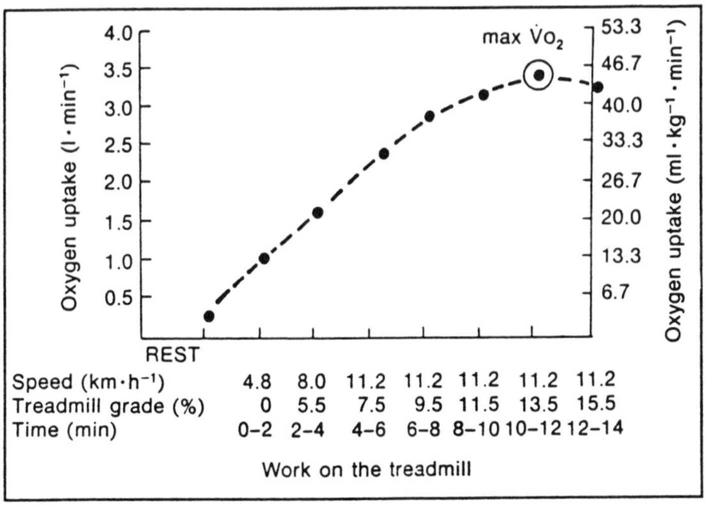

Fig. 10–7. $\dot{V}O_2$ increases linearly with work. (From McArdle, W.D., Katch, F.I., and Katch, V. L. *Exercise Physiology*, 2nd Ed. Courtesy of Lea & Febiger, 1986.)

liters/min. or 80 to 90 ml/kg/min. Female athletes would be about 15 to 20% lower. Sedentary individuals may be as low as 20 ml/kg/min. University students typically range between 30 and 60 ml/kg/min. Like many other functions of the body, $\dot{V}O_2$max decreases with age after about 30 years of age.

CHRONIC ADAPTATIONS TO EXERCISE

One of the most remarkable features of the human body is its ability to adapt to stresses placed upon it. These adaptations occur in almost every tissue or system as a result of training and the changes that result allow the body to perform more effectively because of the change. The purpose of this section is to discuss these changes.

Physiologic Adaptations in Muscle

There are a number of adaptations that occur in the neuromuscular system as a result of various types of training. Since these adaptations are so important in terms of the other systems, they will be discussed first.

Strength. A number of physiologic adaptations occur in muscles with strength training that account for the increase in strength that occurs. These changes can be categorized into two major areas: (1) Nervous adaptations and (2) muscular adaptations. Both of these areas will be discussed below:

Nervous Adaptations. There are numerous situations where feats of strength occur during an intense emotional experience in the absence of any increase in muscular size. The housewife who lifts a fallen tree from her husband, or a small school boy who "flattens" a bully, are examples of how the nervous system can affect strength in times of stress. Even the increase in strength experienced by women who engage in normal weight training programs occurs in the absence of significant hypertrophy.

How are these increases in strength explained? The first explanation relates to motor unit recruitment. It is probably not possible to consciously contract most or all motor units without training. Strength training, as it causes fatigue in motor units normally recruited, probably facilitates recruitment of additional motor units. Second, the role of golgi tendon organs is to protect the muscle and connective tissue from exerting more force than can be tolerated. Training very likely "toughens" the system so that more force is required to stimulate the inhibitory signals from these receptors. Third, gains in strength may be related to an improved coordination in the firing of motor units to allow an increase in strength. There is also the possibility that antagonistic muscles are affected by training to allow a more forceful contraction to occur. In any case, it seems likely that there is a neurogenic component in strength training, especially in the early stages.

Muscle Adaptations. The major, and most noticeable adaptation in muscle as a result of strength training in males is the increased *size* or *hypertrophy* of muscles. Hypertrophied muscle fibers are larger because they contain more actin and myosin (contractile protein). More contractile protein allows for more cross-bridges to form and therefore an increase in force of contraction. Trained muscles also have thicker and tougher connective tissue.

Some scientists have found evidence of an increased number of muscle cells *(hyperplasia)* in hypertrophied muscle. Some athletes have a large muscle mass but normal fiber cross-sectional areas. Other studies have shown "fiber splitting" in trained cats as a result of lifting a weight to get food. Although there is still controversy about this area, hypertrophy of individual fibers is probably the major change that accounts for most muscle hypertrophy.

Anaerobic Adaptations. It is clear that muscles do adapt to anaerobic training by increasing their ability to produce energy more rapidly. Since energy for anaerobic work comes from both ATP-PC stores and glycolysis, changes in the biochemistry of these systems would be expected.

ATP-PC. In one study, a group of men trained one leg for 6 second and the other leg for 30 second maximal exercise bouts. The shorter bouts depended more on ATP-PC as shown by a rise in lactate in the longer bouts but not in the shorter ones. However, the enzymes associated with the ATP-PC system (CPK and MK) were not increased in the shorter bout, but were in the longer one. A similar study using 5-second bouts did show an increase in these enzymes, however. Both of these studies show that the enzymes responsible for ATP resynthesis are adaptable, but not quite as specifically adaptable as might be expected.

Glycolysis. The enzymes of glycolysis (phosphorylase, LDH, PFK) were increased significantly in the 30 second group as described above. However, the ability to resist fatigue during a 60-second performance test was no greater in the group with increased glycolytic enzymes. Since both groups described above (6-second and 30-second groups) increased similarly in strength and in muscle buffering capacity, the researchers suggested that these factors were responsible for the increased performance rather than the increased enzyme levels. Buffering capacity is important because the muscle can work longer before the concentration of hydrogen gets high enough to inhibit the contractile process.

Aerobic Adaptations. There are several major adaptations that occur in muscle as a result of aerobic training. First, the number of capillaries surrounding muscle fibers increases significantly. Endurance athletes may have 50% more capillaries than non-trained individuals. Second, the content of myoglobin, a hemoglobin-like substance responsible for delivery of oxygen from the cell membrane to the mitochondria, goes up significantly. Third, the mitochondrial "reticulum" increases dramatically as a result of endurance training. Some research indicates that mitochondria are interconnected in a network much like sarcoplasmic reticulum. Training apparently increases this "network" of mitochondria into more and more branches. The large increase in the mitochondrial network seen in distance runners probably takes years to occur, but weekly increases of about 5% in the number of mitochondria over a 27-week period was reported and the average size increased about 35% during this time.

As might be expected, the enzymes of oxidation increase during endurance training (Fig. 10–8). SDH (succinate dehydrogenase) increases more than 25% with even moderate activity and may increase by 2.6 times with vigorous training. There is also an increase in the ability of muscles to oxidize fat as a fuel. This response allows endurance athletes to spare glycogen and increase endurance capacity. Interestingly, the amount of increase in the muscle mitochondria and enzyme content is greater than the increase in $\dot{V}O_2max$. This indicates that the two measures are separate and may not indicate an increase in the same factor. Training may increase $\dot{V}O_2max$ by only 10 to 25%, but the ability to endure at submaximal levels may be increased by a much larger margin. Some scientists have found a high correlation between the increase

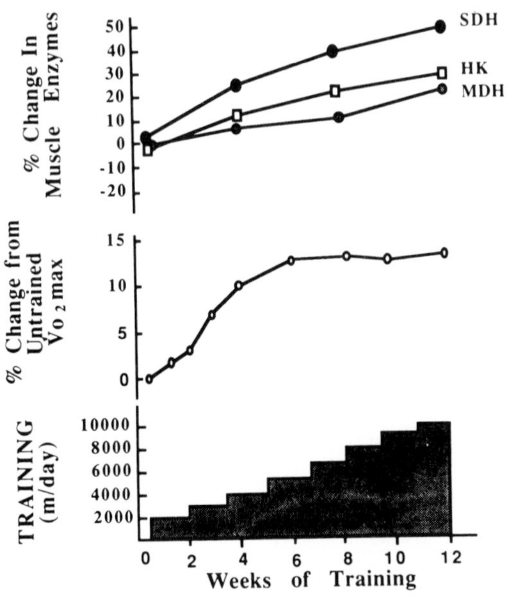

Fig. 10–8. Changes in muscle enzymes and maximal oxygen uptake during 12 weeks of swim training. Note the gradual increase in the oxidative enzymes SDH, HK, and MDH during the gradual increase in the training load. (From Wilmore, J.H., and Costill, D.L. *Training for Sport and Activity,* 3rd Ed. William C. Brown, 1988.)

in mitochondrial content and the increase in enzyme activity. This may mean that endurance training yields more mitochondrial material whose enzyme activity is about the same as before training. Of course the total amount of enzyme is increased significantly because of the increase in mitochondrial content.

It should be mentioned that the ability to store muscle glycogen is increased with endurance training. In addition, the amount of fat droplets in the muscle is increased as well. Both of these changes occur to make fuel more readily available to muscle during endurance work.

Physiologic Adaptations of the Cardiovascular System

The cardiovascular system undergoes many changes as a result of exercise. These changes will be discussed below:

Heart Rate. One of the most obvious changes that occurs with endurance training is a decrease in the resting heart rate. Endurance athletes often have heart rates in the high 30's or low 40's. This decrease could be related to either decreased sympathetic or increased parasympathetic activity, most likely, decreased sympathetic activity. There is also the possibility that the intrinsic rate of the pacemaker of the SA node can be decreased. This may be related to increased amounts of acetylcholine or decreased sensitivity to catecholamines, both of which have been reported as a result of exercise training.

Training also decreases the heart rate response to any given submaximal level of exercise. This decrease is due to the increase in SV which allows the same $\dot{Q}$ with fewer beats of the heart. Maximal heart rate is changed only a little, decreasing slightly with training.

Stroke Volume. One of the most important changes related to endurance exercise is the increase in stroke volume (SV). Most studies indicate the magnitude of the change to be up to about 20%. The increased SV is related to a small but significant increase in left ventricular end diastolic dimension and an increased total blood volume. Contractility also increases as a result of increased calcium flux and calcium myosin-ATPase activity. Increased SV, and the resulting decrease in HR, make the heart more efficient in terms of energy utilization.

Since world-class endurance athletes often have stroke volumes in a range near 200 ml/beat or more, it is unlikely that training could cause enough change in normal hearts to reach the levels needed for this level of competition. Genetics surely play a role in the massive SV seen in these athletes.

Cardiac Output. Resting cardiac output is approximately the same for trained and nontrained subject. Therefore, cardiac output is maintained by an increase in resting stroke volume since resting heart rate is lower. This increase in stroke volume is more pronounced in endurance athletes who experience a volume overload (increased venous return). Strength athletes have normal internal ventricular dimensions, but a thicker than normal ventricular muscle that hypertrophies to about the same extent as their skeletal muscle. This change may be due to the pressure overload experienced by these athletes as they strain against high loads as they develop their strength.

Maximum cardiac output is increased about the same extent as maximum stroke volume by exercise, because maximum heart rate changes very little. Cardiac output for any given submaximal work load changes very little with exercise training, but the heart rate is decreased due to the increase in SV.

Arteriovenous Oxygen Difference (a-$\bar{v}O_2$ diff). Arteriovenous oxygen difference increases only slightly with exercise training. Increased capillary density results in a shorter diffusion distance between the blood and the muscle cell. However, the increased mitochondrial density is even greater than the increased blood flow, so blood coming from the muscle bed is still fairly depleted, even with a greater flow. This blood then mixes with blood from less active areas to show little change in the mixed venous blood returning to the heart.

Blood Flow. Training increases the blood flow to muscles during exercise because of the increased $\dot{Q}$ and the increased number of capillaries in the muscle. The absolute flow to inactive or less active organs is also increased, but not if expressed as a percentage of total blood flow. Blood flow to the heart is slightly less during submaximal exercise because the heart is more efficient when it beats at a lower rate.

Blood Pressure. Endurance training tends to reduce resting systolic, diastolic, and mean blood pressure. Both diastolic and mean pressure is reduced during maximum work. The mechanism for this reduction is not known.

Physiologic Adaptations to the Respiratory System

Static lung volumes change little with endurance training. However, vital capacity may increase some at the expense of residual volume. There is little difference in resting $\dot{V}_E$, but maximum values can increase dramatically. Tidal volume is changed little at rest and at submaximal work, but is increased during maximum levels of work. Frequency of breathing decreases slightly at any given submaximal work load, but may be increased substantially during max work.

Pulmonary blood flow is increased following training and may be greater in the upper lobes of the lung. Lung diffusion is unaltered at rest and during submaximal work, but may increase during maximum work as a result of training.

Physiologic Adaptations to Metabolism

Oxygen consumption during rest is about the same before and after training. Oxygen consumption at a given level of submaximal exercise is the same following training as before, although there may be a slight decrease due to improvement in mechanical efficiency of the activity (skill). Even though submaximal $\dot{V}O_2$ does not change at a given workload, it is important to realize that the *relative* $\dot{V}O_2$ at a given submaximal workload is less due to the increased $\dot{V}O_2max$.

Significant increases in $\dot{V}O_2max$ occur as a result of training. The amount of increase is still unclear, but studies have reported levels from 4 to 93%. However, increases of 20 to 30% seem reasonable. It is not uncommon to see an increase from 32 to 40 ml/kg/min. in untrained adult subjects. This increase is significant because both the max level and the percent of usable $\dot{V}O_2$ increases. Larger changes are sometimes seen in young healthy college students, but even these subjects are far from the 80 to 90 ml/kg/min. seen in world-class endurance athletes. Interestingly, these athletes may train for years after their initial increase without changing their $\dot{V}O_2max$ significantly. Some of them perform better several years later despite the lack of increased $\dot{V}O_2max$.

The increase in $\dot{V}O_2max$ associated with training is related to both increased oxygen delivery to the muscles ($\dot{Q} = HR \times SV$) or by an increased oxygen extraction from the blood by the muscles related to increased mitochondria and enzyme content of the muscles. Which of these factors actually limit $\dot{V}O_2max$ is still a major unanswered question. However, a recent review article concludes that blood flow is by far the most important factor. The adaptations that occur in muscle (increased mitochondria and oxidative enzymes), appears to be more closely related to the ability to perform prolonged high-intensity exercise (endurance).

SELECTED READINGS

1. Adams, T.D., Yanowitz, F.G., Fisher, A.G., Ridges, J.D., Lovell, K., Pryor, T.A.: Noninvasive Evaluation of Exercise Training in College-age Men. Circ., *64*, No. 5:958–965, 1981.

2. Atha, J.: Strengthening muscle. Exerc. Sport Sci. Rev., *9*:1–73, 1982.
3. Astrand, P.O., and Rodahl, K.: *Textbook of Work Physiology.* 3rd ed. New York: McGraw-Hill Book Co., 1986.
4. Baldwin, K.M., Klinkerfuss, G.H., Terjung, R.L., et al.: Respiratory capacity of white, red and intermediate muscle: Adaptive response to exercise. Am. J. Physiol., *222*:373–378, 1972.
5. Berger, R.A.: Comparison of static and dynamic strength increases. Res. Q., *33*:329, 1962a.
6. Berger, R.A.: Effect of varied weight training programs on strength. Res. Q., *33*:168, 1962b.
7. Berger, R.A.: Leg extension at three different angles. Res. Q., *37*:560, 1966.
8. Costill, D.L., Coyle, E.F., Fink, W.F., et al.: Adaptations in skeletal muscle following strength training. J. Appl. Physiol., *46*:96–99, 1979.
9. Costill, D.L., Fink, W.J., Ivy, J.L., et al.: Lipid metabolism in skeletal muscle of endurance-trained males and females. J. Appl. Physiol., *28*:251–255, 1979.
10. Davis, J.A., Frank, M.H., Whipp, B.J., et al.: Anaerobic threshold alterations caused by endurance training in middle-aged men. J. Appl. Physiol., *46*:1039–1046, 1979.
11. Ekblom, B., Astrand, P., Saltin, B., Stenberg, J., and Wallstrom, B.: Effect of training on circulatory response to exercise. J. Appl. Physiol., *24*:518–528, 1968.
12. Eriksson, B., Gollnick, P., and Saltin, B.: Muscle metabolism and enzyme activities after training in boys 11–13 years old. Acta Physiol. Scand., *87*:485–497, 1973.
13. Fortney, S.M., Nadel, E.R., Wenger, C.B., et al.: Effect of acute alterations of blood volume on circulatory performance in humans. J. Appl. Physiol., *50*:292–298, 1981.
14. Foster, C., Anholm, J.D., Hellman, C.K., et al.: Left ventricular function during sudden strenuous exercise. Circ., *63*:592–596, 1981.
15. Fox, E., Bartels, R., Billings, C., Mathews, D., Bason, R., and Webb, W.: Intensity and distance of interval training programs and changes in aerobic power. Med. Sci. Sports, *5*:18–22, 1973.
16. Gollnick, P., Armstrong, R., Saltin, B., Saubert, C., Sembrowich, W., and Shepherd, R.: Effect of training on enzyme activity and fiber composition of human skeletal muscle. J. Appl. Physiol., *34*:107–111, 1973.
17. Gonyea, W.J.: Role of exercise in inducing increases in skeletal muscle fiber number. J. Appl. Physiol., *48*:421–426, 1980.
18. Gonyea, W.J., Ericson, G.C., and Bonde-Petersen, F.: Skeletal muscle, fiber splitting induced by weight-lifting exercise in cats. Acta Physiol. Scand., *19*:105–109, 1977.
19. Gonyea, W.J., Sale, D.G., Gonyea, F.B., et al.: Exercise induced increases in muscle fiber number. Europ. J. Appl. Physiol., *55*:137–141, 1986.
20. Hermansen, L., Hultman, E., and Saltin, B.: Muscle glycogen during prolonged severe exercise. Acta Physiol. Scand., *71*:129–139, 1967.
21. Hettinger, T.: *Physiology of Strength.* Springfield, Charles C Thomas, 1961.
22. Holloszy, J.O.: Adaptations of muscular tissue to training. Prog. Cardiovasc. Dis., *18*:445–458, 1976.
23. Holloszy, J.O.: Biochemical adaptations in muscle. Effects of exercise on mitochondrial oxygen uptake and respiratory enzyme activity in skeletal muscle. J. Biol. Chem., *242*:2278–2282, 1967.
24. Holloszy, J.O., Oscai, L.B., Mole, P.A., et al.: Biochemical adaptations to endurance exercise in skeletal muscle. In B. Pernow and B. Saltin (Eds.), *Muscle Metabolism During Exercise.* New York: Plenum Press, 1971.
25. Johnson, B.L., et al.: A comparison of concentric and eccentric muscle training. Med. Sci. Sports, *8*:35–38, 1976.
26. Jokl, E.: *Physiology of Exercise.* Springfield, Ill., Charles C Thomas, 1964.
27. Karlsson, J., Nordesjo, L., Jorfeldt, L., and Saltin, B.: Muscle lactate, ATP, and CP levels during exercise after physical training in man. J. Appl. Physiol., *33*:199–203, 1972.
28. Larsson, L., and Tesch, P.A.: Motor unit fibre density in extremely hypertrophied skeletal muscles in man. Europ. J. Appl. Physiol., *55*:130–136, 1986.
29. Lesmes, G.R., Costill, D.L., Coyle, E.F., et al.: Musclestrength and power changes during maximal isokinetic training. Med. Sci. in Sports, *10*:266–269, 1978.
30. Mathews, K.D., and Fox, E.L.: *The Physiological Basis of Physical Education and Athletics.* Philadelphia: W.B. Saunders Co., 1976.
31. McDonagh, M.J.N., and Davies, C.T.M.: Adaptive response of mammalian skeletal muscle to exercise with high loads. Europ. J. Appl. Physiol., *52*:139–155, 1984.
32. Mole, P.A., Oscai, L.B., and Holloszy, J.O.: Adaptation of muscle to exercise. Increase in levels of palmityl CoA synthetase, carnitine palmityltransferase, and palmityl CoA dehydrogenase and in the capacity to oxidize fatty acids. J. Clin. Invest., *50*:2323–2330, 1971.
33. Morganroth, J., Maron, B., Henry, W., and Epstein, S.: Comparative left ventricular dimensions in trained athletes. Ann. Intern. Med., *82*:521–524, 1975.
34. Nutter, D., Gilbert, C., Heymsfield, S., Perkins, J., and Schlant, R.: Cardiac hypertrophy in the endurance athlete. Physiologist, *18*:336, 1975.
35. Pette, D.: Activity -induced fast to slow transitions in mammalian muscle. Med. Sci. Sports Exerc., *16*:517–528, 1984.
36. Saltin, B., and Astrand, P.-O.: Maximal oxygen uptake in athletes. J. Appl. Physiol., *23*:353, 1967.
37. Saltin, B., and Rowell, L.B.: Functional adaptations to physical activity and inactivity. Fed. Proceed., *39*:1506–1513, 1980.
38. Saltin, B., and Karlsson, J.: Muscle ATP, CP, and lactate during exercise after physical conditioning. In B. Pernow and B. Saltin (Eds.), *Muscle Metabolism During Exercise.* New York: Plenum Press, 1971.
39. Saltin, B., Nazar, K., Costill, D.L., et al.: The nature of the training response: Peripheral and central adaptations to one-legged exercise. Acta Physiol. Scand., *96*:289–305, 1976.
40. Sanders, M., White, F.C., Peterson, T.M., et al.: Effects of endurance exercise on coronary collateral blood flow in miniature swine. Am. J. Physiol., *234*:H614–H619, 1978.
41. Scheuer, J., and Tipton, C.M.: Cardiovascular adaptation to physical training. Am. Rev. Physiol., *39*:221–251, 1977.
42. Scheuer, J. and Tipton, C.M.: Cardiovascular adaptations to physical training. Ann. Rev. Physiol., *39*:221–251, 1977.

43. Scholander, P.F.: Oxygen transport through hemoglobin solutions. Science, *131*:585–590, 1960.
44. Sharp, R.L., Costill, D.L., Fink, W.J., et al.: Effects of eight weeks of bicycle ergometer sprint training on human muscle buffer capacity. Internat. J. Sports Med., 7:13–17, 1986.
45. Snoeckx, L., Abeling, H., Lambregts, J., et al.: Echocardiographic dimensions in athletes in relation to their training programs. Med. Sci. Sports Exerc., *14*:428–434, 1982.
46. Suga, H., Hisano, R., Hirata, S., et al.: Mechanism of higher oxygen consumption rate. Pressure-loaded vs. volume-loaded heart. Am. J. Physiol., *242*:H942–H948, 1982.
47. Taylor, A., Thayer, R., and Rao, S.: Human skeletal muscle glycogen synthetase activities with exercise and training. Can. J. Physiol. Pharmacol., *50*:411–412, 1972.
48. Tesch, P.A., and Larsson, L.: Muscle hypertrophy in bodybuilders. Europ. J. Appl. Physiol., *49*:301–306, 1982.
49. Thorstensson, A., Sjodin, B., and Karlsson, J.: Enzyme activities and muscle strength after "spring training" in man. Acta Physiol. Scand., *94*:313–318, 1975.
50. Wilkerson, J.E., and Evonuk, E.: Changes in cardiac and skeletal muscle myosin ATPase activities after exercise. J. Appl. Physiol., *30*:328–330, 1971.

Part III

Factors Affecting Performance

After all of the correct training principles have been used (based on the physiologic principles contained in Part I), there are still other factors that affect performance. For instance, the type of food eaten before certain events can make a significant difference to the athlete's ability to compete. Many misunderstandings exist concerning this important topic. Too many athletes search for and use substances and techniques to improve performance not based on scientific fact. Ergogenic aids must be understood to make intelligent decisions concerning their use. In addition, the environment affects performance and its effect must be taken into account. The final chapter in this part discusses the physiologic differences between males and females which account for the differences in their ability to perform certain activities. All of these factors need to be understood to comprehend the scientific basis of athletic conditioning.

11

Nutrition and Performance

Part I concerned itself with the various systems that allow movement to occur. Energy was shown to be essential to the contractile process, and the various systems that support energy production were discussed. Oxygen was shown to be an essential element for metabolism, and the role of the lungs and circulation in providing oxygen for this purpose was described in some detail. As important as oxygen is to the metabolic processes, there could be no energy production without *fuel*, and the fuel for these processes comes from the food we eat. Because of the relationship between food and energy production, basic nutrition principles are often discussed with the other topics in Part I. However, since Part I is more "system oriented," we chose to place this chapter later in the book to be read along with other topics which affect performance.

The question of what to eat to improve performance is as old as the history of sports. The Greeks ate large quantities of meat to replenish the loss of "muscle substance." Primitive tribes often developed food taboos as success or failure followed certain eating habits. Modern athletes have ingested large quantities of substances such as vitamins and protein powders to improve performance.

The question is: Are there really "miracle foods" that when eaten by athletes improve performance? The answer is: No! A good diet, based on a large variety of foods from each of the basic food groups, will meet all of the basic nutritional requirements of the athlete and non-athlete alike. However, this does not mean that performance cannot be affected by the way an athlete eats. The purpose of this chapter is to look objectively at the factors relating to nutrition that can be used to provide fuel in such a way as to optimize energy production for any given event.

WHAT IS A GOOD DIET?

In 1957, the U.S. Department of Agriculture suggested that Americans include foods from four basic food groups in their daily diet. The four basic foods groups were: (1) milk and dairy products, (2) meat and protein foods, (3) breads and cereals, and (4) fruits and vegetables (Fig. 11–1). In recognition of the need for more fruits, vegetables, and whole-grain cereal in the diet, the basic four groups were expanded to eight: (1) milk, (2) meat (including fish, poultry, cheese, eggs), (3) dark green or deep yellow vegetables, (4) citrus fruits, (5) other fruits and vegetables, (6) bread (consisting of whole-grain or enriched flour), (7) cereal and potatoes, and (8) fats (butter, margarine, etc.). The goal of these later guidelines was to decrease the amount of meat, fat, and refined carbohydrates (sugars) in the diet and increase the amount of vegetables, grains, and fruits. These guidelines can surely be recommended in terms of the guidelines from the American Heart Association and more recently, from the American Cancer Society, which both suggest a decrease in the total fat intake and an increase in fiber containing foods, especially vegetables and fruits for a healthier, longer life. These are also the guidelines that should be used by athletes as the basis for a well-rounded, nutritious diet for everyday life. However, because of the way the metabolic systems work, some foods are more important

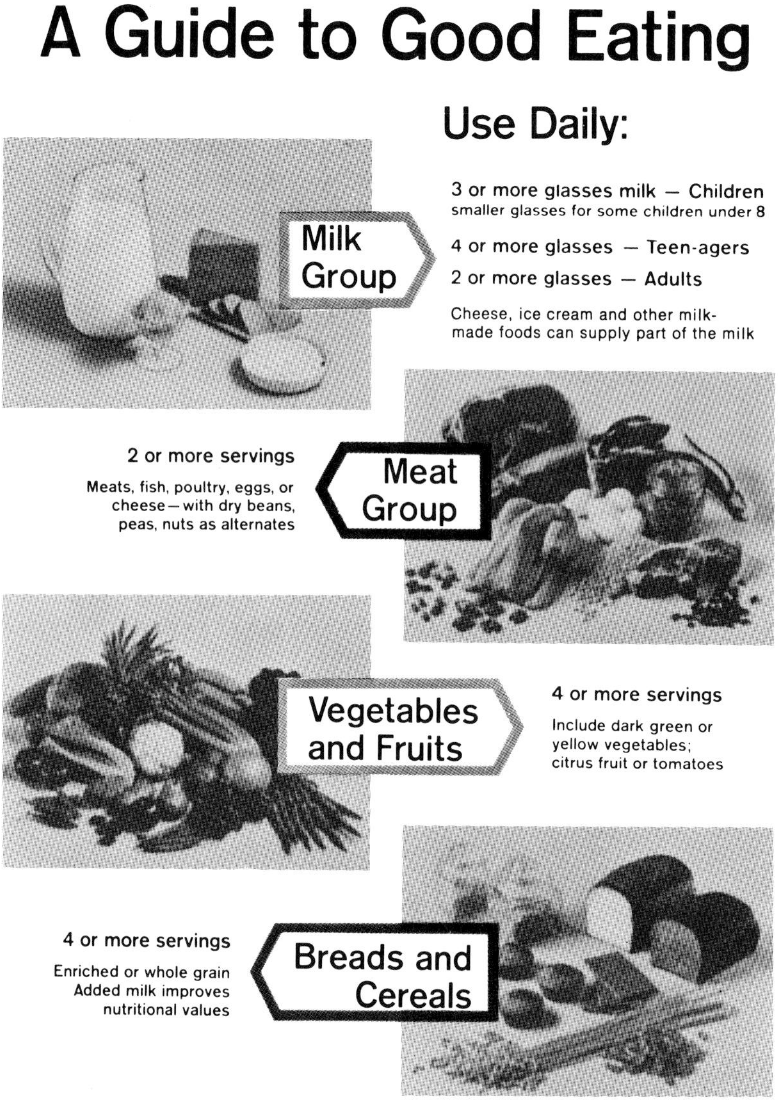
A Guide to Good Eating
Use Daily:
Milk Group
3 or more glasses milk — Children
smaller glasses for some children under 8
4 or more glasses — Teen-agers
2 or more glasses — Adults
Cheese, ice cream and other milk-made foods can supply part of the milk
Meat Group
2 or more servings
Meats, fish, poultry, eggs, or cheese—with dry beans, peas, nuts as alternates
Vegetables and Fruits
4 or more servings
Include dark green or yellow vegetables; citrus fruit or tomatoes
Breads and Cereals
4 or more servings
Enriched or whole grain
Added milk improves nutritional values

Fig. 11–1. The four basic food groups. (Courtesy of the National Dairy Council.)

at certain times and for certain activities than others. For instance, at rest the body gets about equal energy from fats and carbohydrates. Once exercise starts, carbohydrates contribute more of the energy as the intensity of activity increases. In long-term activity, fats may again begin to play a more major role. In addition, other nutrients (water, minerals, and vitamins) contribute to the body's ability to perform and must be considered in any discussion of this type.

BASIC NUTRIENTS

Water

Although water contains no calories, it is necessary for digestion, absorption, and to maintain normal circulatory volume. If fluid volume diminishes during exercise, the transportation of oxygen and nutrients to the cell is impaired and waste products begin to accumulate.

The intake of water is controlled by centers

in the hypothalamus, which are activated by increased concentrations of certain particles in the fluids of the body. Interestingly, thirst mechanisms rarely keep up with the body's need for fluid during work. Since large volumes of sweat can be lost, especially when working in the heat, it is critical to maintain proper fluid intake. Many coaches have athletes weigh themselves before and after workouts to insure that proper rehydration has occurred.

Minerals

Minerals are basic "inorganic" substances that are needed by the body for proper function. Some minerals are needed in fairly large amounts (macrominerals) and other in small amounts (microminerals or trace elements). *Calcium* is probably the most abundant mineral in the body, most being found in the bones and teeth. It is also essential for muscle contraction, blood clotting, cell membrane permeability, and control of the heart.

Phosphorus is also essential and most is found in the form of calcium phosphate to give strength to bones and teeth. It is also used in the metabolic processes, in cell membranes, and in the buffering system. The mineral *iron* plays an important role in the transportation of oxygen. Oxygen is carried primarily by hemoglobin, an iron-containing protein. Women generally have less hemoglobin than men and therefore carry less oxygen per liter of blood. If deficient in this mineral, performance suffers.

Sodium, potassium, and *chloride* are "electrolytes" which help the body maintain cell membrane potential, normal acid-base balance, and normal water balance. A brief description of the minerals, their function and food source is found in Table 11–1.

Vitamins

Vitamins are small organic compounds that function primarily as catalysts in chemical reactions within the body. Because they are so important to proper functioning of metabolism, they are often taken by athletes in large quantities. This practice is seldom helpful and can be dangerous. Water soluble vitamins (the B-complex and vitamin C) can be "washed out" of the system with little damage. However, the fat-soluble vitamins (A, D, E, and K) are less labile and can build up to toxic levels if too much is taken. The major vitamins are shown in Table 11–2 along with their function, source, and recommended daily allowance.

Carbohydrates

Carbohydrates (CHO) get their name from the basic arrangement of the molecules where each carbon (carbo) contains a water molecule (hydrate). A simple sugar such as glucose has the formula $C_6H_{12}O_6$, and is called a *monosaccharide* because it is not connected to other basic sugar molecules. Sucrose and maltose are *disaccharides* because they contain two simple sugars "hooked" together. More complex units are called *polysaccharides* because they are composed of more than two simple sugars. Examples of polysaccharides are starches (in plants) or glycogen (in animals).

The carbohydrates eaten in the diet are broken down by digestion to glucose, which is a major source of energy (fuel) for muscular work. As mentioned in Chapter 3, circulating glucose can be stored by both the liver and muscle using a process called glycogenesis. This process can be reversed (glycogenolysis) to allow the liver to release glucose into the circulation to maintain normal blood sugar levels, or in muscle, to provide energy for muscle contraction through glycolysis.

At rest, carbohydrates supply about half of the energy used by the body. As intensity increases, the body becomes more dependent on these molecules because they can release energy *anaerobically* through the glycolytic pathways. They also release more energy than fat per liter of oxygen, so are more efficient as an energy source for performance requiring oxidative pathways.

Many studies have shown the importance of CHO in endurance events, and it is clear that higher muscle glycogen concentrations are related to increased endurance capacity (Fig. 11–2). Glycogen is important because it is a primary source of energy during high intensity athletic performances, especially those that last for extended periods. Muscle glycogen is used at a higher rate during the first part of activity periods, and then declines at a fairly consistent rate. Blood glucose is

Table 11–1. The Important Minerals in the Body, Their Recommended Daily Intake, Dietary Sources, Major Bodily Functions, and the Effects of Deficiencies and Excesses[a,b]

Mineral	*Amount in Adult Body (g)*	*RDA for Healthy Adult Male and Female[c] (mg)*	*Dietary Sources*	*Major Body Functions*	*Deficiency*	*Excess*
Calcium	1,500	800 800	Milk, cheese, dark-green vegetables, dried legumes	Bone and tooth formation Blood clotting Nerve transmission	Stunted growth Rickets, osteoporosis Convulsions	Not reported in man
Phosphorus	860	800 800	Milk, cheese, meat, poultry, grains	Bone and tooth formation Acid-base balance	Weakness, demineralization of bone Loss of calcium	Erosion of jaw (fossy jaw)
Sulfur	300	(Provided by sulfur amino acids)	Sulfur amino acids (methionine and cystine) in dietary proteins	Constituent of active tissue compounds, cartilage and tendon	Related to intake and deficiency of sulfur amino acids	Excess sulfur amino acid intake leads to poor growth
Potassium	180	1875–5625	Meats, milk, many fruits	Acid-base balance Body water balance Nerve function	Muscular weakness Paralysis	Muscular weakness Death
Chlorine	74	1700–5100	Common salt	Formation of gastric juice Acid-base balance	Muscle cramps Mental apathy Reduced appetite	Vomiting
Sodium	64	1100–3300	Common salt	Acid-base balance Body water balance Nerve function	Muscle cramps Mental apathy Reduced appetite	High blood pressure
Magnesium	25	350 300	Whole grains, green leafy vegetables	Activates enzymes. Involved in protein synthesis	Growth failure Behavioral disturbances Weakness, spasms	Diarrhea
Iron	4.5	10 18	Eggs, lean meats, legumes, whole grains, green leafy vegetables	Constituent of hemoglobin and enzymes involved in energy metabolism	Iron-deficiency anemia (weakness, reduced resistance to infection)	Siderosis Cirrhosis of liver
Fluorine	2.6	1.5–4.0	Drinking water, tea, seafood	May be important in maintenance of bone structure	Higher frequency of tooth decay	Mottling of teeth Increased bone density Neurologic disturbances
Zinc	2	15	Widely distributed in foods	Constituent of enzymes Involved in digestion	Growth failure Small sex glands	Fever, nausea, vomiting, diarrhea

Copper	.1	2 2	Meats, drinking water	Constituent of enzymes associated with iron metabolism	Anemia, bone changes (rare in man)	Rare metabolic condition (Wilson's disease)
Silcon Vanadium Tin Nickel	.024 .018 .017 .010	Not established	Widely distributed in foods	Function unknown (essential for animals)	Not reported in man	Industrial exposures: Silicon—silicosis Vanadium—lung irritation Tin—vomiting Nickel—acute pneumonitis
Selenium	.013	.05–.02	Seafood, meat, grains	Functions in close association with Vitamin E	Anemia (rare)	Gastrointestinal disorders, lung irritation
Manganese	.012	Not established (Diet provides 6–8 per day)	Widely distributed in foods	Constituent of enzymes involved in fat synthesis	In animals: poor growth, disturbances of nervous system, reproductive abnormalities	Poisoning in manganese mines: generalized disease of nervous system
Iodine	.011	.15	Marine fish and shellfish, dairy products, many vegetables	Constituent of thyroid hormones	Goiter (enlarged thyroid)	Very high intakes depress thyroid activity
Molybdenum	.009	Not established (Diet provides .4 per day)	Legumes, cereals, organ meats	Constituent of some enzymes	Not reported in man	Inhibition of enzymes
Chromium	.006	.05–.2	Fats, vegetable oils, meats	Involved in glucose and energy metabolism	Impaired ability to metabolize glucose	Occupational exposures: skin and kidney damage
Cobalt	.0015	(Required as vitamin B_{12})	Organ and muscle meats, milk	Constituent of vitamin B_{12}	Not reported in man	Industrial exposure: dermatitis and diseases of red blood cells
Water	40,000 (60% of body weight)	1.5 liters per day	Solid foods, liquids, drinking water	Transport of nutrients Temperature regulation Participates in metabolic reactions	Thirst, dehydration	Headaches, nausea Edema High blood pressure

[a]From Scrimshaw, N.S., and Young, V.R.: The requirements of human nutrition. Sci. Amer. *235*:50–73, 1976.
[b]Recommended Dietary Allowances, Revised 1980. Food and Nutrition Board, National Academy of Sciences—National Research Council, Washington, D.C.
[c]First values are for males.

Table 11–2. Water- and Fat-soluble Vitamins, Their Recommended Daily Intake, Dietary Sources, Major Bodily Functions, and Effects of Deficiencies and Excesses[a,b]

Vitamin	*RDA for Healthy Adult Male and Female[c] (mg)*	*Dietary Sources*	*Major Body Functions*	*Deficiency*	*Excess*
Water-soluble					
Vitamin B-1 (Thiamine)	1.4–1.5 1.0–1.1	Pork, organ meats, whole grains, legumes	Coenzyme (thiamine pyrophosphate) in reactions involving the removal of carbon dioxide	Beriberi (peripheral nerve changes, edema, heart failure)	None reported
Vitamin B-2 (Riboflavin)	1.6–1.7 1.2–1.3	Widely distributed in foods	Constituent of two flavin nucleotide coenzymes involved in energy metabolism (FAD and FMN)	Reddened lips, cracks at corner of mouth (cheilosis), lesions of eye	None reported
Niacin	18–19 13–14	Liver, lean meats, grains, legumes (can be formed from tryptophan)	Constituent of two coenzymes involved in oxidation-reduction reactions (NAD and NADP)	Pellagra (skin and gastrointestinal lesions, nervous, mental disorders)	Flushing, burning and tingling around neck, face, and hands
Vitamin B-6 (Pyridoxine)	2.2 2.0	Meats, vegetables, whole-grain cereals	Coenzyme (pyridoxal phosphate) involved in amino acid metabolism	Irritability, convulsions, muscular twitching, dermatitis near eyes, kidney stones	None reported
Pantothenic acid	4–7 4–7	Widely distributed in foods	Constituent of coenzyme A, which plays a central role in energy metabolism	Fatigue, sleep disturbances, impaired coordination, nausea (rare in man)	None reported
Folacin	0.4 0.4	Legumes, green vegetables, whole-wheat products	Coenzyme (reduced form) involved in transfer of single-carbon units in nucleic acid and amino acid metabolism	Anemia, gastrointestinal disturbances, diarrhea, red tongue	None reported
Vitamin B-12	0.003 0.003	Muscle meats, eggs, dairy products (not present in plant foods)	Coenzyme involved in transfer of single-carbon units in nucleic acid metabolism	Pernicious anemia, neurologic disorders	None reported

Biotin	0.10–0.20 0.10–0.20	Legumes, vegetables, meats	Coenzyme required for fat synthesis, amino acid metabolism, and glycogen (animal-starch) formation	Fatigue, depression, nausea, dermatitis, muscular pains	None reported
Vitamin C (Ascorbic acid)	60 60	Citrus fruits, tomatoes, green peppers, salad greens	Maintains intercellular matrix of cartilage, bone, and dentine. Important in collagen synthesis	Scurvy (degeneration of skin, teeth, blood vessels, epithelial hemorrhages)	Relatively nontoxic. Possibility of kidney stones
Fat Soluble					
Vitamin A (Retinol)	1.0 0.8	Provitamin A (beta-carotene) widely distributed in green vegetables. Retinol present in milk, butter, cheese, fortified margarine	Constituent of rhodopsin (visual pigment). Maintenance of epithelial tissues. Role in mucopolysaccharide synthesis	Xerophthalmia (keratinization of ocular tissue), night blindness, permanent blindness	Headache, vomiting, peeling of skin, anorexia, swelling of long bones
Vitamin D	0.075 0.075	Cod-liver oil, eggs, dairy products, fortified milk, and margarine	Promotes growth and mineralization of bones. Increases absorption of calcium	Rickets (bone deformities) in children. Osteomalacia in adults.	Vomiting diarrhea, loss of weight, kidney damage
Vitamin E (Tocopherol)	10 8	Seeds, green leafy vegetables, margarines, shortenings	Functions as an antitoxidant to prevent cell-membrane damage.	Possibly anemia	Relatively nontoxic
Vitamin K (Phylloquinone)	0.07–0.14 0.07–0.14	Green leafy vegetables. Small amount in cereals, fruits, and meats	Important in blood clotting (involved in formation of active prothrombin)	Conditioned deficiencies associated with severe bleeding; internal hemorrhages	Relatively nontoxic. Synthetic forms at high doses may cause jaundice

[a]From Scrimshaw, N.S., and Young, V.R.: The requirements of human nutrition. Sci. Amer. *235*:50, 1976.
[b]Recommended Dietary Allowances. Revised 1980. Food and Nutrition Board, National Academy of Sciences—National Research Council, Washington, D.C.
[c]First values are for males.

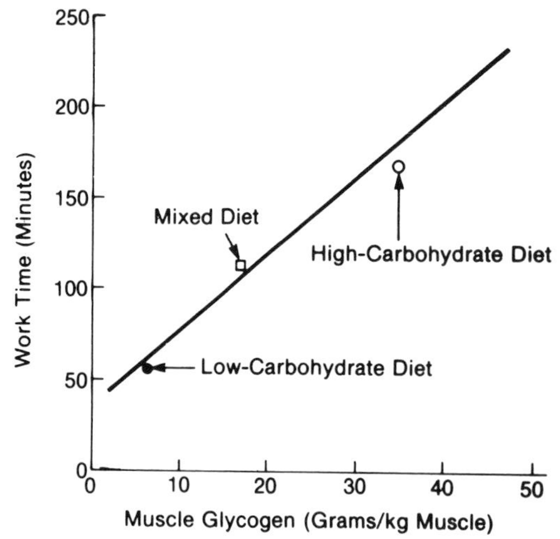

Fig. 11–2. Effects of a mixed diet, a low-carbohydrate diet, and a high-carbohydrate diet on the initial glycogen content of the quadriceps femoris muscle and the duration of exercise on a bicycle ergometer, the higher the initial muscle glycogen content, the longer the duration of exercise. (From Mathews, D.K., Fox, E.L., Bowers, R.W., Foss, M.L. *Physiological Basis of Physical Education and Athletics,* 4th Ed. Courtesy of W.B. Saunders Co., 1988.)

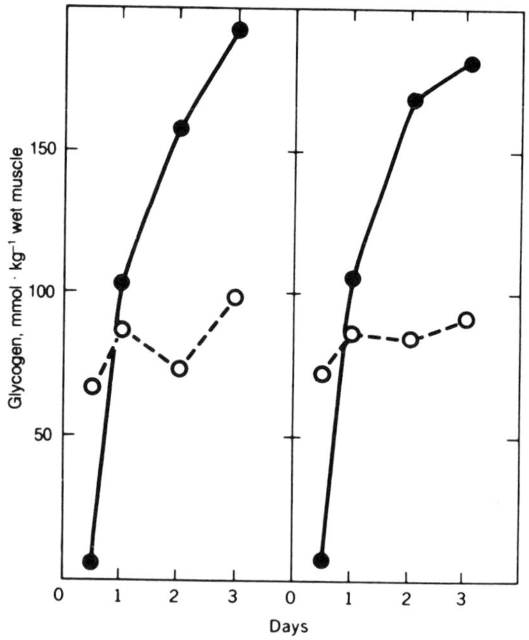

Fig. 11–3. Two subjects were exercised on the same cycle ergometer, one on each side exercising with one leg, while the other leg, rested (dashed line). After exercising to exhaustion the subjects' glycogen content was analyzed in specimens from the lateral portion of the quadriceps muscle. Thereafter a carbohydrate-rich diet was taken for 3 days. Note that the glycogen content increased significantly in the leg that had been previously emptied of its glycogen content. (Modified from Astrand, P.O., and Rodahl, K. *Textbook of Work Physiology: Physiological Basis of Exercises,* 3rd Ed. Courtesy of McGraw Hill, 1986.)

supplied by the liver. In the early stages, little blood sugar is used for muscle contraction. As glycogen stores decrease, blood glucose makes a larger and larger contribution to the energy needs of the muscles. However, since the liver is limited in how much glucose it can produce using gluconeogenic sources, the muscles rely more and more on their glycogen reserves resulting in an acceleration of muscle glycogen use and an earlier onset of fatigue.

It is also clear that certain techniques can increase the concentrations of glycogen in the muscle. In a classic study, Bergstrom and Hultman exercised two cyclists to exhaustion using only one leg on a cycle ergometer. After the work bout, subjects rested and ate a high-carbohydrate diet. Several important ideas came from this experiment. First, only the leg that was used was depleted of glycogen, which showed that glycogen in an inactive muscle cannot be used as energy for an active muscle. Second, depletion of glycogen in a muscle allows it to *supercompensate* upon refeeding and fill to much higher levels. Note that the non-exercised limb was not affected much by refeeding (Fig. 11–3).

Studies showing the importance of glycogen to performance and studies showing the potential of the body to supercompensate led athletes to the technique of "carbohydrate loading." Early guidelines suggested a "depletion" run about 7 days prior to the event, followed by a *low* carbohydrate, *high* fat/*high* protein diet for several days, and then a *high* carbohydrate diet for the last 3 days prior to the event with little activity during the refeeding days. However, little evidence exists that the carbohydrate starvation period was beneficial and many athletes found it most uncomfortable.

A more moderate approach has since been recommended for carbohydrate loading. Using this approach, the athlete exercises to exhaustion 3 or 4 days prior to the event. The exhaustive exercise should include hard interval work if the white fibers are to be exhausted. He then tapers his work, eating a balanced diet containing a substantial level of carbohydrate, to allow the muscles to supercompensate. This technique has proven to be as good as the old approach and much more comfortable. Some researchers have suggested doing away with the depletion run (a modified regimen) with the athlete simply reducing the training intensity several days prior to competition while eating a diet at least 55% carbohydrates. This technique has also proved to be effective (Fig. 11–4).

There are several factors to consider when using carbohydrate loading techniques: First, some individuals do not respond to the procedure and others get less able to respond after using it routinely. Second, some athletes eat such a terrible diet while loading that their basic nutritional balance may suffer. Third, about 3 grams of water is stored with each gram of glycogen. In some events, this extra weight would be a liability rather than a help. For endurance activity, the extra water is great because it can help prevent dehydration. Fourth, initial speed is not influenced by increased glycogen, only the amount of time that this best speed can be maintained (Fig. 11–5). From these data, it appears that carbohydrate loading is probably needed for only those events that are longer than an hour.

Athletes who train at high intensities day after day deplete their glycogen reserves automatically and must be extremely careful to eat enough carbohydrate to maintain normal levels. Figure 11–6 shows the effect of heavy training with a low and a high carbohydrate diet. Consistent heavy work can often result in chronic fatigue because of glycogen depletion and coaches must be sure that sufficient carbohydrates are available in the diet to maintain normal levels. If the diet available to the athlete has enough carbohydrate (from 50 to 70%), the natural increase in calories associated with training will insure sufficient carbohydrate to maintain glycogen stores.

Fats

Fats are long-chain hydrocarbons which contain little oxygen and therefore contain much more energy per gram than carbohydrates. Fat supplies about 40% of the calories of the average American diet and these levels have been associated with increased risk from both heart disease and cancer.

Fat provides a little more than half of the energy at rest and becomes a major source of energy during long-term activity of low to moderate intensity. Whereas glycogen can provide between 1200 and 1500 calories of energy, fat stores in the average person are

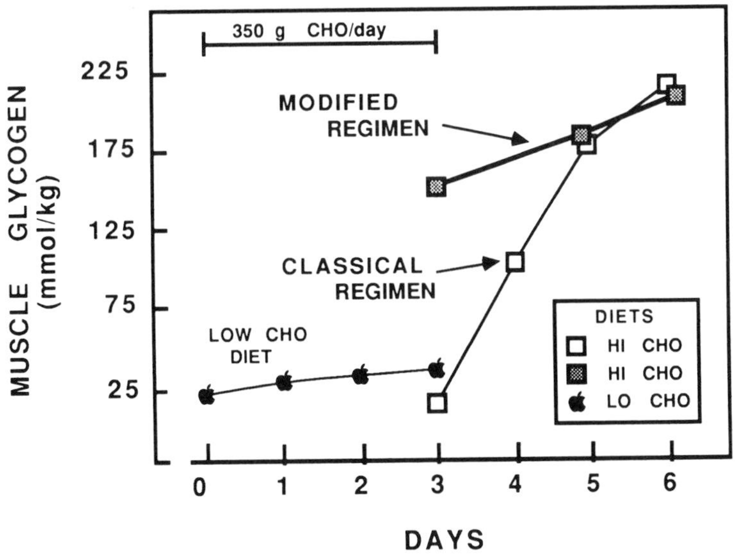

Fig. 11–4. A comparison of the results of the modified glycogen loading regimen described by Sherman, et al. (1981) and the results of the classic method of glycogen loading developed by Scandinavian researchers. (From Sherman, W.M. et al.: Effects of exercise-diet manipulation muscle glycogen and its subsequent utilization during performance. Int. J. Sports Med., 2:114, 1981.)

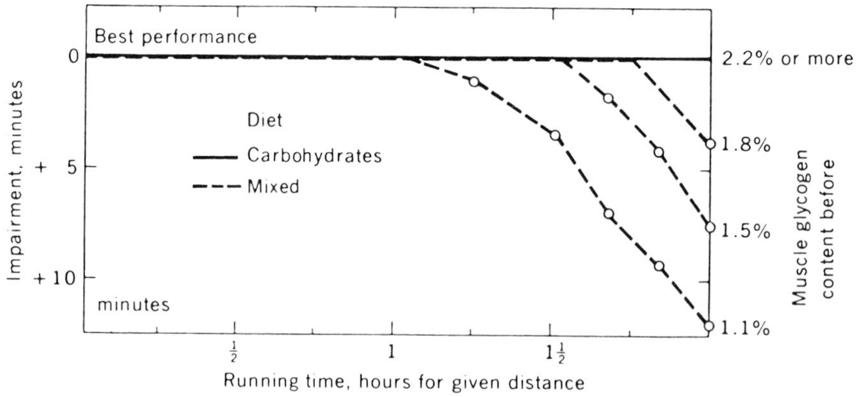

Fig. 11–5. Schematic illustration of the importance of a high glycogen content in the muscle before a 30-km race. The lower the initial glycogen store, the slower the speed at the end of the race, compared with the race during which the muscle glycogen content was 2.2 g of more per 100 g muscle at the start of the race. For the first hour, however, no difference in speed was observed. (From Astrand, P.O., and Rodahl, K. *Textbook of Work Physiology: Physiological Basis of Exercises*, 3rd Ed. Courtesy of McGraw Hill, 1986.)

in excess of 100,000 calories. Fat has value not only in energy supply, but also for protection of the internal organs and for insulation. Dietary fat also provides the fat soluble vitamins, A, D, E, and K and essential fatty acids which are not synthesized by the body. Provided these basic dietary requirements can be met, a diet high in fat is not essential and indeed, can be harmful in terms of overall health.

Since muscle and liver glycogen stores are limited, using more fat for energy could be helpful to "spare" the glycogen stores. Fortunately, the body can increase its ability to use fat for energy through training. Endurance athletes actually do use a higher per-

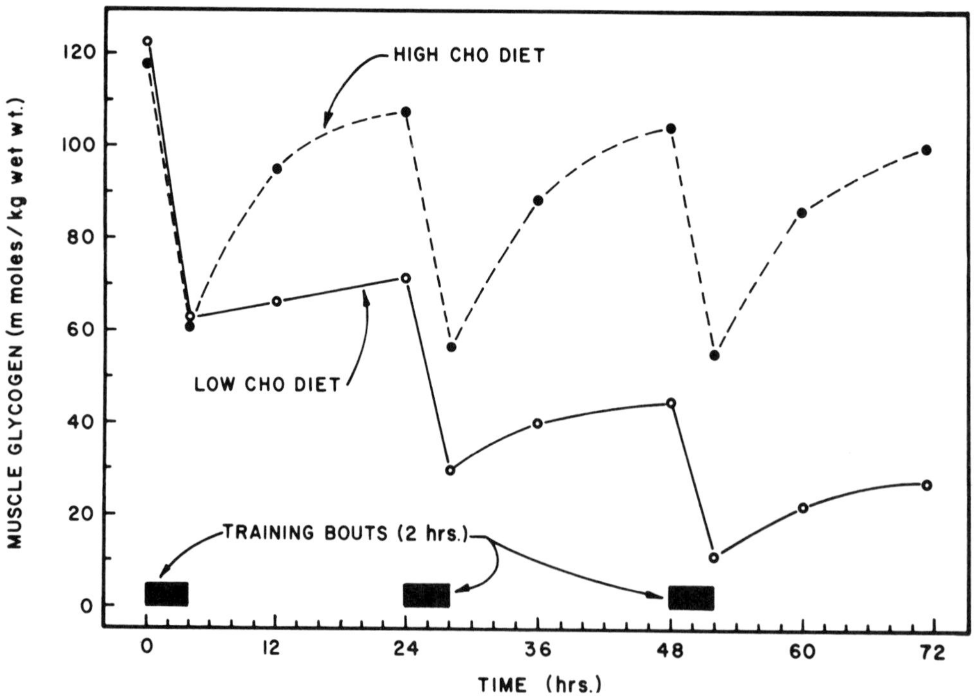

Fig. 11–6. Muscle glycogen content of the vastus lateralis (thigh) during 3 successive days of heavy training with diets whose caloric compositions were 40% carbohydrate (low CHO) and 70% carbohydrate (high CHO). (From Costill, D.L., and Miller, J.M.: Nutrition for endurance sport: carbohydrate and fluid balance. Int. J. Sports Med., *1*:12, 1980.)

centage of fat during endurance work, probably by increasing the mitochondrial and enzyme content of the muscle. This adjustment allows them to go longer at a faster pace before glycogen depletion causes muscular fatigue.

Other than this natural adaptation from training, the only way to increase fat usage is to increase the FFA levels in the blood. In the laboratory, injecting heparin raises blood FFA and increases the contribution of fat to the total energy need. Caffeine has been shown to have similar effects in many people. Since increased levels of blood FFA increase their uptake, it might be tempting to eat more fats. Unfortunately, eating more fat does not stimulate the body to burn more fat because ingested fat is carried as triglycerides. Increased endurance, with the associated increase in mitochondria and enzyme content is still the best way to spare glycogen during work.

Some interesting studies have been done using a diet where 85% of the total calories come from fat. After 4 weeks of "training" on this diet, the R dropped from 0.83 during submaximal exercise (about 64% $\dot{V}O_2max$) to 0.72 with a 4-fold reduction in muscle glycogen use. Some of these studies show an increase in endurance time after fat adaptation. It is unknown whether this adaptation would work to increase endurance at higher intensities of work. There were problems associated with this diet, including lethargy, mild constipation, etc. There is also the problem relating to the health consequences of such a diet for a long period of time. What these studies do indicate, however, is the body's adaptability in the face of strange treatments.

Proteins

Proteins are nitrogen containing carbon compounds formed from amino acids that are used as the major structural components of cells, antibodies, many hormones, and enzymes, as well as for growth, repair and maintenance of body tissue, and many other functions associated with normal living. There are over 20 different amino acids (the small basic components of protein) and 8 are considered to be "essential," meaning that they must be ingested in the food we eat because the body cannot produce them from scratch. Animal products are the best sources of essential or complete protein (proteins that contain all of the essential amino acids). Vegetables and grains often lack one or more of these important structures. Protein constitutes from 10 to 15% of the caloric intake of the average diet, and the recommended daily allowance (RDA) for protein is about .8 g per kg of body weight.

Since muscle is protein, many athletes have increased their intake of this substance to help muscle growth. Large quantities of eggs and meat or amino acid supplements are common "training aids" for strength athlete. Are these practices necessary for muscle growth? Many studies have used protein supplementation to evaluate its effect on muscle hypertrophy, strength, or work performance. Most have found little positive effect from increasing protein intake during training. However, more recent studies which have examined nitrogen balance (a way of telling if the body is getting enough protein for its needs) have found evidence of an increased need for protein, especially during the early stages of training. Based on these studies, it might be a good idea for both endurance and strength athletes to increase their protein intake during the first 2 to 3 weeks to about 2.0 g per kg per day.

The contribution of protein to the overall energy needs of the body is not great, probably in the range from 5 to 10%. However, this contribution could be significant in high level competition and should not be overlooked. Proteins are also important to the smooth running of the energy systems and particpate in several roles to help maintain proper metabolic activity.

EATING GUIDELINES BASED ON RESEARCH

General Guidelines

Studies evaluating athlete's diets have found them to be similar in composition to normal diets except that more calories are consumed to support the needs of training and performance. It is likely that any increased need for vitamins and other nutrients are met by the increased intake of total calories. Based on these facts, athletes should probably use the guidelines for healthy eating mentioned at the beginning of this chapter as the model for obtaining basic nutrients they need. Further they should probably lower the total fat intake to less than 30% of total calories not only for performance, but also for health. The ideal balance of nutrients would be approximately as follows: Protein, 15%; Carbohydrate, 50 to 65%, and fat, no more than 30%.

Pre-Competition Meal

There are probably no foods eaten before a competition that will result in an increased performance. However, certain foods (such as foods high in fat, highly seasoned foods, or gas-forming foods) may hinder performance and these foods should be avoided. The goals for the pre-competition meal are to: (1) provide enough energy to preclude hunger or weakness during the competition, (2) provide enough carbohydrate of the proper type (complex) to load the liver and muscles to the desired level without stimulating excessive insulin response, (3) provide food that can be easily digested to avoid upsetting the gastrointestinal tract during the activity and which will allow the stomach and upper bowel to be fairly empty by competition time, and (4) provide food that is acceptable to the athlete based on his past experience and background.

Based on these recommendations, the meal could consist of many different combinations of foods and still be acceptable. For instance, if the athletes are used to steak prior to a game, you could provide a small, lean steak, a large baked potato, some easily digested vegetables, rolls and a beverage. This meal emphasizes carbohydrates, but would be acceptable to the athlete used to eating steak before the game. Some athletes might be more comfortable with pasta dishes such as spaghetti; others with tacos or tortillas. These main dishes could be supplemented with a salad, rolls and drink to make an acceptable pre-event meal.

It is important to eat from 3 to 4 hours prior to the event to allow time for digestion to occur. It is also important to avoid a large dose of simple carbohydrate just prior to the event. Simple sugars are rapidly digested, but they cause an increase in insulin which could clear the sugar from the bloodstream followed by a fall in blood sugar just when you need it most. High levels of insulin also inhibit the release of FFA and cause an increased use of glycogen during the initial stages of exercise.

Eating During Competition

Interestingly, whereas a simple sugar solution may be detrimental just before competition, this same solution may enhance performance if consumed during the performance. When sugar solutions are taken during exercise, they do not elicit the same response as before exercise. Thus, the fuel becomes available to the muscle without lowering blood sugar level. A highly concentrated solution may delay stomach emptying, but in long-term events, this delay may not be detrimental because of the continuing need for energy. In events such as the triathalon, which can last for 10 to 14 hours, it is essential to take energy on a regular basis. This is usually taken in the form of a sugar drink to maintain proper water balance at the same time. The newer *polyglucose* drinks are excellent for maintaining both energy and water balance during long-term events. It is important to remember that the thirst mechanisms do not usually keep up with the need, so weighing an athlete during heavy training can give a good indication of the ongoing needs in terms of liquid during competition. The athlete can then take the required fluid load and maintain a normal hydration state and at the same time keep blood glucose levels in a normal range.

Eating After Competition

Just as carbohydrates are needed before and during competition, they must be available after as well. Studies have shown that muscle glycogen was restored to muscle within 24 hours if athletes ate a carbohydrate-rich diet after exhaustive exercise. Other research has shown the need to begin repletion of carbohydrate stores within 30 minutes of the completion of exercises. It is a good idea to lower the work load following competition and maintain a fairly high carbohydrate level to allow muscles to regain a normal glycogen level.

Making Weight

One of the most serious problems of athletic competition is the problem of "making weight." This problem exists in sports where weight classifications make it possible to gain advantage over an opponent by getting to an extremely low weight during the weigh in and then competing at a higher, more normal weight (wrestling is probably the worst offender in this category). Many athletes in these sports use crash diets or dehydration (including rubberized sweat suits, steam or sauna baths, spitting to lose saliva, restricting water intake, and using diuretics) to make their weight. Other athletes, such as gymnasts, worry about weight because excess weight affects their ability to perform certain movements not only in terms of strength, but with balance as well. Some of these athletes become anorexic or bulimic because of the pressure to meet certain weight demands set by themselves or their coaches. One study showed that 32% of 182 female collegiate athletes practiced at least one of the weight-control behaviors defined as pathogenic, which included self-induced vomiting, eating binges more than twice weekly, and the use of laxatives, diet pills, and/or diuretics. Any of the procedures mentioned are potentially dangerous and will often actually decrease the performance of those using them.

What can be done to help prevent these abuses to the body? The key to proper nutritional practices in athletics is a wise and well-trained coach. A coach who understands the dangers of improper weight control techniques will teach his/her charges properly and many of the problems will disappear. Another important step would be for professional organizations to establish *standards* for various activities. These standards could be based on lean body mass evaluation and require that athletes maintain a certain weight based on a realistic lean body mass. For men, the minimal competition weight might realistically require at least 5% fat. This means that the minimum weight would be their lean body mass (LBM) divided by 0.95 (Minimum weight = LBM/0.95). For women, this value could be 90 (at least 10% fat). Other suggestions include weighing in immediately before the contest. Athletes who had depleted their weight incorrectly would be unable to compete effectively in that state and would soon begin competing at a state where strength and endurance were normal.

The potential health hazards of incorrect weight loss practices led the American College of Sports Medicine to publish a position stand on *Weight Loss in Wrestlers.* This statement basically re-emphasized the need for a more moderate and healthful approach as follows:

1. Prolonged fasting and diet programs that severely limit caloric intake are scientifically undesirable and can be medically dangerous.
2. These programs result in mostly a loss of water, electrolytes, minerals, glycogen stores, and other fat-free tissue with minimum fat loss (in other words, they do not work).
3. Mild caloric restriction approaches are healthier.
4. Dynamic exercise can be used to lose weight and at the same time conserve LBM.
5. A sound diet and a good exercise program is the best approach for losing weight. Weight loss should not exceed 2 pounds per week.
6. To maintain proper weight requires a lifetime commitment to proper eating habits and regular physical activity.

SELECTED READINGS

1. Ahlborg, B., Berstrom, J., Ekelund L., et al.: Muscle glycogen electrolytes during prolonged physical exercise. Acta Physiol. Scand., *70*:129–142, 1967.
2. American College of Sports Medicine: Weight loss in wrestlers. Med. Sci. Sports, *8*:xi–xiii, 1976.
3. Bergstrom, J., Hermansen, L., Hultman, E., et al.: Diet, muscle glycogen and physical performance. Acta Physiol. Scand., *71*:140–150, 1967.
4. Bergstrom, J., and Hultman E.: Muscle glycogen synthesis after exercise: An enhancing factor localized to the muscle cells in man. Nature, *210*:309–310, 1967.
5. Brownell, K.D., and Foreyt, J.P.: *Handbook of Eating Disorders: Physiology, Psychology, and Treatment of Obesity, Anorexia, and Bulimia.* New York: Basic Books, Inc., 1986.
6. Conlee, R.K.: Muscle Glycogen and Exercise Endurance: A Twenty-Year Perspective. Exer. Sport Sci. Rev., *15*:1–28, 1987.
7. Costill, D.L., Coyle, E., Dalsky, G., et al.: Effects of elevated plasma FFA and insulin on muscle glycogen usage during exercise. J. Appl. Physiol., *43*(4):695–699, 1977.
8. Fisher, G., Remington, D., and Parent, E.: *How to*

Lower Your Fat Thermostat. Provo: Vitality House, 1983.
9. Foster, C., Costill, D.L., and Fink, W.J.: Effects of pre-exercise feedings on endurance performance. Med. Sci. Sports, *11*(1):1–5, 1979.
10. Fox E. (ed.): *Report of the Ross Symposium on Nutrient Utilization During Exercise.* Columbus, Ohio, Ross Laboratories, 1983.
11. Fox, E.L., Bowers, R.W. and Foss, M.L.: *The Physiological Basis of Physical Education and Athletics.* Philadelphia: W.B. Saunders Co., 1988.
12. Girandola, R.N., Bulbulian R., Hecker, A., et al.: Effects of liquid and solid meals and time of feeding on VO_2max. Med. Sci. Sports, *11*(1):101, 1979.
13. Jette, M., Pelletier, O., Parker, L., et al.: The nutritional and metabolic effects of a carbohydrate-rich diet in a glycogen supercompensation training regime. Am. J. Clin. Nutri., *31*(2):2140–2148, 1978.
14. Gontzer, I., R. Sutzescu, and S. Aumitrache: The Influence of Adaptation to Physical Effort on Nitrogen Balance in Man. Nutr. Rep. Inter., *11*:231–236, 1975.
15. Karlsson, J., and Saltin, B.: Diet, muscle glycogen and endurance performance. J. Appl. Physiol., *31*(2):203–206, 1971.
16. McArdle, W.D., Katch, F.I., and Katch, V.L.: *Exericse Physiology; Energy, Nutrition, and Human Performance.* Philadelphia: Lea & Febiger, 1986.
17. Mirkin, G.: Carbohydrate loading: a dangerous practice. JAMA, *223*(13):1511–1512, 1973.
18. Nelson, R.A.: Nutrition and physical performance. Physician Sports Med., *10*(4):55–59, 1982.
19. *Nutrition for the Athlete.* Washington D.C., American Association for Health, Physical Education and Recreation, 1971.
20. Parizkova, J., and V.A. Rogozkin: *Nutrition, Physical Fitness, and Health.* Baltimore: University Park Press, 1978.
21. Pavlou, K.N., W.P. Steffee, R.H. Lerman, et al.: Effects of dieting and exercise on lean body mass, oxygen uptake, and strength. Med. Sci. Sports Exerc., *17*:466–471, 1985.
22. Rosen, L.W., D.B. McKeag, D.O. Hough, et al.: Pathogenic weight-control behavior in female athletes. Physician Sports Med., *14*(#1):79–86, 1986.
23. Saltin, B., and Karlsson, J.: Muscle glycogen utilization during work of different intensities. Adv. Exper. Med. Biol., *11*:289–299, 1971.
24. Sherman, W.M., D.L. Costill, W.J. Fink, et al.: Effects of exercise-diet manipulation on muscle glycogen and its subsequent utilization during performance. Internat. J. Sports Med., *2*:1–15, 1981.
25. Willmore, J.H., and D.L. Costill: Training for Sport and Activity, the physiological basis of the conditioning process, 3rd Ed., Dubuque: William C. Brown Co., 1988.
26. Sherman, W.M.: Carbohydrates, muscle glycogen, and muscle glycogen supercompensation. In *Ergogenic Aids in Sport,* by Williams M.H. (ed). Champaign: Human Kinetics Publishers, 1983.
27. Stamford, B.: Does carbohydrate loading really work: Physician Sports Med., *12*(9):196, Sept 1984.
28. Williams, M.: Nutritional aspects of human physical and athletic performance. Springfield, Charles C Thomas, 1976.

12

Ergogenic Aids

Since the beginning of athletic competition, athletes have searched for some easy ways to improve their performance, whether by the magical potions used by medieval warriors or the countless drugs and nutrients employed by modern day athletes. In the 1880s, the Kaffiers of Southeast Africa used a hard liquor called "dop" as a stimulant to enhance performance. The term "doping" was coined to refer to the use of substances alien to the body, or of physiologic substances in abnormal amounts with the exclusive aim of attaining an artificial and unfair advantage over other athletes.

Coaches and athletes are still searching for ways to gain the "competitive edge." If an athlete uses some substance or treatment and performs well, he may give credit to this substance (called an *ergogenic aid*) for his success. This may lead to other athletes trying the same substance or treatment. Whether the substance or treatment really helps performance or not, depends on how it affects the athlete either physiologically or psychologically. The purpose of this chapter is to discuss the commonly used ergogenic aids and evaluate their effectiveness and/or danger so that the reader can better evaluate the substances or treatments available in terms of their real effects.

The purpose of ergogenic aids is to improve performance, speed recovery, or both. This may be accomplished by: (1) increasing the efficiency of the circulatory system and facilitating the transport of oxygen, fuel, and wastes, (2) counteracting the CNSs' inhibitory effect on a muscle's maximal contraction, thus allowing development of greater force, (3) directly affecting muscle fibers, (4) altering the supply of muscular fuel, or (5) delaying the onset of feeling of fatigue by acting on the nervous system. Ergogenic aids are usually nutritional, pharmacologic, physiologic, or psychologic.

The following ergogenic aids are commonly used:

VITAMINS

The known role of vitamins in the metabolic pathways relates to their use as components of coenzymes, the important carriers in the metabolic pathways. These critical molecules serve about the same role in all forms of life, but higher animals have lost the capacity to synthesize them, so they must be ingested in the food we eat. The critical role of vitamins in the metabolic pathways has led to the misconception that excess vitamin supplementation would help the metabolic pathways work more effectively with a concomitant increase in performance. In addition, it was once believed that the need for vitamins in the metabolic pathways increased out of proportion to the increase in metabolism caused by increased exercise. However, there is little evidence that "extra" vitamins help metabolism in any way and most research shows that vitamin needs increase in about the same proportion as does metabolism. This would suggest that the increased vitamin intake associated with increased food intake automatically provides all the vitamins needed by most athletes.

Van Huss compared the recovery rate of laboratory animals that received vitamin C before exercising with animals that received no supplements. Those that received vitamin C recovered more quickly. Counsilman agreed, stating that, "all research seems to indicate an increasing need for vitamin C during the stress of a training program." He further pointed out that vitamin C cannot be stored in the body, and moderate excesses are harmless and will be excreted.

Conversely, it has been found that excessive vitamin C supplementation contributes to destruction of natural sources in the body, and can contribute to malnutrition after the supplementation is discontinued. Rhead and Schrauzer found that the vitamin C level in the blood of persons who consumed 5 g of vitamin C per day were no different from the levels in the blood of those who ate a similar diet but took no vitamin C. This suggests that the increased rate of destruction of natural vitamin C produced by the supplementation counteracted the effect of the supplementation itself. Further, Herbert and Jacob found the excessive dose of vitamin C taken with food destroys vitamin B_{12}.

Other vitamins have been used to increase performance, but little evidence exists to support their use. If taken in moderate amounts, vitamins are probably harmless and could be beneficial if the diet is not nutritionally balanced. However, large quantities of fat soluble vitamins (A, D, E, and K) can be toxic if consumed in excess since these vitamins are stored primarily in the liver. The water soluble vitamins (C and B complex) generally do not have adverse effects since any excess is excreted by the kidneys. However, long-term vitamin supplementation can eventually create an unnatural adaptation-dependence. Information from the American Medical Association's Division of Foods and Nutrition indicates that a balanced diet is still the best method of obtaining adequate vitamins.

BLOOD DOPING

One of the great success stories of the 1984 Summer Olympic Games in Los Angeles was the achievements of the U.S. cyclists. Unfortunately these accomplishments were tainted when 7 members of the team, 4 of whom were medalists, admitted receiving red blood cell transfusion (blood doping) several days prior to competing. In essence, blood doping refers to the process of infusing blood, either whole or packed red blood cells, into an athlete before competition. Most often the athlete's own blood is withdrawn several weeks before the event, stored and then reinfused just prior to the event. Once blood is withdrawn, the athlete's body will regenerate new blood cells to restore normal hemoglobin levels. Upon reinfusion, there will be an increase in total blood volume as well as an increase in RBC concentration. Approximately 45% of the volume of normal blood is red blood cells (RBC). These cells contain hemoglobin (Hb) which has an affinity for oxygen of approximately 1.34 ml oxygen/g Hb. The greater the Hb concentration the greater the oxygen carrying capacity of blood. During heavy exercise, muscles require a great deal of oxygen and any increase in the oxygen carrying capacity of the blood can affect the ability of the muscle to produce energy.

The three main factors governing maximal oxygen uptake (and therefore endurance) are ventilation ($\dot{V}_E$), gas transportation ($\dot{Q}$), and the metabolic processes in the cell (tissue respiration). Some evidence suggests that gas transportation by the blood is the main limiting factor rather than either respiration or metabolic processes. If this is the case, increasing the amount of oxygen carried by blood doping could increase the ability of the body to produce energy and therefore affect performance.

There is no question about the effects of reduced oxygen carrying capacity *(anemia)*. Anemics demonstrate a pronounced reduction in $\dot{V}O_2max$ compared to normal healthy individuals. Reductions in performance also occur following blood withdrawal. This may be due to blood volume changes as well as reduced oxygen carrying capacity. Since decreases in Hb and the resultant decrease in oxygen transport reduce $\dot{V}O_2max$, it is reasonable to assume that an increase in Hb would augment performance.

In the early 1970s, Dr. Bjorn Ekbolm reported an increased endurance time (25%) in athletes whose blood was withdrawn and later reinfused. Since 1972 when these results were first reported, many researchers have tried to reproduce these results without success. However, a review of these studies reveals that their failure was due to; (1) too little infused blood, or (2) insufficient time between the time of withdrawal and reinfusion to allow the body to fully recover.

The first factor is critical because red blood cells are fairly fragile and have a life span of only 120 days and many RBCs are lost in the storage and reinfusion procedure. Blood reinfused after 3 weeks of cold storage is only about 60% viable. Modern technology has increased storage time to between 6 to 8 weeks with an 85% recovery of RBC.

Recovery time between removal and reinfusion of blood also is an important factor. Research has shown that it requires 3 to 4 weeks for Hb concentrations to return to normal after a 400-ml phlebotomy and 6 to 10 weeks when 900 ml are withdrawn. If blood Hb concentrations are allowed to return to normal before reinfusion, Hb concentrations may remain elevated for several days or weeks. However, if the reinfusion occurs before Hb concentrations are back to normal, the effect would be greatly diminished, especially if there has been a 15 to 40% loss in viable RBC's.

Table 12–1 summarizes the blood-doping research from 1966 to 1982. The common thread through all the studies that were successful in increasing $\dot{V}O_2$ max and/or endurance time was that the blood volume infused ranged from 800 to 1200 ml and reinfusion was between 4 to 6 weeks after withdraw. From these studies, an increase of about 10% in $\dot{V}O_2$ max and a 20% increase in endurance time could be expected using blood doping techniques. The increase in VO_2max consequent to increased Hb supports the hypothesis that blood doping really works. It also adds credence to the idea that the oxygen transport system is the limiting factor to exercise.

One major concern with blood doping is the problem of increased viscosity, which could decrease cardiac output. However, Gledhill reported an actual increase in cardiac output after reinfusion with no increase in blood pressure. The increased cardiac output is probably facilitated by the extra oxygen supply to the myocardium.

Some athletes have been transfused with matched blood from other donors. Although blood transfusions from matched donors is routine in medical and therapeutic applications, there is a definite risk-benefit ratio associated with this procedure that is acceptable in medical situations but not in research or in athletics. Inherent dangers involved in using cross-matched blood include contracting hepatitis, mononucleosis, AIDS, or a simple flu virus. In fact, 4 of the 1984 Olympic U.S. cyclists actually became ill from receiving cross-matched blood or blood from their relatives. Gledhill states that "even for research purposes, it's completely unethical to use someone else's blood."

Detection methods for blood doping are difficult. Obviously, if the hematocrit of an

Table 12–1. Summary of Blood Doping Research from 1966 to 1982, Indicating the Amount of Blood Infused, the Time Between Withdraw and Infusion, and Percent Increase in $\dot{V}O_2$ and Endurance Time

Researchers	*Date*	*Amount of Blood*	*Time*	$\dot{V}O_2$	*Endurance*
Robinson, Epstein	1966	100–1200 ml	21 days	No effect	No effect
Williams et al.	1973	500 ml	21 days	No effect	No effect
Frye and Ruhling	1977	500 ml	17 days	No effect	No effect
Videmann and Rytoma	1977	400–600 ml	14–21 days	No effect	No effect
Pate, Macfarland et al.	1979	450 ml	21 days	No effect	No effect
Ekbolm et al.	1972	800–1200 ml	4 wks	1.6–5%	15.6–25.1%
Van Rost, Hullman et al.	1975	900 ml	4 wks	9%	37%
Ekbolm et al.	1975	800 ml	30–35 days	6%	no record
Moore and Perry	1979	405 ml	63 days	—	1–5%
Buick et al.	1980	900 ml	immediate*	increase	increase
Spriet, Gledhill et al.	1980	800 ml	immediate*	increase	increase
Williams et al.	1981	920 ml	immediate*	increase	increase
Goforth, Campbell et al.	1982	760 ml	immediate*	increase	increase
Ekbolm, Wilson et al.	1976	800 ml	5 weeks	8%	—

*No time frame is indicated since the blood infused was cross-matched.

athlete registers over 50, some type of doping can be suspected. But individual hematocrits vary greatly from values as low as 40 to values as high as 47 in males. It would be difficult to detect blood doping in an individual when their normal level is 41 and they increased it to 47. Hopefully a procedure to expose doping will be developed, but currently a process does not exist. Surely, blood doping is not only potentially dangerous, but also unethical and should not be used to improve performance.

SODA LOADING

During high levels of work, the body depends heavily upon anaerobic processes to provide energy for muscular contraction. The by-product from these processes, lactic acid, must be buffered by the blood to prevent a severe decrease in blood pH. This buffering action depends mainly upon the blood alkaline reserve. Acids (lactic acid) are neutralized by alkali, much like the antacid buffers that neutralize the acid in the stomach. The idea behind soda loading is that if the blood was more alkaline before work, more lactic acid could be produced and therefore more energy produced prior to fatigue. Therefore, if the blood bicarbonate reserves were raised by simply ingesting sodium bicarbonate, it could delay the onset of fatigue.

Early research found little effect from ingestion of an alkalizer such as sodium bicarbonate in either cross-country runners or treadmill running. However, the amount or dose of sodium bicarbonate ingested was too low to elicit any significant change in the bicarbonate reserve.

Apparently, the quantity of bicarbonate ingested and the amount of time between ingestion and performance must be balanced properly to receive benefits from this procedure. Jones reported that 0.3 g of sodium bicarbonate per kg of body weight was an effective dosage. Thus a 70-kg man must ingest 21 g of sodium bicarbonate to be effective (about eleven 2.0 g Alka-Seltzer tablets). The total amount of bicarbonate prescribed must also be ingested within a 2-hour period with the performance taking place within ½ hour after ingestion is completed. One main drawback to this type of therapy is that one-half of the subjects studied suffered from "urgent" diarrhea 3 hours after the beginning of the ingestion. If the ingestion time is shortened from 2 hours to under 1½ hours, the gastrointestinal problems increased, but if they were lengthened to 3 hours no buffering effect was observed. Fortunately, analysis of urine samples is an easy and effective method of detecting elevated bicarbonate concentrations, so this type of doping can be controlled.

More recent evidence shows a dramatic effect with proper dosage. In one study, six 800 meters runners increased their average time by 2.9 seconds, which represents a distance of 19 meters, and reported that these runners felt like they had not performed well because they did not feel as fatigued. The two proposed mechanisms for this delay in fatigue are first, the alkalizers buffer the effect of lactic acid; and second, that the higher pH in the blood stream promotes the removal of lactate from the muscle, promoting an increase in muscle pH.

Athletes have also tried a technique called *phosphate loading*. There are two arguments for their use. First, since phosphates can act as buffers, their consumption could have an acid-neutralizing effect during activities in which lactic acid is being produced. Second, one author found that phosphate loading increased 2,3-diphosphoglycerate content in blood and that this increase was associated with an increased $\dot{V}O_2max$. Curiously, their data also revealed that exercise alone raised 2,3-diphosphoglycerate content without phosphate supplementation, and yet this did not effect $\dot{V}O_2max$. A carefully controlled, double blind study looking at these questions found no improvement in either aerobic or anaerobic performance from using phosphates.

OXYGEN INHALATION

It is unusual to think of oxygen as an ergogenic aid, but if the delivery of oxygen to active muscle is a limiting factor to performance, it seems reasonable that increasing the amount of oxygen available to the lungs would increase performance. However, since most oxygen is carried by Hb, and since Hb is normally about 97% saturated, oxygen inhalation has not been as effective as might be thought.

Ever since the 1932 Olympic Games where the successful Japanese swim team attributed their success to breathing pure oxygen before racing, athletes have used oxygen prior to and after almost any type of activity. It is common to see basketball and football players with oxygen masks during time-outs hoping to decrease recovery time.

Oxygen inhalation has proved to be of little value in athletics, whether oxygen is administered before, during, or after performance. Experiments show that oxygen inhaled *before* a contest has little effect, because oxygen cannot be stored successfully by the body. Any increase in oxygen saturation in the blood or lungs is quickly diluted by atmospheric air before the athlete can begin competing.

Increasing the supply of oxygen *during* work does increase the maximal oxygen uptake, and reduces pulmonary ventilation, and the amount of work is significantly increased. Unfortunately, applying this principle to any practical situation is impossible, since carrying an oxygen tank out on the football field or strapping it to your back during a run is unreasonable.

Oxygen consumed *after* the contest does not seem to speed up the elimination of anaerobic by-products, so is of little value. Almost every researcher who has investigated oxygen as an ergogenic aid has shown that oxygen breathed after a contest does little to speed up the elimination of anaerobic by-products, and is probably helpful only from a psychologic standpoint.

ANABOLIC STEROIDS

In 1937, Adolf Hitler commissioned his scientists to develop two drugs, a non-addictive pain killer as powerful as morphine and a drug that would make his feared SS Troops more aggressive. The first drug developed is commonly known today as methadone. The second drug synthesized by the scientists was very similar to the male sex hormone testosterone which is now called *androgenic-anabolic steroids*. This drug was successful in creating the overly-aggressive behavior characterized by the SS. Steroids were used after WWII to help malnourished people regain weight. Since that time, they have been used clinically as an anti-inflammatory agent and for the treatment of osteoporosis, fracture healing, burns, protein tissue building, myotrophy, and muscular dystrophy. They are useful in these areas because they increase nitrogen retention in the form of protein synthesis, and because they decrease the rate of catabolism of amino acids.

Because of their effects on clinical patients, it seems logical that steroids could stimulate muscle growth and strength in normal subjects. Since many athletic events require increased muscular strength, athletes in these events have taken steroids in non-medically approved dosages.

Modern day steroids have been altered in an attempt to reduce the androgenic effects (the kinds of changes that occur to young men at puberty—masculinization), and increase the anabolic effects (the effects that cause an increase in muscle mass only) to avoid the negative changes associated with the drug while increasing muscle mass. The abuse of anabolic steroids by athletes attempting to develop high strength levels has become all too common at the professional, amateur, and collegiate levels, and has now filtered into high school athletics. The reported benefits of anabolic steroids are certainly attractive to the young athlete as well as the older athlete trying to maintain competitiveness. Perhaps the sector of athletes which have the highest use of anabolic steroids is the professional bodybuilders. A 1981 report by the Alcohol and Drug Addiction Research Foundation claimed that 99% of male and 10% of female bodybuilders use steroids.

There is apparently a wide range of individual responses to the different kinds of steroids. Because of this, athletes often "shop around" for the most effective brands. Are anabolic steroids effective? Do they really increase muscle size and strength? Lamb did a careful review of the research on this topic, and found that there was about an equal number of studies which furnished evidence against and in favor of administration of anabolic steroids as an aid to increasing strength. He found that the differences in the research

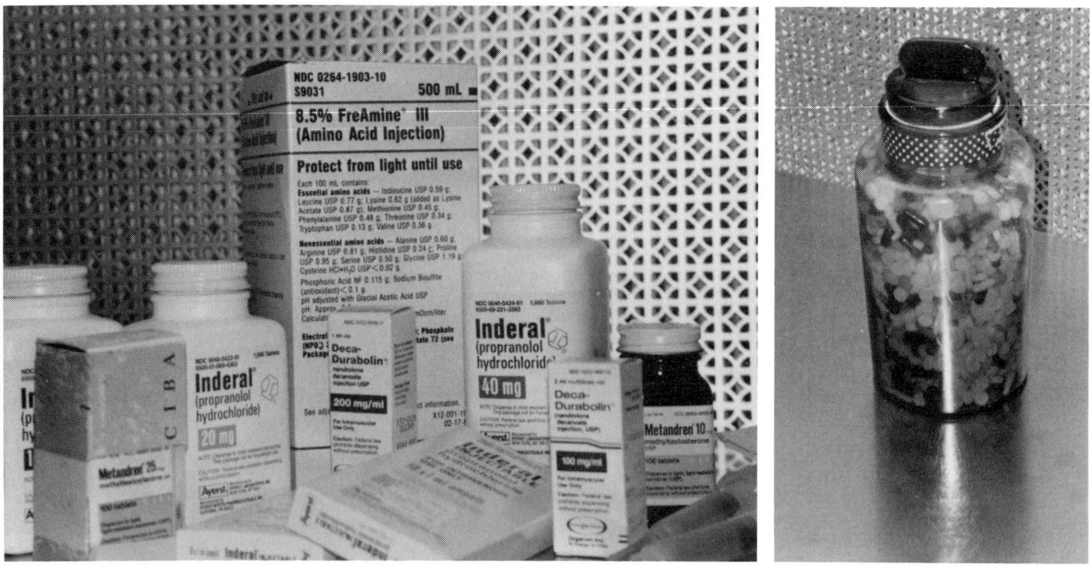

Fig. 12–1. Whether prescribed by a physician or through the black market, about every type of drug is available to athletes.

results related to several associated factors: (1) the psychologic conditioning of the subjects, (2) the level of protein in the diet, (3) the level of dosage, (4) the duration of the experiment, and (5) the individual reactions to the drug. Even though some of the studies did not furnish evidence in favor of anabolic steroids for building of strength, none reported negative results.

Johnson and O'Shea found that strength, body weight, oxygen uptake, and blood nitrogen retention were significantly increased in healthy subjects who were administered anabolic steroids in connection with strength training. Fowler reported no effects of steroids on strength. Casner reported no significant increase in strength from the steroid treatment. Ariel and Saville noted a "psychological enhancement" of performance by those who took steroids. This, combined with strength training produced favorable effects on the development of strength.

A normal prescribed therapeutic dose of anabolic steroids is approximately 0.5 to 1.0 mg/kg body weight or between 70 to 100 mg/day. At this level, only minor differences may exist between treated and untreated subjects as a result of strength training. However, in "real life" situations, athletes often use up to 100 times the normal therapeutic dose and the effects of these doses have as yet not been studied.

When all of the objective evidence is considered, along with the mass of testimonial evidence, it would appear that mega doses of steroids administered for 3 to 6 weeks often contribute to extra gains in strength, body weight, and lean body mass, if the recipients participate simultaneously in a program of intensive strength training.

Most specialists advocate a protein-rich diet along with the training. Why the strength training and high-protein diet are necessary for effectiveness has not been answered satisfactorily.

The potential detrimental effects of steroids have long been a legitimate concern. The elevated levels of steroid suppress the production of natural testosterone by the testis, resulting in testicular atrophy and possible sterilization. Other possible side effects include enlargement of the prostate gland, liver damage, early coronary heart disease, and closure of the epiphyseal plate which stunts growth in younger athletes. For this reason steroid use at the high school level is extremely detrimental. Steroids also seem to influence behavior. Athletes taking steroids are more aggressive and thus may train and compete at higher intensities. However, depres-

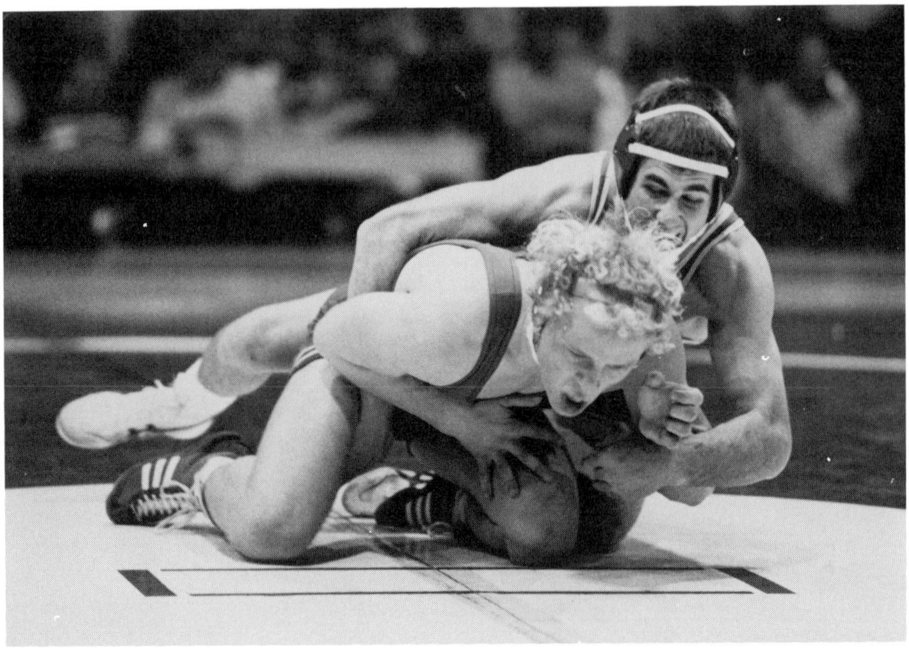

Fig. 12–2.

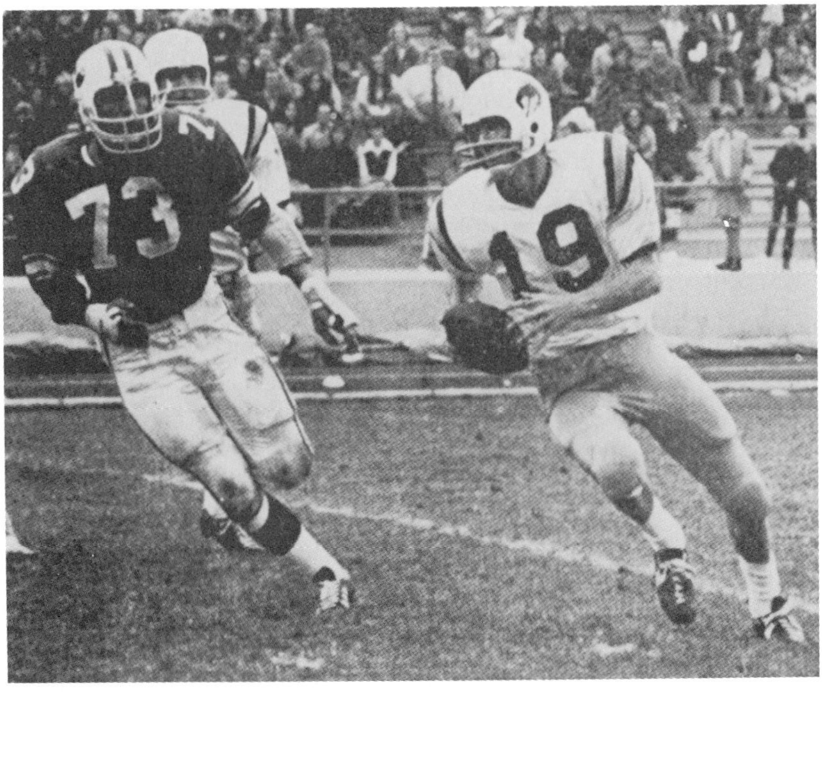

Fig. 12–3.

sion is often experienced when steroid use is stopped. A list of possible detrimental side effects is shown in Table 12–2.

The American College of Sports Medicine has taken a stand on the steroid issue. The following is a brief summary of their statement:

1. With an adequate diet, anabolic steroids can contribute to increased body weight and lean body mass.

2. Gains in muscular strength achieved by training and proper diet can be increased by the use of steroids in some individuals.

3. Steroids do not improve aerobic power or capacity for muscular exercise.

4. Anabolic-androgenic steroids have been associated with adverse effects on the liver, cardiovascular system, reproductive system, and psychological status. Until further research is completed, the potential hazards must be recognized.

5. The use of steroids by athletes is contrary to the rules and ethical principles of athletic competition as set forth by many of sports' governing bodies. The American College of Sports Medicine supports these ethical principles and deplores the use of these substances by athletes.

It should be pointed out that much of the research using steroids to date has been nonconclusive due to the fact that it is impossible and unethical to conduct research on human subjects using 5 to 15 times (some athletes have reported using near 100 times) the normal therapeutic dose, the amount commonly consumed by athletes who are such staunch advocates of steroid use. Within the next decade, any long-term ill effects of steroid abuse will become more apparent in these athletes. Until longitudinal studies are conducted we cannot condone or encourage athletes to put themselves at risk solely for the purpose of gaining an athletic advantage over their opponents. Steroids should be used only for medical reasons and then under the supervision of a qualified physician.

GROWTH HORMONE

Another relatively new ergogenic aid used by athletes, power lifters, and body builders to increase strength and muscle mass is *growth hormone (GH)*. Normally this hormone is secreted from the anterior pituitary gland and regulates the growth of the skeletal system. Like anabolic steroids, GH produces a positive nitrogen balance and facilitates the transport of amino acids into the cell, which is evidenced by increased protein synthesis and increased muscle hypertrophy. However, the use of growth hormone by any athlete without the supervision of a physician is unwise. Large doses of GH are known to cause enlargement of the heart with accelerated atherosclerosis, acromegaly (characterized by large facial features), osteoporosis, and heart disease which are all irreversible. In young athletes, an excess of GH could produce giantism.

To date, no research has been conducted on the effects of GH on endurance and strength gains. However, any advantage that could be perceived would surely be outweighed by the known dangers of its use. With the recent advances in genetic engineering, growth hormone is now more accessible and cheaper and will most likely be found in more and more athletes' lockers, even though severe side effects have already been documented.

AMPHETAMINES

Amphetamines (trade names: Benzedrine, Dexedrine, Desamine, and Methedrine) are

Table 12–2. Reported Side Effects of Anabolic Steroids

Liver toxicity	Prostatic hypertrophy
Elevated blood pressure	Prostatic cancer
Edema	Increased aggressiveness
Clitoral enlargement in women	Decreased HDL levels
Elevated cholesterol and triglycerides	Lowered voice in women and children
Elevated blood glucose	Reduced LH and FSH production
Increased nervous tissue	Acne
Masculinization/menstrual irregularities	Depressed spermatogenesis
Lowered testosterone production	Increased or decreased lipids
Premature closure of epiphyses in children	Testicular atrophy

prescription drugs that produce effects similar to those caused by the activity of the sympathetic nervous system. Amphetamines are "sympathomimetic" in that their action mimics that of the sympathetic hormones epinephrine and norepinephrine. The immediate effects are elevated blood sugars, increased metabolism, increased heart rate, increased blood pressure, increased cardiac output, increased vasoconstriction, decreased sense of fatigue, and increased muscle tension. A decreased sense of fatigue is thought to allow for increased performance. With amphetamines there is an increased feeling of alertness and faster reaction times, which appear to be ideal for enhancing performance.

Numerous double-blind studies have been conducted to determine if amphetamines can increase endurance time. Although there do appear to be many beneficial physiologic responses, there is no conclusive evidence that amphetamines increase performance. It is interesting to note that amphetamines may actually distort an athlete's perception, of his performance. Cooper noted that when cyclists were tested for amphetamines, that athletes that tested positive were ones that finished near the end of the race, but felt that their performance was outstanding.

Using amphetamines is not without risk. In addition to the probability of death or addiction caused by excessive use, amphetamines are known to reduce blood flow, cause disorientation, confusion, hallucination, increase anxiety, and damage to the heart and liver. As with other dangerous drugs, the use of amphetamines is illegal unless prescribed by a physician. The dangers of using amphetamines far outweigh any potential benefit in improvement of athletic performance, and we discourage their unsupervised use.

CAFFEINE

Caffeine is an alkaloid consumed daily by millions of individuals in coffee, tea, and cola drinks. It is a mild stimulant and moderate intakes of caffeinated beverages are apparently harmless. However, caffeine is a toxic drug. Even a small amount injected directly into the blood stream, can prove fatal. When injected into a muscle, it causes temporary paralysis, and when injected directly into the brain, a single drop can cause severe convulsions. Fortunately, since the caffeine in soft drinks is diffused into the blood stream and then carried to the kidneys for excretion, these severe toxic effects seldom occur.

Caffeine affects primarily the blood vessels, heart, and nervous system. A mild dose may cause general vasoconstriction with simultaneous dilation of the coronary artery, increase the contractile force of the heart, increase heart rate and mobilize free fatty acids. Mild doses may also increase the metabolic rate up to 25%, stimulate the central nervous system, and accelerate the respiration rate. Small doses may act beneficially upon the psychic processes for a short time and have been associated with aiding memorization.

There is a conflict among researchers regarding the effect of caffeinated drinks on work output and fatigue. At this point, the answer to this question is not clear. Caffeine ingestion of 4 to 5 mg per kg of weight lessens the subjective feeling of effort during exercise, and foods or drinks containing caffeine consumed an hour before a prolonged, exhaustive exercise may improve performance due to its effect on increasing blood FFA. There is also some evidence that caffeine has a direct effect on muscle tension. One study showed an increase in muscle tension in both a fatigued and non-fatigued state, but no change has been shown in maximal short-term exercise bouts. Despite the potential "unnatural" advantages of caffeine ingestion, at least in endurance events, its use must be questioned on an ethical basis.

COCAINE

At this time, little is known concerning the effects of cocaine on performance. However, there is no question about the health risks associated with its use. Cocaine addiction has ruined the careers and taken the lives of many outstanding athletes who became addicted and its use and should not be encouraged even if it had a positive effect on performance.

Research shows that cocaine does have the effect of stimulating lipolysis and glycolysis. However, cocaine is also a potent vasoconstrictor and the ability to use substrate is severely limited. Preliminary studies with rats injected with cocaine shows a substantial decrease in endurance performance on the treadmill. There are surely no positive reasons for cocaine use at this time and athletes should avoid this substance completely.

ALCOHOL

Alcohol has long been on the athlete's taboo list, but strict enforcement is difficult because many "social drinkers" argue that moderate drinking is unlikely to have a negative effect on general health or life span. The coach should resist such logic because drinking can have a direct negative influence on performance, since alcohol is not a stimulant, but a narcotic which suppresses body functions. It provides a temporary sense of well-being, but in actuality serves as a depressant to both mind and body. Alcohol increases fatigue by slowing the removal of lactic acid from the cells. It seriously interferes with the functioning of the nervous system, slowing reaction time and reducing coordination. Alcohol affects the cerebral portion of the brain which controls thoughts and actions, causing the person to be less coherent and less responsive than normal. It interferes with both voluntary and involuntary reflexes. Use of alcohol can lead to poor eating patterns and eventual malnutrition. It often is associated with loss of sleep and normal inhibitions, both of which are vital to athletes. In addition, its use can become addictive to some people.

Alcohol is absorbed directly from the stomach and its effect is felt quickly. Strong alcoholic drinks are undoubtedly detrimental to both conditioning and performance. Since there are no points in favor of alcohol, coaches ought to prohibit its use either by their athletes or themselves.

HYPNOSIS AND SUGGESTION

Stories of superhuman strength during stress have made researchers wonder if this type of strength could be released during athletic events using hypnosis. However, the use of hypnosis as an ergogenic aid is still unproven.

Much of the disagreement in the literature stems from poorly designed experiments that do not account for the variability of subjects and their responsiveness to suggestion. In fact, several investigators have reported negative effects of hypnosis on muscular strength and performance. It is interesting to note that while hypnotic suggestion seems to have little effect on increasing strength and performance, these same suggestions will almost always have a decreasing effect on strength and performance.

Hypnosis does appear to be effective in releasing the stress and anxiety before a competitive event and in reducing pain. Obviously, all attempts to facilitate muscular performance by using hypnosis have not been failures, but additional research that encompasses the many variables that interact while using human subjects will hopefully shed more light on this type of ergogenic aid.

TEMPOROMANDIBULAR JOINT REPOSITIONING (TMJ)

Another ergogenic aid used by some practitioners relates to aligning the jaw with a dental appliance to correct possible temporomandibular joint (TMJ) imbalances. It is theorized that the malalignment of the jaw causes muscle tension in the cervical region of the spinal cord which results in a loss of muscle strength and endurance. If this is the case, correcting the malocclusion would change the position of the TMJ and relieve the pressure on the auriculotemporal nerve allowing full strength to again be developed.

There are a few studies which show improvement in overall muscle strength on isokinetic devices as a result of TMJ alignment. Although these studies report some type of improvement, they all suffer from two major problems. First, both the investigators and subjects were aware of possible positive effects of TMJ alignment, making the placebo effect a major factor. Second, the studies to date have had poor or no statistical design. Only one study used a double blind TMJ appliance design and reported no change in strength as a result of TMJ alignment.

SELECTED READINGS

1. American College of Sports Medicine: Position Stand on the Use of Anabolic-androgenic Steroids in Sports. Indianapolis, Ind., 1984.
2. Ariel, G., and W. Saville: Anabolic steroids: The physiological effects of placebos. Med. Sci. Sports, *4*, 124–126, 1972.
3. Aronson, V.: Vitamins and minerals as ergogenic aids. Physician Sports Med. *14*(3):209–212, 1986.
4. Barnett, D.W., and R.K. Conlee: The effects of a commercial dietary supplement on human performance. Am. J. Clin. Nutr. *40*:586–590, 1984.
5. Bracken, M.E., D.R. Bracken, A.G. Nelson, et al.: Effect of cocaine on exercise endurance and glycogen use in rats. J. Appl. Physiol. *64*(2):884–887, 1988.
6. Cantwell, J.D., and F.D. Rose: Cocaine and Cardiovascular Events: Physician Sports Med. *14*(11), Nov., 1986.
7. Casner, S.W., Early, R.G., and Carlson, B.R.: Anabolic steroid effects on body composition in normal young men. J. Sports Med. *11*:98–103, 1971.
8. Conlee, R.K.: Muscle Glycogen and Exercise Endurance: A Twenty-Year Perspective. Exerc. Sport Sci. Rev. *15*:1–28, 1987.
9. Cooper, D.L.: Drugs and the Athlete. JAMA, *221*:1007–1011, 1972.
10. Costill, D.L., G.P. Dalsky, and W.J. Fink: Effects of caffeine ingestion on metabolism and exercise performance. Med. Sci. Sports Exerc. *10*(3):155–158, 1978.
11. Counsilman, J.: *The Science of Swimming.* Englewood Cliffs, N.J.: Prentice-Hall, Inc., 1968.
12. Duffy, D.J., and R.K. Conlee: Effects of phosphate loading on leg power and high intensity treadmill exercise. Med. Sci. Sports Exerc. *18*:674–677, 1986.
13. Ekblom, B., G. Wilson, and P-O. Astrand: Central circulation during exercise after venesection and reinfusion of red blood cells. J. Appl. Physiol. *40*:379–383, 1976.
14. Fowler, W.M.: The facts about ergogenic aids and sports performance. J. Health, Phys. Educ. Rec. *40*:37–42, 1969.
15. Fowler, W.M., Jr., Gardner, G.W., and Egstrom, G.H.: Effect of an anabolic steroid on physical performance of young men. J. Appl. Physiol., *20*:1038–1040, 1965.
16. Gledhill, N.: Blood doping and related issues: a brief review. Med. Sci. Sports Exerc. *14*:183–189, 1982.
17. Gledhill, N.: Bicarbonate Ingestion and Anaerobic Performance. Sports Med. *1*:177, 1984.
18. Gledhill, N.: The influence of altered blood volume and oxygen transport capacity on aerobic performance. Exerc. Sport Sci. Rev. *13*:75–93, 1982.
19. Herbert, V., and Jacob, E.: Destruction of vitamin B in ascorbic acid. JAMA, *230*:241–242, 1974.
20. Johnson, L.C., and O'Shea, J.P.: Anabolic steroid: Effects on strength development. Science *164*:957–959, 1969.
21. Jones, N.L., J.R. Sutton, R. Taylor, et al.: Effect of pH on cardiorespiratory and metabolic responses to exercise. J. Appl. Physiol. *43*(6):959–964, 1977.
22. Lamb, D.R.: Androgens in exercise. Med. Sci. Sports, *8*:1, 1975.
23. Lamb, D.R.: Anabolic steroids. In M.H. Williams (Ed.). *Ergogenic Aids in Sports.* Champaign, IL: Human Kinetics Publishers, 1983, pp. 164–182.
24. Lombardo, J.A.: Stimulants and athletic performance: amphetamines and caffeine. Physician Sports Med. *14*(11), 128–142, 1983.
25. Lombardo, J.A.: Stimulants and Athletic Performance: Amphetamines and Caffeine: Physician Sports Med. *14*(11), 128–142, 1986.
26. Lombardo, J.A.: Stimulants and athletic performance: cocaine and nicotine. Physician Sports Med. *14*(12), 85–91, 1986.
27. Miller, A.: Influence of oxygen administration on the cardiovascular function during exercise and recovery. J. Appl. Physiol. *5*:165–168, 1952.
28. Morgan, W.P. (ed): *Ergogenic Aids and Muscular Performance.* New York: Academic Press, 1972.
29. Rhead, W.J., and Schrauzer, G.N.: Risks of long-term ascorbic acid overdosage. Nutr. Rev., *29*:262–263, 1971.
30. Sutton, J.R., D.B. Clement, P.F. Gardiner, et al.: Drugs in Sports: A five article symposium. Physician Sports Med. *15*(9), Sept. 1983.
31. Van Huss, W.D.: What made the Russians run? Nutrition Today, *1*:20, 1966.
32. Williams, M.H. (ed): *Ergogenic Aids in Sports.* Champaign: Human Kinetics Publishers, 1983.

13

Environmental Factors

The choice of Mexico City as the site of the 1968 Olympic Games aroused tremendous interest in the effects of altitude on athletic performance. It stimulated much discussion among physiologists and athletic coaches and caused considerable research on problems related to performance at high altitude. Since that time numerous sports enthusiasts have "headed to the hills" to backpack, ski, and hang-glide to altitudes well over 10,000 feet. Other sportsmen have gone to the seas, experiencing the effects of the increased pressures (hyperbaria) associated with underwater sports. Since all athletes experience changes in temperature, as well as changes in pressure, the study of environmental factors becomes important. The purpose of this chapter is to discuss the effects of various environmental factors on the body during exercise.

EFFECTS OF LOW PRESSURE

Atmospheric pressure is produced by the layer of air surrounding the earth. As man ascends to higher and higher altitudes, the total pressure of the atmosphere decreases because of the decreased weight of the column of air above him. Although the total pressure decreases as man ascends to higher altitudes, the percentage of each of the gases in the atmosphere remains the same. Since the partial pressure of any gas is its percent concentration times the total pressure, the partial pressure of each gas decreases in proportion to the decrease in total pressure.

As mentioned in Chapter 5, the three major gases of the atmosphere are oxygen, carbon dioxide, and nitrogen (an inert gas which is not used in the body). At sea level where the atmospheric pressure is 760 mm Hg, the partial pressures of each gas are presented in Table 13–1.

If a man were to climb to 2,000 meters (6,560 feet), the atmospheric pressure is about 600 mm Hg and PO_2 would decrease to 125 mm Hg. When the partial pressure of oxygen is reduced, the availability of oxygen to support work is reduced, and this decreases aerobic work capacity. This decreased work capacity can be demonstrated by comparing the performance in the 1968 Olympics at Mexico City (elevation: 7,400 feet) with previous Olympic and world records (Table 13–2). No new records were set in events requiring individual efforts of over 1 minute's duration.

From these figures it is apparent that altitude has its greatest effect upon endurance (aerobic) events, and the longer endurance events are affected more than the shorter

Table 13–1. Partial Pressures of Major Atmospheric Gases at Sea Level

Gas		*Pr*		*% Gas*		*Partial Pressure*
Oxygen	=	760 mm Hg	×	.2093	=	159.07 mm Hg
Carbon Dioxide	=	760 mm Hg	×	.0004	=	0.30 mm Hg
Nitrogen	=	760 mm Hg	×	.7903	=	600.63 mm Hg

Table 13–2. Comparison of Performances at Mexico City and Elsewhere

Performance	*800 meter*	*1500 meter*	*5000 meter*	*10,000 meter*
World Record	1:44.3	3:33.1	13:16.1	27:39.4
Olympic record before 1968	1:45.1	3:35.1	13:39.6	28:24.4
1968 Olympic Performance	1:44.3	3:34.9	14:05.0	29:27.4

ones. (The world 800-meter run record was equaled at Mexico City, but the 10,000-meter run was about 2 minutes slower than the world record.)

The cause of the reduced performance in endurance events is the reduced oxygen pressure which decreases the arterial saturation of the blood. This in turn decreases the amount of oxygen available to the cells to be used for the production of energy (Table 13–3).

Luckily, the arterial oxygen saturation does not decrease at the same rate as the alveolar partial pressure because of the flattening of the oxygen dissociation curve (see Chapter 5). The percent saturation of the blood remains fairly high to about 3,050 meters (10,000 feet), then falls fairly rapidly (70% at 6,100 meters [20,000 feet], 50% at 7,012 meters [23,000 feet], and only about 20% at 9,150 meters [30,000 feet]. Because unconsciousness usually occurs between 25 to 50% saturation, pilots and mountain climbers are required to use oxygen at altitudes over 6,100 meters.

The lack of oxygen associated with high altitudes is called *hypoxia.* The earliest effect of hypoxia on bodily function is a decrease of the ability to see at night (night vision). Hypoxia also stimulates pulmonary ventilation at elevations above 8,000 feet, and can cause drowsiness, mental fatigue, headache, occasional nausea, and sometimes euphoria at altitudes above 12,000 feet. The body makes several adjustments to acute and chronic exposure to altitude for the purpose of increasing the amount of oxygen delivered to the cells. These adjustments or adaptations will be discussed in more detail in sections to follow.

Physiologic Adaptations to Altitude

Several changes occur to the physiologic systems of the body which help it adjust to the decreased atmospheric pressure at high altitude. Some of these changes take place immediately; others require several weeks. The net effect of these changes counters the negative effects caused by the decrease in oxygen pressure by increasing both O_2 carrying capacity and cellular metabolic efficiency.

When a person travels from sea level to high altitude (2,440 meters/8,000 ft) the oxygen saturation of hemoglobin changes very little (97 to 92%), but the PaO_2 (arterial saturation) drops from 94 mm Hg to 60 mm Hg. If the tissue pressure in the muscle is 20 mm Hg, the diffusion gradient for oxygen is 74 mm Hg at sea level and only 40 mm Hg at 2,440 meters (8,000 feet), a reduction of nearly 50%. This reduction in diffusion gradient decreases diffusion capacity. A reduction in diffusion capacity and a decreased maximum heart rate seems to be the two major factors in reducing $\dot{V}O_2$max or aerobic

Table 13–3. Effects of Altitude on Alveolar Gas Concentrations and Arterial Oxygen Saturation

			Breathing Air		
Altitude (feet)	*Barometric Pressure (mm Hg)*	*pO_2 in Air (mm Hg)*	*pCO_2 in Alveoli (mm Hg)*	*pO_2 in Alveoli (mm Hg)*	*Arterial Oxygen Saturation (%)*
0	760	159	40	104	97
10,000	523	110	36	67	90
20,000	349	73	24	40	70
30,000	226	47	24	21	20
40,000	141	29	24	8	5
50,000	87	18	24	1	1

work capacity. It has been calculated by some researchers that each 1,000 foot rise in elevation (above 5,000 feet) yields a 3% reduction in $\dot{V}O_2max$ and some decrement even at altitudes below 5,000 feet. Interestingly, the $\dot{V}O_2max$ of highly fit mountain climbers ($\dot{V}O_2max$ around 60 ml/kg/min.) at a base testing site just below the crest of Mt. Everest was only about 7 to 10 ml/kg/min (Figs. 13–1 and 13–2).

Mountain climbers have subjected themselves to extreme altitudes such as Mount Everest (8,848 meters), and several groups have reached the summit without the use of external oxygen. These climbers have tremendous climbing skill and physical strength with a high power/weight ratio. They also have a relatively high sea level $\dot{V}O_2max$ and a low ventilatory response to hypoxia. They must also take sufficient time at several different intermediate altitudes for acclimatization to take place.

The time it takes for acclimatization to occur is dependent on the altitude and the individual. At 2,744 meters (9,000 feet) about 7 to 10 days are required for acclimatization,

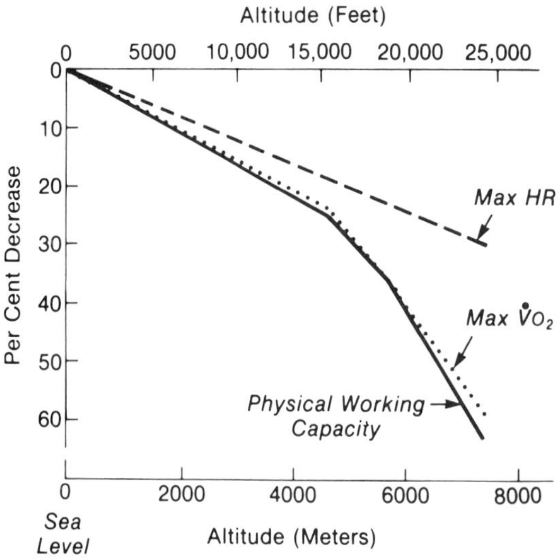

Fig. 13–1. At altitudes of over 5000 ft., the ability to perform physical work is affected. In general one can expect a reduction in max $\dot{V}O_2$ of 3 to 3.5% for every 1000 ft. ascended above the 5000 ft. level. Physical working capacity and max $\dot{V}O_2$ are reduced by 60% or more at extremely high altitudes. (From Mathew, D.K., Fox, E.L., Bowers, R.W., Foss, M.L. *Physiological Basis of Physical Education and Athletics*, 4th Ed. Courtesy of W.B. Saunders Co., 1988.)

at 3,660 meters (12,000 feet) 15 to 21 days, and for 4,575 meters (15,000 feet) 21 to 25 days. Some individuals never adjust to high altitudes and suffer from a condition called *acute mountain sickness* (AMS). AMS is related to the altitude one ascends to and is more common at altitudes above 10,000 feet (3,000 m). How rapidly a person goes to altitude also affects the occurrence of this problem. Symptoms include headache, anorexia, nausea, vomiting, dizziness, insomnia, breathlessness at rest, reduced urine output, and weakness. These symptoms usually occur within a day or two of arrival and may last for several days, or get progressively worse.

Treatment of AMS consists of rest, aspirin, and fluid replacement. Some persons do not respond and should be returned to more normal altitudes.

Several techniques can be used to help avoid AMS. First, going to altitude for a limited time (as to ski) but returning to a lower altitude at night is usually an effective avoidance procedure. If long-term altitude living is required (as in backpacking, hunting, or job requirement), it helps to ascend slowly, spending some time at intermediate altitudes. Taking the drug Diamo can be helpful for persons forced to go to high altitude quickly. This drug elevates the blood CO_2 levels and reduces pH. To be effective it must be taken the day before ascent. Other techniques include increasing fluid intake to keep urine from becoming too concentrated and eating more carbohydrates to increase the production of CO_2.

Acute Adaptations. Hypoxia itself probably stimulates the acclimatization mechanisms. The most noticeable response to acute exposure to altitude is hyperventilation. The chemoreceptors in the aortic arch and carotid sinus are sensitive to decreased O_2 pressure and stimulate ventilation upon exposure to reduced oxygen pressure at high altitudes in an attempt to provide sufficient O_2 to the alveoli. This response occurs within a few hours. However, hyperventilation tends to "blow off" CO_2, causing the blood to become more alkaline (higher pH), and lowers the partial pressure of carbon dioxide (PCO_2). This decrease in PCO_2 inhibits rather than aids the hyperventilatory response. There-

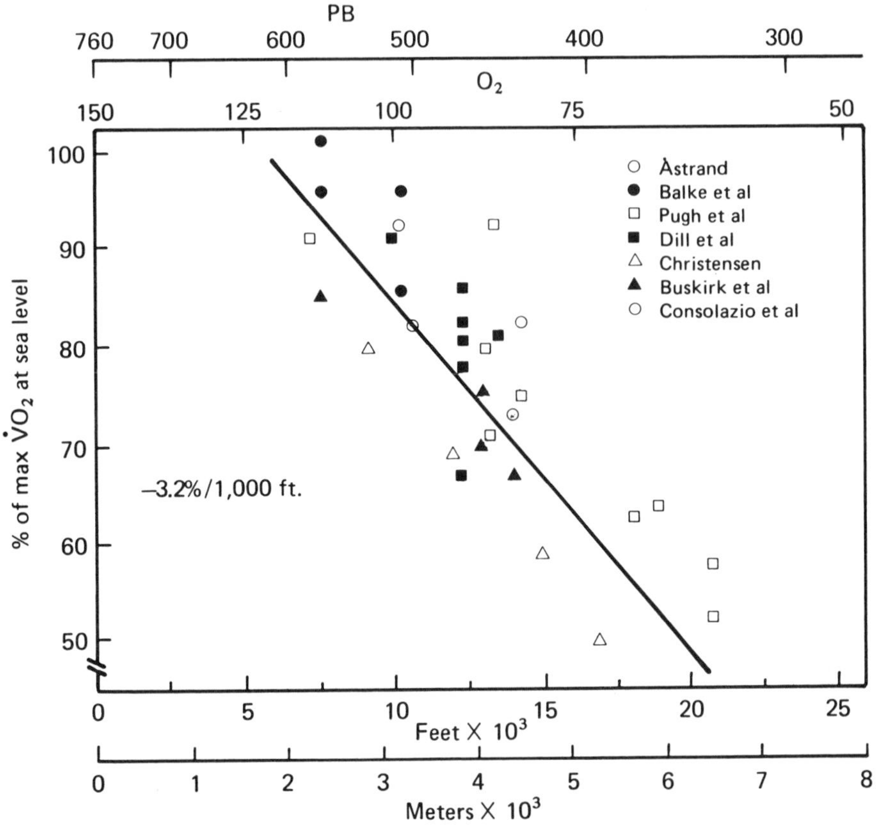

Fig. 13–2. Reduction in maximal oxygen uptake in relation to increases in altitude, and a decrease in the barometric pressure (BP) and partial pressure of oxygen in the ambient air (PO_2). The symbols represent data of various authors. (From Buskirk, E.R., et al.: Physiology and performance of track athletes in U.S. and Peru. *In* The Effects of Altitude on Physical Performance. Edited by R.F. Goddard. Courtesy of Chicago Athletic Institute, 1967.)

fore, at altitude there are two mechanisms working against each other to regulate ventilation.

When an athlete moves from sea level to an intermediate altitude, there is a significant increase in heart rate at rest and during submaximal work. This is followed by a steady decline over a 10-week period to normal sea level rates. The heart rate pattern is followed closely by the cardiac output, except that sea level values usually will not be reached, even after a 10-week adjustment period. These adjustments are necessary to maintain cellular oxygen levels with the decreased alveolar oxygen tension.

The large increase in respiratory rate increases alveolar oxygen pressure, which increases the diffusion of oxygen to the blood from the alveoli. However, blood O_2 saturation levels never reach those experienced at lower altitude.

Chronic Acclimation to Altitude. A major adaptation after prolonged exposure to altitude is the reestablishment of normal ventilatory control. Within a week or two, the body begins to reduce the levels of bicarbonate (HCO_3^-) in the blood and cerebrospinal fluid and excess bicarbonate is disposed of by the kidneys. There is also a progressively increased ventilatory sensitivity to CO_2. These changes help to make normal the pH levels of the blood which were altered during initial exposure to altitude. The oxygen dissociation curve shifts back to the right once normal respiration is established restoring normal binding of oxygen to hemoglobin.

After only a few days at moderate altitude, the hemoglobin concentration increases due to a decrease in plasma volume. Later, a real increase occurs in both hemoglobin and hematocrit, which increases the amount of oxygen the blood is able to carry per unit volume.

Hemoglobin has been known to increase from 14 to 16 g/dl to as high as 35 g/dl at high altitudes. Of course, the increased red blood cell percentage (hematocrit) also increases the viscosity of the blood which, in turn, increases the cardiac work at a given heart rate.

During extended periods of exposure to high altitude there seems to be an increase in the concentration of muscle and tissue capillaries. There is also a vasodilation in those areas where gas exchange is needed for optimal functioning. This provides a source of oxygen closer to each cell even with a relatively lower oxygen tension. There may also be an increase in myoglobin, mitochondria density, and enzymes that enhance the aerobic capacity.

The cardiac output and heart rate will be greater at altitude for any given submaximal work load than for corresponding work at sea level. Although the initial adjustment in cardiac output is brought about primarily by an increased heart rate, stroke volume takes on a greater portion of the cardiac output as the intensity of work increases.

Maximal cardiac output, stroke volume, and heart rate are affected little at intermediate altitudes (4,000 meters/13,000 feet), but the maximal heart rate is reached at a lower work level. In one study, maximal oxygen uptake was reduced to 72% of sea level VO_2max when the arterial oxygen content was reduced to 74% of normal.

At extremely high altitudes, the cardiac output may be reduced significantly, with the decrease due primarily to decreased heart rate. Pugh and associates reported decreases in cardiac output from 22 to 25 liter/minute at sea level to 16 to 17 liter/minute at 19,000 feet. This reduction occurred because of a reduction in heart rate from 192 to 135 beats/minute and a small reduction in stroke volume. This decrease in heart rate is probably associated with a lack of O_2 to the myocardium.

In a summary statement at an altitude symposium, Dr. Bruno Balke mentioned the following compensating mechanisms which are used by the body to restore "normal" aerobic capacity: (1) an increase in pulmonary ventilation for any given level of work; (2) an increase of cardiac output for any submaximal work load brought about primarily by increased heart rate; (3) reduced maximal oxygen uptake, usually related to the reduction in arterial oxygen content; (4) initial hemoconcentration because of reduction in plasma volume; (5) a gradual increase in red blood cell count and hemoglobin content in the blood; (6) an increase in myoglobin, the oxygen-carrying pigment in the muscle; (7) a vasodilation in the areas where oxygen is needed for optimal performance; and (8) an increase in the number of capillaries per unit of tissue.

Effect of Altitude on Competitive Performance

Studies have shown that both conditioned and unconditioned subjects are affected equally upon initial exposure to altitude. The fit individual will be able to do more work than the unfit person, but the work will be diminished for both.

Not all the effects of altitude are detrimental to athletic performance. The reduced density of the air decreases the resistance to the flow of air into and out of the lungs. This allows larger volumes of air to be breathed during work with no significant increase in ventilatory cost. Of course, this does not make up for the reduced partial pressure of oxygen, but it does allow the body to adjust somewhat to the requirements for more oxygen during heavy work.

The positive effects of decreased air resistance are also noticeable on sprinting activities, jumping events, and other high-velocity events which do not require extensive aerobic involvement. Performers in these activities are sometimes phenomenal. Take, for example, the long jump record of 29 feet 2¼ inches set by Bob Beamon in Mexico City at the 1968 Olympics. This performance might not have been achicved at a lower altitude.

Air is usually cooler and dryer at high altitude. Cooler temperatures can aid performances involving prolonged heavy work, but at the same time, the dryer air and increased hyperventilation can increase the water loss from the respiratory system, causing discomfort to the performer.

There is no doubt that aerobic capacity is reduced with increased altitude. This was clearly demonstrated at the Olympic Games in Mexico City in 1968. At 7,400 feet, running times were about 10% longer than at sea level for distances over 1,500 meters. There seemed to be no effect on the events under 400 meters. These findings are logical in terms of our understanding of the anaerobic energy schemes discussed in Chapter 3. The body is able to provide energy for short periods of time without large quantities of oxygen. Any activity that can be completed before the depletion of readily available energy stores in the body will not be affected by the decreased oxygen pressure at high altitude. Events requiring energy from the oxidative systems are affected significantly.

An excellent example of how altitude affects performance, was conducted on five athletes from Lexington, Kentucky (altitude 1,000 ft) and five athletes from Leadville, Colorado (altitude 10,200 feet). After 12 days of acclimation to the Colorado altitude a track meet was held and then the process was repeated in Lexington. The results show that the hypoxia affected both teams equally, and that the faster times in the 220 and 440 meter are probably due to decreased air resistance. It was concluded that highly trained athletes will probably be equally successful at either altitude (Table 13–4).

One of the main reasons that $\dot{V}O_2$ max and performance time does not improve with altitude training is that the training intensity maintained at sea level (approx. 75 to 80%) cannot be sustained at high altitudes. A given workout which at sea level may be 80% of $\dot{V}O_2$max may be only 50% of sea level $\dot{V}O_2$max at 10,000 feet. The reduction in training intensity may result in an overall "detraining" or decrease in peak performance time (see Table 13–5).

Training at Altitude

Four years after the Mexico City Olympics, the 1972 Olympics in Munich revealed some interesting facts. Every gold medalist in endurance events from the 1,500 meters to the marathon had altitude-trained prior to competing. Whether this was a response to the 1968 Olympics or whether altitude training actually helped increase endurance performance is not known. Training at higher altitudes may produce faster physiologic adaptations than training at sea level especially in unconditioned individuals. First, training at altitude evokes a tissue hypoxia which is thought to be essential in stimulating the conditioning responses of the body. Second, the increased red blood cell count and hemoglobin concentration would increase O_2 carrying capacity. Third, altitude training also increases 2,3-DPG, the enzyme responsible for lowering oxyhemoglobin affinity. Fourth, there is a definite increase in maximum ventilation volume. Theoretically, the net effect of all these adaptations could give an athlete a distinct advantage when returning to sea level. Unfortunately studies have not substantiated a benefit of high altitude training to sea level performance. Because highly trained individuals would be unable to maintain the same intensity training, it is unlikely that altitude training of these subjects would improve sea level performance.

Comments on Training at Altitude

The following comments can be made about altitude training:

1. No acclimatization is necessary for athletes involved in anaerobic events, such as short races, jumping, and throwing events.
2. There seems to be no evidence that per-

Table 13–4. Running Times for Track Events at 300 and 3100 Meters*

Running Distances		*Lexington Team*		*Leadville Team*	
		Altitude (meters)		*Altitude (meters)*	
		300	*3100*	*300*	*3100*
Yards	*Meters*	*Time (min:sec)*		*Time (min:sec)*	
220	201	0:24.0	0:22.4	0:25.7	0:27.0
440	402	0:54.0	0:51.0	1:03.5	0:52.5
880	804	2:10.0	2:11.5	2:24.7	2:30.0
1760	1608	4:49.0	5:10.9	5:23.5	5:35.0

*From Grover, et al.: Muscular exercise in young men native to 3,100 m altitude. J. Appl. Physiol. *22*(3):555–564, 1967.

Table 13–5. Effect of Altitude on Training Intensity of Six Collegiate Athletes[a]

	Altitude (m)			
	300	*2300*	*3100*	*4000*
Intensity of Workout (% of max $\dot{V}O_2$ at 200 M)	78	60	56	39

[a]From Kollias, J., and Buskirk, E.R.: Exercise and altitude. In Science and Medicine of Exercise and Sports, 2nd ed. Edited by W.R. Johnson, and E.R. Buskirk. New York, Harper and Row, 1974.

formance is improved by training at a higher altitude for a performance at a lower altitude, with the possible exception that the anaerobic processes of the body may be improved slightly by high-altitude training.

3. Athletes who live and train at high altitude do not perform better at high altitude than athletes who train at sea level and then acclimatize themselves to the high altitude. Athletes who train at high altitude train at a lower $\dot{V}O_2$max and thus do not perform better at sea level than athletes who train at sea level.

4. There may be individual differences in ability to acclimatize. Some athletes may be more vulnerable to the effects of high altitude than others. Some athletes will require longer periods of time to adjust.

5. The time necessary to acclimatize is related to the fitness level of the individual athlete; a well-trained athlete will acclimatize more quickly than an untrained person. As a general rule, however, the acclimatization period should probably start 2 to 3 weeks prior to the competition in aerobic (endurance) events.

6. Training programs similar to those used at sea level can be used for training at high altitude. However, the coach and athlete should be aware that fatigue will set in earlier. Less intense workouts of shorter duration will stress the system maximally at high altitude.

7. Man has the ability to adjust to higher altitudes and can perform more successfully after a period of acclimatization. Pugh states that man can probably acclimatize to altitudes in excess of 23,000 feet if sufficient time and proper procedures are used. However, performance of aerobic activities will always suffer at high altitude no matter how well acclimatized the athlete becomes.

EFFECTS OF HIGH PRESSURE

With the interest in water sports and scuba diving, the principles of exercise under increased pressures need to be explored. In fact, underwater diving is about the only environment where an individual can experience 3 to 5 atmospheres of pressure, unless one happens to be a caisson worker or have access to a decompression chamber. The weight of 33 feet (10 meters) of fresh water (31 feet of salt water) causes an increased pressure of 1 atmosphere (760 mm Hg). This means that a person diving to 66 feet experiences 2 atmospheres of water pressure, plus 1 atmosphere of air pressure above the water or a total of 2,280 mm Hg. This amount of pressure is enough to require special care to avoid serious health consequences.

The body can tolerate high pressures fairly well as long as the pressure inside the body is the same as the pressure outside the body. This principle is apparent when flying or driving up mountainous terrain. As the air pressure decreases on the outside of the body, a person must allow pressure to equalize in the middle ear through the eustachian tubes or suffer great pain. The potential pressure differences are much greater when diving, and can become a problem at a depth of only a few meters. If the lungs are connected to a long snorkel tube above the water, the difference in pressure between the water and the lungs will become so great even at 1 meter that the muscles of inspiration will be unable to overcome it, and normal breathing will be impossible. Therefore air must enter the lungs under pressure (from either a pressurized air tank or pressurized hose) to equalize the pressure gradient established by the water.

A much greater problem exists at greater depths. A person taking a large breath of air from a scuba tank and holding it while ascending may explode the alveoli. Since gas expands as pressure decreases, a fully inflated lung at 99 feet would expand to 4 times the original volume by the time the diver reached the surface. Even at 5 or 6 feet of water, a full breath held to the surface of the water may over-distend the lungs and may lead to pulmonary hemorrhage. Air must always be released by the diver as he ascends from a dive (Table 13–6).

Dangers Inherent in a High Pressure Environment

Most diving problems occur because pressure increases so rapidly during descent. At sea level, nitrogen is an inert gas and passes through the body with little effect. As pressure increases nitrogen diffuses into the various tissues of the body, and once in the tissues, it affects the central nervous system, and causes symptoms much like those of drinking alcoholic beverages. This phenomenon is called *nitrogen narcosis* or "rapture of the deep." The effects are related to the depth and duration of the dive. As a general rule, scuba diving should be limited to depths of less than 200 feet, with a practical depth of around 100 feet to decrease the effects of nitrogen narcosis.

Nitrogen also causes problems if a diver surfaces rapidly after being under water for some time. In this situation, the nitrogen which diffused into the tissues is released as insoluble gas bubbles, much like the CO_2 in bottled carbonated drinks when the lid is removed. These bubbles congregate in the small blood vessels, where they obstruct the flow of blood and cause pain, or they may even become trapped in the brain and cause paralysis. Pain is felt in the joints, ligaments, and tendons first, usually within about 4 hours, and causes what is commonly known as *decompression sickness* or the *bends* (Fig. 13–3).

Bends can be prevented by surfacing slowly so that the tissues can get rid of the excess nitrogen without the formation of bubbles. Another way to prevent the bends is to breathe a helium-oxygen mixture of gas. Helium is less easily dissolved in the body tissues than nitrogen, and once dissolved, can diffuse out of the tissues more easily when normal pressures are restored. Breathing a helium and oxygen mixture decreases the likelihood of having the bends and decreases the chance of nitrogen narcosis.

Once a diver has the bends, the only treatment is to subject the body to high pressure (using a decompression chamber) to force the bubbles back into solution. The diver is then brought back to normal pressure slowly, allowing the nitrogen to diffuse normally out of the tissues.

When pure oxygen is breathed under high pressure, the amount of oxygen in solution is increased to such a high level that carbon dioxide cannot be accepted by the red blood cells, causing a buildup of CO_2 in body tissues. This disturbs cerebral blood flow and results in the symptoms of *oxygen toxicity* or *poisoning* (tingling of appendages, visual problems, noise in the ears, confusion, muscle twitching, and convulsions). Oxygen toxicity may occur at any depth greater than 10 meters, but there is a large range of individual sensitivity to oxygen under pressure. The onset of most high pressure problems are hastened by physical activity.

Dangers of Rapid Decompression and Breath-Holding

Since the tissues of the body are composed mostly of water, they are relatively unaffected or damaged by the compressive weight of the column of water above the diver. However, there are many hollow chambers in the body such as the lungs, sinuses, middle ear, and the face mask where pressure must be equalized. For example, the tympanic membrane will rupture, the sinuses will fill with blood, or the

Table 13–6. Relationship of Pressure and Volume to Depth of Dive

Depth (feet)	Depth (meters)	Pressure (atm)	Pressure (mm Hg)	Hypothetical Lung Volume (liters)
Sea Level		1	760	6
33	10	2	1520	3
66	20	3	2280	2
99	30	4	3040	1.5
132	40	5	3800	1.2
165	50	6	4560	1

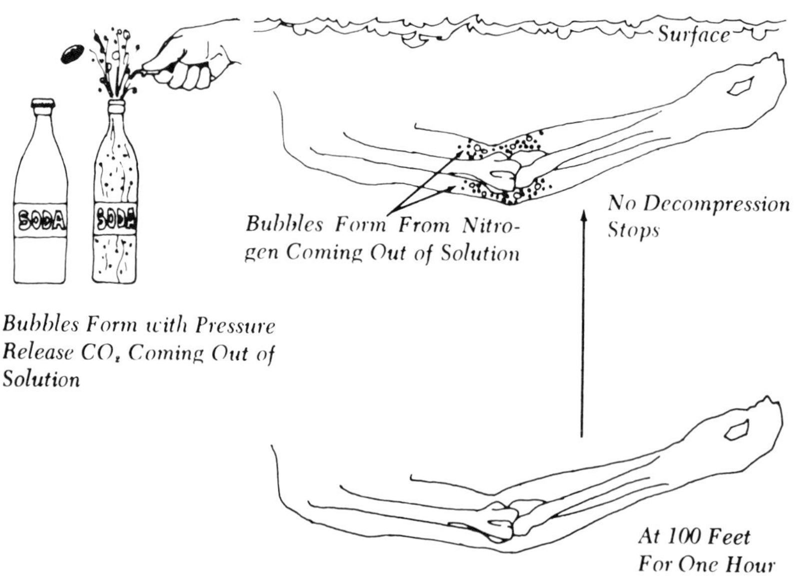

Fig. 13–3. The bends. (From Harper, D.D. *Skin and Scuba Diving.* Courtesy of Charles E. Merrill Publishing Co.)

pressure may "squeeze" the blood vessels in the eye. Figure 13–4 illustrates the hazards of not equalizing pressure while diving.

Breath-Holding

A serious problem exists when swimmers hyperventilate before an extended dive. The fallacy behind this practice is that the swimmer believes he is super-saturating his blood with oxygen so that the duration of the dive can be extended. In fact there is little increase in oxygen tension. The major effect of hyperventilation is that it blows off large amounts of circulating CO_2 and thus lowers PCO_2. Under normal conditions, carbon dioxide is the main stimulus for respiration and will override any voluntary suppression of breathing when the PCO_2 levels rise to about 50 mm Hg. However, with hyperventilation the PCO_2 can be lowered to about 20 mm Hg. This causes two problems: (1) the O_2 dissociation curve shifts to the left and makes it difficult to release O_2 into the tissue. (2) If the oxygen that can be released is utilized before enough carbon dioxide is produced, the swimmer may pass out from lack of oxygen and drown without even feeling the need to breathe.

TEMPERATURE REGULATION

Often athletes are required to train and compete in severe weather conditions, such as the sub-zero temperatures of the Rocky Mountain winters, the blistering heat of the desert Southwest, or the tropical humidity of the Southeast. These athletes must learn how to adjust to these conditions and also understand the potential dangers. Although exercising in either heat or cold presents special problems, hot weather poses by far the greatest concern in terms of overall temperature regulation.

There are two measures of temperature of concern to an athlete: the ambient temperature (the temperature around the body) and the internal temperature (the core or internal temperature of the body). The athlete has little or no control of his environment, but is capable of regulating his own core temperature within a narrow range independent of the ambient temperature. This regulatory ability resides in the hypothalamus, which operates much like a thermostat that controls the temperature in a house. If the internal temperature of the body rises or lowers from the set temperature (set-point), the hypothalamus responds to either increase heat production or to decrease core temperature by carrying heat to the surface of the body. The

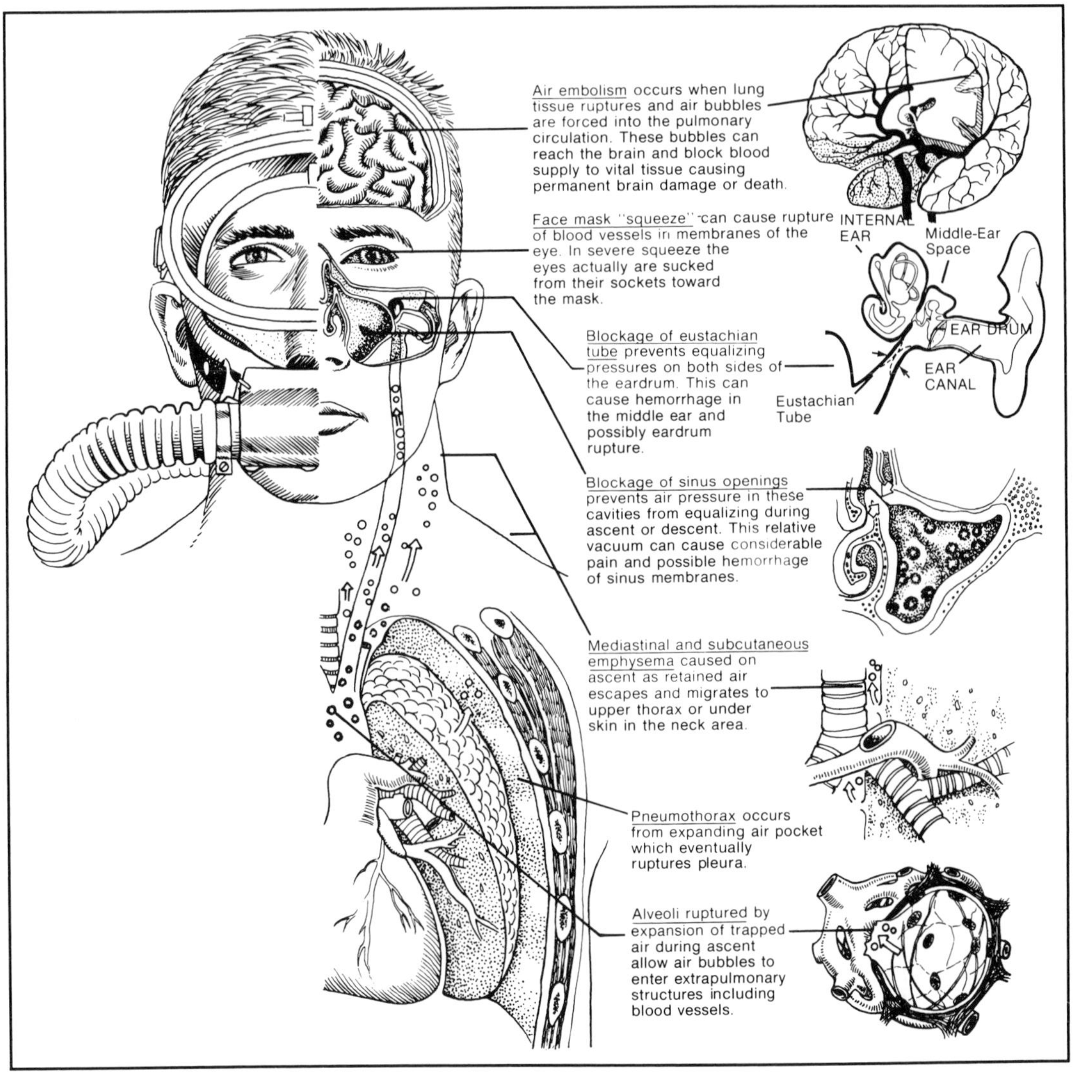
Air embolism occurs when lung tissue ruptures and air bubbles are forced into the pulmonary circulation. These bubbles can reach the brain and block blood supply to vital tissue causing permanent brain damage or death.
Face mask "squeeze" can cause rupture of blood vessels in membranes of the eye. In severe squeeze the eyes actually are sucked from their sockets toward the mask.
INTERNAL EAR
Middle-Ear Space
EAR DRUM
EAR CANAL
Blockage of eustachian tube prevents equalizing pressures on both sides of the eardrum. This can cause hemorrhage in the middle ear and possibly eardrum rupture.
Eustachian Tube
Blockage of sinus openings prevents air pressure in these cavities from equalizing during ascent or descent. This relative vacuum can cause considerable pain and possible hemorrhage of sinus membranes.
Mediastinal and subcutaneous emphysema caused on ascent as retained air escapes and migrates to upper thorax or under skin in the neck area.
Pneumothorax occurs from expanding air pocket which eventually ruptures pleura.
Alveoli ruptured by expansion of trapped air during ascent allow air bubbles to enter extrapulmonary structures including blood vessels.

Fig. 13–4. Hazards in scuba diving due to the inability to equalize internal external pressure. (From McArdle, W.D., Katch, F.I., and Katch, V.L. *Exercise Physiology*, 2nd Ed. Courtesy of Lea & Febiger, 1986.)

sensors for heat are thought to be located in the preoptic region of the anterior hypothalamus, while the cold sensitive neurons are controlled by the posterior hypothalamus. There are probably peripheral receptors (free nerve endings) located in the skin, but these are only capable of modifying core temperature to a small degree (Fig. 13–5).

There is a critical temperature threshold that must be reached before afferent signals are sent to the hypothalamus. As core temperature increases, the hypothalamus compensates by stimulating the sweat glands, reducing the vasoconstrictive tone to the skin, and shunting blood to the skin through vasodilation. As the cooling process proceeds the afferent signals from the heat-sensitive sensors subside, which in turn restores the hypothalamus to its normal activity.

The body's response to cold is similar to the heat response but almost exactly reversed. With cold, the hypothalamus *increases* heat production by stimulating the shivering centers and reduces heat loss by vasoconstricting the blood vessels that supply the skin. This in essence creates a thicker layer of tissue to insulate the body as the blood pool is concentrated in central regions.

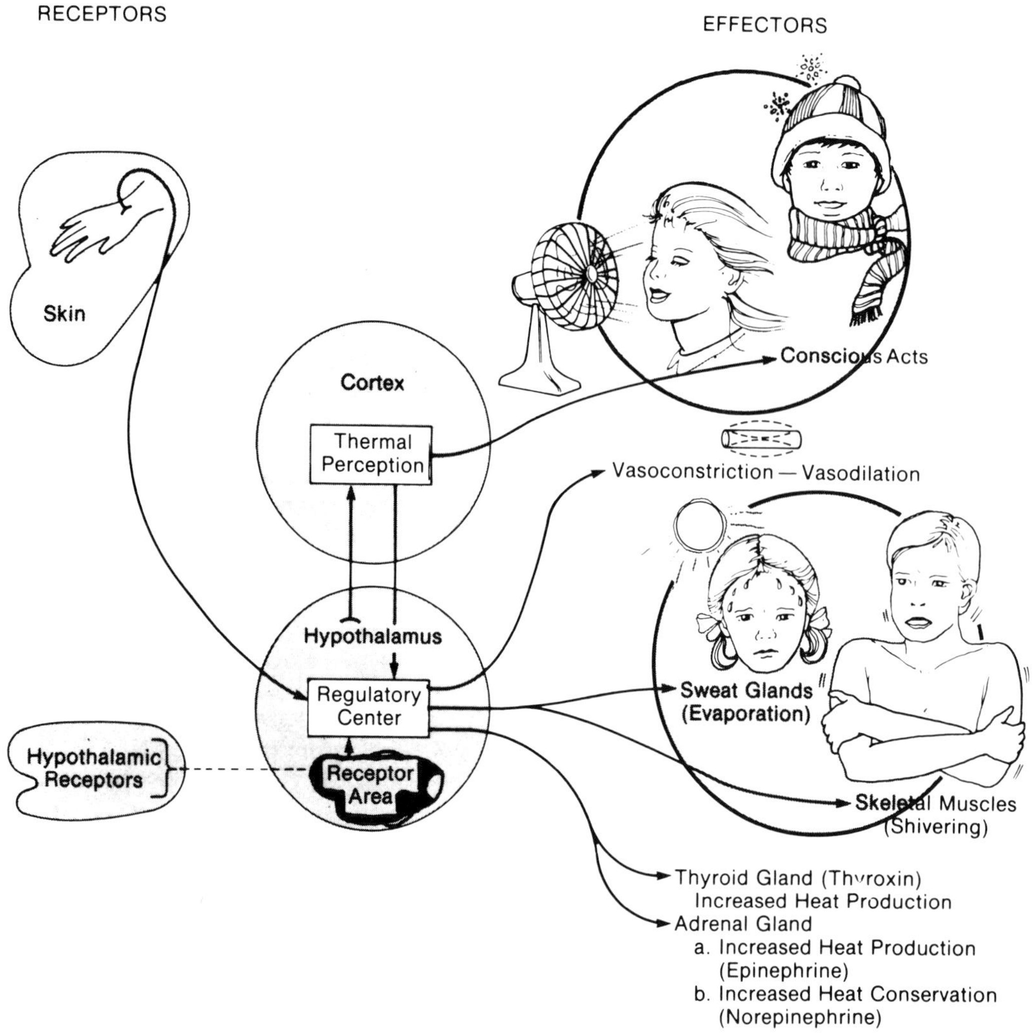

Fig. 13–5. Summary of the thermoregulatory system. (From Fox, E.L., Bowers, R.W., Foss, M.L. *Physiological Basis of Physical Education and Athletics*, 4th Ed. Courtesy of W.B. Saunders Co., 1988.)

HEAT PRODUCTION AND HEAT LOSS

The body gains or loses heat through four separate processes, *conduction, convection, radiation,* and *evaporation. Conduction* is the process whereby heat is lost or gained by direct contact with a cooler or hotter object. An example of this process is when deep muscle loses heat by direct contact with the cooler tissues towards the surface of the body or when you lean against a warm brick wall on a cold day and the heat warms your body. *Convection* involves the transfer of heat from one place to another by the motion of a heated substance. For example, riding a bike can cool the body because the air flow removes air warmed by the body and replaces it with cooler air. Convection is the process that allows blood to release heat at the skin if the air near the skin is cooler than the blood. The amount of convection depends on the temperature difference between two areas. Water can absorb several thousand times more heat than air. Swimming pools often feel cold even though the water temperature is the same as the ambient air. Because of the heat absorption qualities of water, wetness becomes a major contention when exercising in the cold. *Radiation* is the loss of heat transmitted from electromagnetic waves emitted from the body to cooler objects in the surroundings. Our body also absorbs heat from the sun by radiation. The principle of radiation is based on the fact that molecules within a body are constantly vibrating, and as a result, heat is given off in the form of electromagnetic waves. We gain heat from radiation when surrounding objects are warmer, and lose heat if these objects are cooler.

The major factor in heat loss from our bodies is the process of *evaporation*. Evaporation is the process of changing a liquid to a vapor. This process requires energy (heat), and this heat comes from the body. For every liter of water that evaporates from the body, approximately 580 Kcals of heat are lost into the environment. In the summer, evaporation is the major defense to overheating. In the winter, evaporation must be controlled to balance the heat gain and heat loss. As sweat and water are evaporated from the skin, the cooling process helps cool the blood that is flowing through the periphery. If humidity is high, it is difficult for sweat to evaporate because the air is already full of water vapor and the sweating process is inefficient in terms of cooling the body (Fig. 13–6).

EXERCISE IN THE HEAT

Essentially, all metabolic activity ends up as heat. At rest, the heat production is small (only about 75 kcals/hour). During exercise, the heat production can increase 15 to 20 times. This excess heat could pose a real problem for the body, because if not removed, the body temperature would continue to rise until death occurred. The ability of an athlete to successfully perform in the heat depends on many factors (air temperature, humidity, intensity, duration of effort), but in the final analysis, the body must take heat that is produced as a result of metabolic activity and carry it to the surface where it can be released. One of the primary responsibilities of the circulatory system is to transport heat from the muscles to the skin so that heat can be transferred to the environment. Since the volume of blood is limited, exercise in the heat is a problem for circulation because there is simply too little blood to service the needs of the muscles and cool the body at the same time. In addition, during exercise, nearly 80% of the body's cooling is accomplished by evaporation. Since a high percentage of the fluid lost in sweat comes from blood plasma, the cardiovascular system suffers another setback and the body may become *dehydrated.*

Humans are able to sweat at the rate of about 2 liters an hour for short periods of time and can sweat over 1 liter an hour for 3 to 4 hours. This kind of water loss could be extremely dangerous because it has been estimated that deep body temperature will rise from 0.3° to 0.5°F for every 1% loss in body weight due to water loss. Consistent water loss could quite quickly lead to hyperthermia if not replaced.

Although most of the water loss comes from the cells and the interstitial fluid, the fluid loss from plasma is critical because it affects the total circulating blood volume and therefore cardiac output. This in turn impairs not only the transport of heat to the periphery, but also the supply of blood to the exercising muscles. One researcher found losses in running performance from 4 to 7% from a 3% loss in body weight due to dehydration. In addition to these problems, exercise in the heat reduces the temperature gradient between the skin and environment and between the body core and the skin. As these gradients are decreased, heat loss becomes more difficult. In fact, the body gains heat when environmental conditions (temperature and humidity) are such that heat is lost at slower rates than heat is produced. Of more serious concern are the heat disorders that can occur to the body (these will be discussed later in this chapter).

Fortunately, the circulatory system in conjunction with the sweating mechanism has great capacity to dissipate body heat. As exercise intensity increases, the active muscle tissue produces heat which is collected by the venous blood and distributed to various parts of the body increasing the overall core temperature. Thermal sensors in the hypothalamus sense the increased blood temperature, and adjust nervous activity appropriately. Blood vessels in the skin dilate shunting blood to the skin to be cooled, either through sweating (evaporation), convection, radiation, or a combination of all three. If the rate of heat dissipation matches production, the internal temperature remains steady; if there is an imbalance, there is a danger of heat cramps, heat

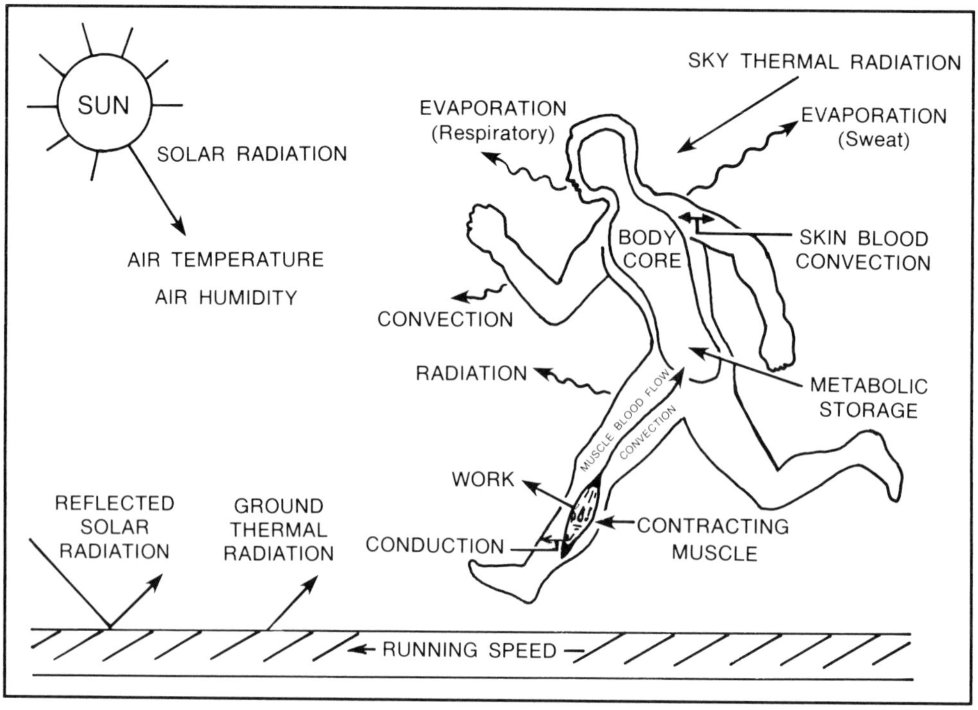

Fig. 13–6. Schematic diagram showing heat production within working skeletal muscle, its transport to the body core and to the skin, and its subsequent exchange with the environment. (From Gisolfi, C.V., and Wegner, C.B.: Temperature regulation during exercise: old concepts, new ideas. Exer. Sport Sci. Rev., *12*:339, 1984. Edited by Tergung, R.L. Courtesy of Macmillan Publishing Co.)

stroke, heat exhaustion, or even death. The human body can withstand a gain in temperature of only about 5°C. It is necessary to have both a large blood flow to the working muscle to carry the heat from the deep muscles and core to the periphery, and in the skin to dissipate the heat to the environment. Because of the limited supply of blood, the excess requirement for blood negatively affects performance.

Moderate exercise in the heat requires an increased cardiac output due to the increased need for blood in the periphery. This is supplied mostly by an increased heart rate. Blood lactate and sub-maximal $\dot{V}O_2$ are not changed. Submaximal heart rate increases in response to heat stress in order to maintain cardiac output. Submaximal oxygen consumption is a function of exercise intensity and therefore would not be expected to increase as a result of heat stress. Maximum exercise is limited because of the decreased heart rate reserve.

All these thermal regulatory systems are useless if the transfer of heat is blocked by excessive layers of clothing or equipment (e.g., football players and exercisers trying to lose weight by wearing vinyl sweat suits), or if athletes voluntarily dehydrate themselves trying to "make weight" before competition. These factors can lead to several serious heat disorders (these will be discussed later in the chapter). From 1960 to 1984, there were 73 heat stroke deaths reported among high school athletes, all because the coaches and trainers failed to take the necessary precautions to prevent their athletes from becoming victims of heat illness.

Acclimatization

Some of the negative problems associated with exercise in the heat can be decreased by acclimatization. Acclimatization is best accomplished by progressively increasing the duration and intensity of exercise in the heat over a 2-week period. However, major changes in the physiological response to heat stress begin to occur within the first 4 to 5 days of exercise in a hot environment. It appears that physical training itself produces some degree of acclimatization, even in the absence of heat. However, athletes who live in a moderate climate and know that they will need to compete in a hot climate should either go to a hotter site and train, or at least train in the hottest part of the day. Care should be taken during the first few days of training in a hotter environment to avoid heat injury. In team sports, athletes should refrain from wearing full uniform until after the first week. Appropriate fluids should always be available. The following changes have been reported as a result of acclimatization to the heat:

1. *Improved heat tolerance.* The body begins to sweat at a lower temperature. Because of this, skin temperatures are lower and less blood is needed in the skin to transfer body heat.

2. *Improved distribution of sweat.* The amount of sweat is not necessarily less, but the distribution is better over the body, so the efficiency of the mechanism is better.

3. *Improved conservation of minerals in sweat.* The sweat that is produced is a more dilute sweat and the mineral content is conserved.

4. *Lower skin and body temperature.* A lower skin and body temperature for a given level of work decreases the amount of blood needed for cooling and yields a lower heart rate.

Table 13–7 contains a list of changes associated with acclimatization.

GUIDELINES FOR EXERCISE IN THE HEAT

The following guidelines will be helpful for coaches or athlete who must participate in activity in the heat:

Table 13–7. Physiological Adjustments Following Acclimatization

Circulatory system
Increased plasma volume
Increased blood volume
Decreased heart rate
Increased stroke volume
Cooling system
Decreased sweating threshold
Increased rate of sweating
Increased evaporative heat loss
Decreased Na^+ loss

1. Gradually acclimatize to hot weather by slowly increasing intensity and duration. Usually after a week to 10 days a person will be 80% acclimated.

2. Since increased sweating leads to dehydration, fluid replacement is a necessity. Drink more fluids than thirst dictates. The body normally takes in and eliminates from 2.0 to 2.5 liters of water per day. Sweating can increase fluid loss to 10 or 15 liters. Weigh before and after exercise to ensure complete rehydration and have fluid immediately available to the practice area and stop at regular intervals for rehydration. Since there is usually a 1% decrease in overall weight with each liter of water lost through sweat, a decrease of 5 to 7% body weight represents a dangerous threshold where the individual should stop any activity until completely rehydrated.

Weigh during training sessions to get an idea of how much fluid should be replaced during any given event. Then drink enough during the event to stay up with the water needs.

During activity, use a cold drink to help cool the body. Either water or "aid" drinks may be used. If "aid" drinks are used, they should be fairly dilute in glucose content (3 to 10 g per 100 ml solution) to avoid slowing the emptying process, or use a polyglucose drink. Any drink that contains more than 2.5 g glucose/dl will probably slow stomach emptying, but this has not proven to be a problem and higher concentrations are being used. Some athletes are using "polyglucose" drinks to decrease this problem. About 200 to 300 ml (½ pint) of glucose-electrolyte solution will be needed every 15 to 20 minutes during the exercise session, but this level will depend on temperature, humidity, and type and intensity of activity (check the body weight for more exact figures).

3. Electrolytes loss is decreased in acclimatized athletes, but any loss must be replaced. The best way to replace electrolytes is through a balanced diet containing a wide variety of food from all of the basic food groups and using salt liberally. However, the "aid" drinks do contain a good balance of the essential minerals and can be beneficial to the athlete during hot weather.

4. Salt tablets should be prohibited, since as

fluids are lost from the body there is actually a concentrating of the salt contained within the body. The only time salt tablets would be considered necessary is if one is required to perform heavy work in an extremely hot environment for an extended period of time.

5. Schedule exercise sessions for the cooler times of the day unless games or competition will be held in the heat. If practice or games must be held in the heat, be aware of the humidity since it decreases the effectiveness of evaporation. The higher the humidity or saturation of air, the more difficult it becomes for the sweat to evaporate and cool the body. Obviously, a 5 to 20% humidity reading common to the deserts of the Western United States is more advantageous than the 95% humidity typical of the Southeast since there is more dry air to pick up the moisture. There have been many scales developed to determine the heat/humidity levels that are safe for exercise. A simplified and easy way of estimating these levels is presented in Table 13–8.

6. Reduce the amount of clothing worn to compensate for hot/humid conditions. Be concerned about sunburn.

7. *Never* use rubberized clothing, even though they claim to accelerate weight loss. The only thing that is lost is water. These suits are also dangerous since they inhibit the corrective, convective, and evaporative actions necessary to dissipate heat.

8. Athletes should be taught how to recognize the early warning signals that precede heat injury, such as piloerection on the chest and upper arm, chilling, throbbing pressure in the head, nausea, dry skin, and be familiar with emergency procedures. A brief discussion of the various levels of heat injury follows.

Related Heat Problems

As the internal core temperature rises, the body either successfully handles the thermal stress or suffers from possible disorders such as heat cramps, heat stroke, and heat exhaustion.

Heat Cramps. Heat cramps are characterized by excessive sweating which depletes water and salt from the muscles causing a fluid-electrolyte imbalance. This results in involuntary cramping and spasms. This condition is usually not serious and can be reversed by drinking large amounts of water. It is not necessary to take salt tablets, since the kidneys and sweat glands become efficient salt conservers. Most people will automatically eat more salt with meals when working in the heat.

Heat Exhaustion. Another form of heat illness which is more severe than heat cramps is heat exhaustion. Heat exhaustion is characterized by extreme weakness, a rapid and weak pulse, headaches, dizziness, fainting, profuse sweating, cold and clammy skin, with a near-normal temperature. All of these symptoms stem from dehydration, salt depletion, and an elevated core temperature (usually less than 39.5°C) resulting in a blood volume loss and the inability of the circulatory system to maintain its normal function.

Treatment is relatively easy, the individual should lie down in a cool shady area and drink cool liquids. Excessive clothing should be removed, and the person should avoid stressful activity for at least 24 hours. On occasion, hospitalization and intravenous fluid replacement may be necessary, but this is the exception, not the rule.

Heat Stroke. Heat stroke is the most serious of the heat illnesses and is due to the failure of the hypothalamic temperature-regulatory control center. It is characterized by a high rectal temperature, warm/dry skin, lack of sweating, rapid pulse, delirium, vomiting, diarrhea, liver damage, unconsciousness, and an extremely high core temperature (41.5°C).

If heat stroke occurs, there is a strong pos-

Table 13–8. Determining Risk of Heat Injury

Temperature	*Humidity Level*	*Recommended Precautions*
less than 80°F	Less than 70%	No precautions necessary
80–90°F	Less than 70%	Caution to sedentary and untrained individuals
90–100°F	Less than 70%	Drink plenty of water, change T-shirt when wet
80–90°F	Greater than 70%	Drink plenty of water, change T-shirt when wet
90–100°F	Greater than 70%	Move session to cooler times of the day
Above 100°F	Greater than 70%	Cancel exercise session

sibility of cerebral or organ damage, and emergency measures to cool the body should be taken immediately. Such measures include immersing the body in cool water, packing the body in ice, wrapping the body in wet towels and transporting the athlete to the nearest hospital.

Some people are extremely susceptible to heat illness, and must take extra precautions to ward against possible problems.

EXERCISING IN THE COLD

There are fewer problems related with exercising in the cold than in the heat for two reasons: (1) the body produces a significant amount of heat during exercise, and (2) the loss of heat can be regulated easily by the amount of clothing worn. For the nonathlete, the only real dangers related with exposure to the cold are those of frostbite on exposed areas and hypothermia. The added weight of clothing and the numbing effects of the cold on hands and feet serve to impair overall athletic performance.

Physiologic Response to Cold

Exposure to the cold causes peripheral vasoconstriction which reduces the amount of blood circulating to the extremities. This occurs over the entire body with the exception of the head, where the flow remains about the same. For this reason, a great deal of heat is radiated through the head if left uncovered. The purpose of vasoconstriction during exposure to the cold is to maintain body core temperature. Vasoconstriction shunts the blood to the core where proper temperature of vital organs is maintained.

Hypothermia. At extremely low core temperature, the hypothalamus ceases to control body temperature, which results in the depression of the central nervous system. It is characterized by the absence of shivering, low body temperature (below 30.2°C), sleepiness, slurring of speech, possible ventricular fibrillations, and eventually coma. Young children who have fallen through the ice into the super-cooled water have survived with no long term after-effects, even though they were submerged for 20 to 30 minutes. These children survived because the extreme cold depressed all their body functions to the point that little oxygen was needed. The treatment for hypothermia involves slowly rewarming the body, and transporting the person to the nearest hospital where blood gases, urine and liver functions can be monitored during the rewarming process. Fatter people are less susceptible than thin people to hypothermia because of the insulation role of fat. Clothes are valuable since they increase the body's insulative layer, which reduces the heat loss due to convection and radiation while allowing evaporation of sweat. As exercise increases it may be necessary to remove several layers of clothing to allow excess heat to escape.

Temperature and Wind-Chill

The absolute temperature reading alone is not a valid criterion to estimate the effects of the environment on athletes. Twenty degrees below zero is very cold, but with a 40 mph wind, it can freeze a truck's radiator while running on the freeway. On the other hand, a temperature of 10°F, with 70% humidity and a small breeze, will feel almost as cold as the 30° below with no wind. The effect wind has on overall temperature is referred to as the *wind-chill*. Listed in Figure 13–7 are the equivalent temperatures at various temperature and wind conditions, and the relative danger of each.

Frostbite

Over-exposure to the cold can cause permanent tissue and circulatory damage when frostbite occurs. The areas of the body most vulnerable are those that are most often exposed such as the fingers, toes, and earlobes. Since blood is shunted inwardly to maintain core temperature, those exposed areas cool rapidly and can freeze. Unfortunately, once damaged the tissue will not regenerate and the function to that particular area will be lost.

Dressing for Exercise in the Cold

As "homeotherms," humans are able to function quite well under almost any environmental conditions. In fact, the mean environmental temperature of many areas in the Soviet Union and Canada is less than 0°C and the mean January temperature of Fairbanks, Alaska is about 25°C below zero. It is true that

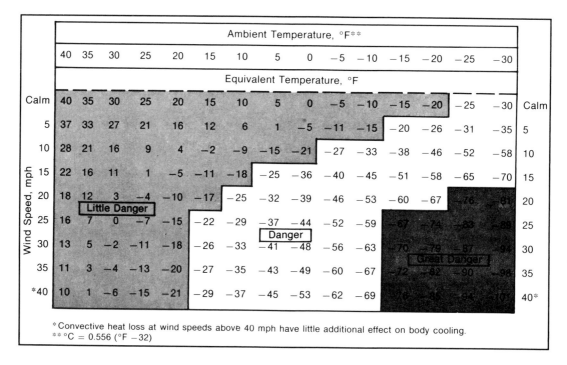

Wind Speed, mph	Ambient Temperature, °F**															
	40	35	30	25	20	15	10	5	0	−5	−10	−15	−20	−25	−30	
	Equivalent Temperature, °F															
Calm	40	35	30	25	20	15	10	5	0	−5	−10	−15	−20	−25	−30	Calm
5	37	33	27	21	16	12	6	1	−5	−11	−15	−20	−26	−31	−35	5
10	28	21	16	9	4	−2	−9	−15	−21	−27	−33	−38	−46	−52	−58	10
15	22	16	11	1	−5	−11	−18	−25	−36	−40	−45	−51	−58	−65	−70	15
20	18	12	3	−4	−10	−17	−25	−32	−39	−46	−53	−60	−67	−76	−81	20
25	16	7	0	−7	−15	−22	−29	−37	−44	−52	−59	−67	−74	−83	−89	25
30	13	5	−2	−11	−18	−26	−33	−41	−48	−56	−63	−70	−79	−87	−94	30
35	11	3	−4	−13	−20	−27	−35	−43	−49	−60	−67	−72	−82	−90	−98	35
*40	10	1	−6	−15	−21	−29	−37	−45	−53	−62	−69	−76	−85	−94	−101	40*

Little Danger

Danger

Great Danger

*Convective heat loss at wind speeds above 40 mph have little additional effect on body cooling.
** °C = 0.556 (°F −32)

Fig. 13–7. Wind-chill-factor chart. (From McArdle, W.D., Katch, F.I., and Katch, V.L. *Exercise Physiology,* 2nd Ed. Courtesy of Lea & Febiger, 1986.)

the body is required to maintain a fairly rigorous control of internal temperature so that it stays within the range of 36° to 40°C (normal body temperature is 37°C). However, the body is well equipped to maintain normal temperature with just a little help in the way it is dressed.

Basically, body temperature is a function of the body's production of heat (metabolic heat production) plus or minus the heat that is gained or lost to the environment. For instance, when exercising outside on a cold day (say 32°F) the body could easily produce 4 to 8 times more heat than at rest, but it could also lose a significant amount of heat to the air by convection, especially if the wind is blowing at all. The wind chill table (Fig. 13–7) helps clarify this relationship. At 32°F, a 15 mile per hour wind would make it feel like a calm day at 13°F. The problem in cold weather is that a person receives little environmental heat gain because the sun is usually low in the sky and/or covered by clouds, but experiences a lot of environmental heat loss because the air is cold and the wind often blows. Therefore, the biggest problem is containing the heat the body produces, and decreasing the heat that is lost to the atmosphere. This is done by proper selection and wearing of clothing.

If too much clothing is worn, there is the potential of becoming a "tropical person" in a cold environment. The solution lies in wearing "layers" of clothing so that the insulation value is increased and so that adjustments can be made as metabolic heat increases. The most important layer is next to the skin. This layer needs to absorb sweat and then "wick" it away to prevent chilling. A new fiber called olefin or polypropylene is excellent for this layer. Wool also has excellent properties, but is usually too itchy to be worn next to the skin. Silk is good, but expensive, and cotton is a fairly poor insulator and absorbs too much water. Because of cost, a cotton tee shirt could be worn next to the skin with a wool sweater over that if the weather is cold enough for two layers under the outer garments.

The best outerwear is Goretex. It is waterproof, windproof, durable, and yet allows sweat to escape. Luckily, the cost of Goretex outerwear is coming down, and most people will be able to afford this material in the future. Nylon is almost as good, but is usually not waterproof without a treatment like Scotchguard or some other waterproofing substance. Cotton and cotton blends can be used for outerwear, but the wind penetrates these too much, and they also get wet easily. The jacket-type coverings are excellent because it is easier to release or contain heat by simply opening or closing the zipper. On colder days, wear long stockings or some other insulator on the legs.

The most important item for exercise in the cold is a hat or head covering. Uncovered, you can lose up to 40% of your body heat. Exposed skin on the hands also needs to be covered not only because of heat loss, but because of the danger of frostbite. Mittens are preferred to gloves because the hands stay warmer, but either may be worn. There is probably no danger in terms of freezing the lungs in cold weather, but wearing a scarf or face mask will warm the air and protect the facial skin from frostbite.

SELECTED READINGS

1. Brooks, G.A., Hittelman, K.J., Faulkner, J.A., et al.: Temperature, skeletal muscle mitochondrial functions, and oxygen debt. Am. J. Physiol. *220*:1053, 1971.
2. Buskirk, E., Kollias, J., Akers, R., et al.: Maximal performance at altitude and on return from altitude in conditioned runners. J. Appl. Physiol. *23*(2):259–266, 1967.
3. Costill, D.L.: Fluids for athletic performance: why and what you should drink during prolonged exercise. In The New Runners Diet. Mountain View, California, World Publications, 1977.
4. Costill, D.L. and Saltin, B.: Factor limiting gastric emptying during rest and exercise. J. Appl. Physiol. *37*(5):679–683, 1974.
5. Daniels, J., and Oldridge, N.: The effects of alternate exposure to altitude and sea level on world class middle distance runners. Med. Sci. Sports *2*(3):107–112, 1970.
6. Faulkner, J.A.: Heat and contractile properties of skeletal muscle. In Horvath, S.M. and Yousef, M.K. (eds). *Environmental Physiology: Aging, Heat and Altitude.* Amsterdam: Elsevier, 1981.
7. Faulkner, J., Daniels, J., and Balke, B.: Effects of training at moderate altitude on physical performance capacity. J. Appl. Physiol. *23*(1):85–89, 1967.
8. Faulkner, J., Kollias, J., Favour, C., et al.: Maximum aerobic capacity and running performance at altitude. J. Appl. Physiol. *24*(5):85–89, 1968.
9. Folk, G.E.: *Textbook of Environmental Physiology.* Philadelphia: Lea & Febiger, 1974.
10. Fox, E.L., Bowers, R.W., and Foss, M.L.: *The Physiological Basis of Physical Education and Athletics.* 4th Ed. Philadelphia: Saunders College Publishing, 1988.
11. Gisolfi, C.V. (ed): Symposium on the thermal effects of exercise in the heat. Med. Sci. Sports *11*(1):30–71, 1979.
12. Gisolfi, C.V. and Cohen, J.S.: Relationships among training, heat acclimatization, and heat tolerance in men and women: the controversy revisited. Med. Sci. Sports *11*(1):56–59, 1979.
13. Grover, R.F., Weil, J.V., and Reeves, J.T.: Cardiovascular Adaptation to Exercise at High Altitude. Exerc. Sports Sci. Rev. *14*:269–302, 1986.
14. Haymes, E.M. and Wells, C.L.: *Environment and Human Performance.* Champaign: Human Kinetics Pub., 1986.
15. Horvath, S.M.: Historical perspectives of adaptation to heat. In Horvath, S.M. and Yousef, M.K. (eds). *Environmental Physiology: Aging, Heat and Altitude.* Amsterdam: Elsevier, 1981.
16. McArdle, W.D., Katch, F.I., and Katch, V.L.: *Exercise Physiology.* 2nd Ed. Philadelphia: Lea & Febiger, 1986.
17. Nadel, E.R.: Recent advances in temperature regulation during exercise in humans. Federation Proc. *44*(7):2286–2292, 1985.
18. Pandolf, K.B., Sawka, M.N., and Gonzalez, R.R.: *Human Performance Physiology and Environmental Medicine at Terrestrial Extremes.* Indianapolis: Benchmark Press, 1988.
19. Pugh, L.G.C.E.: Cardiac output in muscular exercise at 5,800 m (19,000 ft). J. Appl. Physiol. *19*(3):441–447, 1974.
20. Rowell, L.: Human cardiovascular adjustments to exercise and thermal stress. Physiol. Rev. *54*(1):75–159, 1974.
21. Squires, R.W. and Buskirk, E.R.: Aerobic capacity during acute exposure to simulated altitude, 914 to 2286 meters. Med. Sci. Sports Exerc. *14*(1):36–40, 1974.
22. Sutton, J.R.: Exercise at extreme altitudes. In *Exercise: Benefits Limits and Adaptations.* Macleod, D., Maughan, R., Nimmo, M., et al. (eds). London: E. & F.N. Spon. 1987, pp. 313–323.
23. West, J.B., Boyer, S.J., Graber, D.J., et al.: Maximal exercise at extreme altitudes on Mount Everest. J. Appl. Physiol: Respir. Environ. Exercise Physiol. *55*(3):688–698, 1983.
24. Welch, H.G.: Effects of Hypoxia and Hyperoxia on Human Performance. Exerc. Sport Sci. Rev. *15*:191–221, 1987.
25. West, J.B., Hackett, P.H., Maret, K.H., et al.: Pulmonary gas exchange on the summit of Mount Everest. J. Appl. Physiol: Respir. Environ. Exerc. Physiol. *55*(3):678–687, 1983.
26. Wyndham, C.H.: The physiology of exercise under heat stress. Ann. Rev. Physiol. *35*:193–220, 1973.
27. Wyndham, C.H, Rogers, G.G., Senay, L.C., et al.: Acclimatization in a hot humid environment: cardiovascular adjustments. J. Appl. Physiol. *40*:779–785, 1976.

14

Training Considerations for Females

For many years, women have been forced to participate in recreational sports such as swimming and tennis that were considered less strenuous in nature. Women basketball players were restricted to half court games to avoid overtaxing their bodies, and sports such as long distance running were considered to be completely inappropriate.

Women themselves were somewhat to blame for this perception. For example, at the 1928 Olympic games held in Amsterdam, the women's 800 meter run ended in disaster. At the finish line 6 out of 9 runners collapsed from exhaustion. Several of the competitors had to be carried off the track, and even the sturdiest "needed attention before she was able to leave the field." The London Times reported ". . the half dozen prostrate and obviously distressed forms lying in the grass at the side of the track after the race may not warrant a complete condemnation of the girl athletic championships, but it certainly suggests unpleasant possibilities." The media never understood that these women were simply untrained, but the event caused such a stir that the 800 meter event was deleted from the Olympic program and was not reinstated until 1960.

Only recently has the Olympic Committee reversed many of its longstanding attitudes about women's capacity to participate in long distance events by instituting the first women's marathon in the 1984 Summer Olympic Games in Los Angeles. Joan Benoit's decisive win in the marathon and the resurgence of women into almost all aspects of athletic competition should put to rest forever the notion that women are incapable of competing in endurance sports. It is interesting to note that Benoit's world record time of 2:22:43 set at the 1983 Boston Marathon was better than the gold medal time of the men's marathon in 1956. Beginning with Miki Gorman's 1973 world record time for the women's marathon of 2:46:36, to Benoit's 2:22:43 in 1983, and with the advent of Title IX legislation, there has been a major change in the participation and acceptance of women in so-called men's sports (Fig. 14–1).

There has been an abundance of research in recent years concerning women in sports. It seems clear from these data that women are physiologically similar to men, and that training programs that work for men will also work for women. The differences that do exist are those of magnitude, not basic physiologic function. The purpose of this chapter is to discuss both the similarities and the differences between males and females that have a bearing on training and performance.

STRUCTURAL DIFFERENCES

During childhood, there is little difference between girls and boys in either size or performance. The similarity begins to end at the onset of puberty when humans begin to secrete gonadotrophic hormones from the pituitary gland. Which of the hormones and to what degree they are secreted is determined

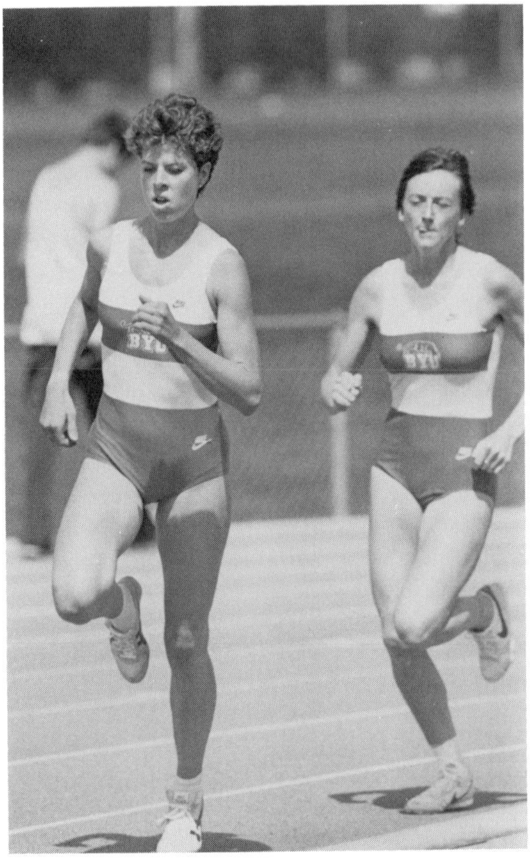

Fig. 14–1.

by the genetic coding located in the chromosomes. In boys, these hormones stimulate the production of androgens; in girls the production of estrogens. It is the hormone *estrogen* that endows girls with more adipose tissue, and reduces the amount of lean body mass. In boys, *testosterone* is responsible for increased muscle mass and retards the deposition of fat. The level of testosterone is the major factor that accounts for the increased muscle mass in men. Before puberty the circulating levels of testosterone in both sexes is about 20 to 60 ng/dl. These levels remain the same in adult women, but are increased to approximately 600 ng/dl in adult men.

As a result of genetic and hormonal differences, women tend to be 3 to 4 inches shorter, 25 to 30 pounds lighter, have 10 to 15 pounds more fat (generally 7% more), and have 40 to 45 pounds less lean body mass than their male counterparts. The effect of this 10 to 15 pounds more adipose tissue and 40 to 45 less pounds LBM is that women have less muscle mass to generate force in situations requiring strength, power, speed, and endurance. Also, because adipose tissue increases the metabolic costs of weight bearing exercise without simultaneously contributing to the production of energy, there is a detrimental influence on performance in endurance events. It should be pointed out that the increased relative fat for women is an advantage in some sports. The greater body fat tends to decrease the total cost of swimming by 10 to 20%.

The amount of fat in some female athletes is much less than normal and lower than most men. For instance, where college-age women have between 22 and 26% fat, well-trained female marathoners often have less than 12% body fat and active women often have less than 16% body fat.

There are moderate structural differences between males and females. Although the width of the female hip is similar to that of the male, the width of other bones and structures is about 10% less in the female. This makes the angle of insertion of the femur more pronounced than in males, and this may increase the amount of pelvic shift necessary to keep the center of gravity aligned during running. Many successful women sprinters seem to have narrow hips. On the positive side, the larger hips lowers the center of gravity, giving women an added advantage in sports which require greater balance (e.g., gymnastics).

With age, both men and women tend to accumulate fat and decrease lean body mass starting in the mid-twenties. The rate of decrease in LBM is about one-half pound a year.

AEROBIC CAPACITY

Twenty-five years ago there existed the popular idea that ". . . at puberty, development of ability for strenuous exercise stops or even declines in girls, while it continues to advance in boys." Over the last decade research has shown that women can improve their aerobic capacity for strenuous exercise to about the same degree as men, but that there is still a significant difference (15 to 25%) in maximal aerobic capacity between men and women. This difference is not ap-

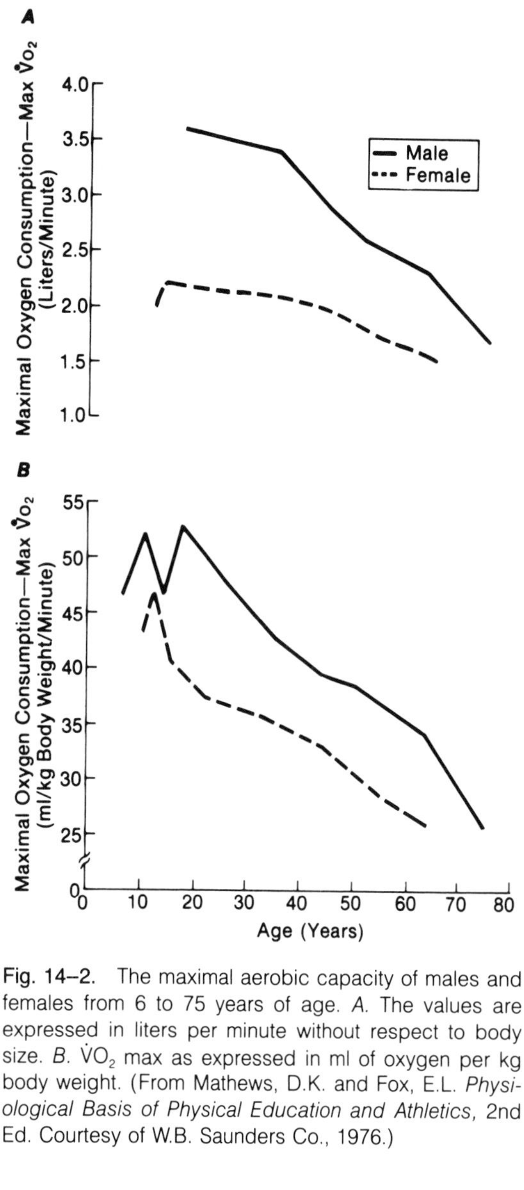

Fig. 14–2. The maximal aerobic capacity of males and females from 6 to 75 years of age. *A.* The values are expressed in liters per minute without respect to body size. *B.* $\dot{V}O_2$ max as expressed in ml of oxygen per kg body weight. (From Mathews, D.K. and Fox, E.L. *Physiological Basis of Physical Education and Athletics*, 2nd Ed. Courtesy of W.B. Saunders Co., 1976.)

parent in younger children when body size and composition differences are minimal, but begins to show up after the size difference becomes a factor during adolescence and adulthood.

The difference in aerobic capacity ($\dot{V}O_2$ max) is greatest when expressed in absolute terms (liters O_2/minute) but decreases when expressed in relative terms (ml/kg/min.). The male-female differences in aerobic power decrease even more when expressed as ml/kg lean body mass/min. or in ml/kg active tissue mass/minute. A compilation of 15 comparative studies of trained and untrained subjects 15 to 36 years of age attempted to quantify the effect of gender (rather than size and body composition) on $\dot{V}O_2$max. When $\dot{V}O_2$max was expressed in absolute terms (l/min.), males were 56% higher than females with 66% of the variance being accounted for by sex. When expressed relative to total body weight (ml/kg/min.), male values were 28% higher than females with 49% of the variance being accounted for by sex. When aerobic capacity was expressed relative to LBM, male values were only 12 to 15% greater than female counterparts and only 35% of the variance was accounted for by sex. Because men on the average are larger than females, these results were not surprising. The larger average body size of men not only requires, but is also capable of using more oxygen.

When extra weight is added to a man to equal the percent body fat of a matched woman, there is a significant decrease in running time as well as $\dot{V}O_2$max. This demonstrates that the extra body fat carried by female athletes induces a greater O_2 cost during submaximal exercise and that any given submaximal workload requires a greater percent of $\dot{V}O_2$max. Maximal capacity is not only reached sooner, but a submaximal pace which can be endured for a long period of time by a lean person is less in an individual carrying more fat.

Although a higher percent fat obviously affects anyone's ability to perform endurance events, the major difference between men and women exists in oxygen transportation. First, women have less hemoglobin (Hb) per liter of blood (13.6 g/dl to 15.3 g/dl from data in Table 14–1). Since each gram of Hb carries 1.34 ml O_2, the total arterial oxygen carrying capacity is decreased.

Females also have a lower total blood volume and a smaller heart than do men of equal size. After both are trained, the differences are somewhat reduced but still significant. The differences in Hb and heart size (volume) are minimal during pre-puberty, and are maximal after puberty.

The relationship between heart size (volume) and $\dot{V}O_2$max is essentially the same for males and females. Because of the smaller heart and decreased Hb in females, a lower $\dot{V}O_2$max is expected. Regardless of how heart

Table 14–1. Normal Values of Hemoglobin ([Hb]), O_2 Carrying Capacity, Blood Volume, and Heart Volume for Trained and Untrained Men and Women

Subjects	*[Hb] g/dl*	*O_2 Capacity (ml/dl)*	*Blood Volume (L)*	*Heart Volume (L)*
Untrained				
Females	13.6	18.22	4.07	560
Males	15.3	20.50	5.25	785
Trained				
Females	14.1	18.89	5.67	790
Males	1.51	20.23	6.58	930

size is expressed (ml, ml/kg, ml/m_2, g/kg) the female heart is about 80% as large as the male counterpart. The larger hearts of men allow for a greater end diastolic volume (EDV) which gives a larger maximal stroke volume and cardiac output. The smaller cardiac output and stroke volume in females also requires a higher heart rate during submaximal exercise as shown in Table 14–2.

Although not as important, women's vital capacity and maximal ventilation volumes are also lower in relation to their size.

Because of the physiologic differences in heart size, blood volume, and hemoglobin content, women cannot realistically expect to compete evenly with men in activities requiring high aerobic capacity. Measures of $\dot{V}O_2$max in athletes confirm these differences. Women endurance athletes routinely measure between 60 and 65 ml/kg/min. as compared to men who measure from 75 to 85 ml/kg/min. The highest level of aerobic fitness recorded by a women was a Russian cross-country skier whose $\dot{V}O_2$max was 77 ml/kg/min.; the highest recorded $\dot{V}O_2$max for a male was 94 ml/kg/min. in a Nordic cross-country skier, a 22% differences. These differences are clearly shown in Figure 14–2. Note that $\dot{V}O_2$max decreases with age for both men and women.

Table 14–2. Two Runners of the Opposite Sex Who Are the Same Size Would Use About the Same Amount of Oxygen and Have a Similar $\dot{V}O_2$. However, Because of the Larger SV, the Male Runner Would Have a Lower Heart Rate at Any Submaximal Work Load

	Female	*Male*
$\dot{V}O_2$	2 liters/min.	2 liters/min.
$\dot{Q}$	15 liters/min.	15 liters/min.
SV	90 ml/beat	120 ml/beat
HR	167 bts/min.	125 bts/min.

Effects of Endurance Training

The large variability of reported gains on $\dot{V}O_2$max due to training is due primarily to the lower initial fitness levels of women. Women of all ages benefit from an aerobic training program, and the changes that occur are similar to those experienced by men. As long as the training intensity is high, both men and women will respond similarly. In one study with women, 7 weeks of training 2 times per week for 30 minutes yielded an increase in $\dot{V}O_2$max from 34.8 ml/kg/minute to 44.2 ml/kg/minute. This was accomplished primarily by an increase in stroke volume which resulted in a larger cardiac output. There were no significant changes in maximal heart rate or in a-$\bar{v}O_2$ diff. It should be noted that significant changes occurred in maximal lactate production.

Young unfit males tend to increase their $\dot{V}O_2$max in response to exercise training by increasing both stroke volume and a-$\bar{v}O_2$ difference. Young unfit females appear to improve aerobic capacity initially by increases in stroke volume. Continued training in females results in a shift from central adaptations to peripheral, and changes in a-$\bar{v}O_2$ difference generally occur after central adaptations. Interestingly, biopsy studies comparing well-trained male and female runners who had similar muscle fiber types and training mileage found a higher level of key oxidative enzymes in the male runners even though both received similar fractions of their energy from lipids during treadmill running at a submax pace. The more sedentary a population prior to engaging in an appropriate exercise training program, the greater the gains expected as a result of the program.

As a result of prolonged exercise training,

any submaximal exercise would yield a lower heart rate due to the increased stroke volume, and a lower percent of $\dot{V}O_2max$. Lactate production would decrease if the original submaximal exercise were near the anaerobic threshold. Females can also expect a decrease in relative fat following endurance training, while experiencing a small increase in lean body mass.

STRENGTH

Human skeletal muscle generates appropriately 4 to 6 kg of force per cm^2, regardless of sex. This would indicate that there is no basic difference in the quality of muscle between men and women. Therefore, two cross-sectional segments of muscle of equal size, one from a male and one from a female would generate approximately the same force. As with aerobic capacity, strength differences between the sexes should be evaluated in terms of absolute strength, strength relative to body size, and strength relative to muscle mass.

In absolute terms (amount of weight lifted) males are about 35 to 50% stronger in both the upper and lower body. Although muscle generates the same force in both men and women, the difference in absolute strength stems from the fact that men are generally larger than women, and thus have more muscle mass to generate force.

There is also a difference among the basic muscle groups. For example, women are weaker than men in absolute strength of all the major muscle groups. However, this difference is greatest in the muscles of the chest, arms, and shoulders, and least in muscles of the legs. This may be due to the fact that even though both sexes use their legs in daily activities, females use upper body muscles less than do males in daily activities and recreation. It is difficult to determine if upper body differences would be less apparent if boys and girls had the same activity profile as they developed, since they start out at the same level as children.

Since women generally average 7% more body fat than males, they are in a sense carrying around more "dead weight." Consequently when strength is expressed in terms of total body weight, the differences mentioned previously are quite large. When strength is expressed in terms of relative strength (weight lifted in relation to muscle mass) the differences in strength are eliminated. This means that a 150-pound woman could theoretically lift as much as a 150-pound man, if both had a similar LBM.

Effects of Strength Training

With the increased interest in fitness and also in female body building, many women are concerned about the effects of strength-training programs on muscle size since large, bulging biceps would not be particularly attractive to some of them. The truth is women can make strength gains with little or no muscle hypertrophy. There are at least three explanations for a strength gain of this type: (1) strength training may increase the ability of the body to recruit extra motor units when lifting. People who have never trained are probably unable to consciously fire all of their motor units. (2) Training could overcome the inhibitory signals sent to muscles from golgi tendon organs. The primary purpose of these receptors is to protect muscle from injury. Training may decrease their sensitivity. (3) Training may allow the muscle to better synchronize the firing of motor units.

Although women have much lower levels of the male hormone *testosterone*, there is some evidence that women experience about the same relative hypertrophy as men in similar training programs. However, the hypertrophy is not as apparent in women because of the smaller muscle mass involved and the increased fat over the muscle. Female bodybuilders use a much higher total work volume than normal and concentrate on specific muscle areas. They also decrease total body fat dramatically so that muscle definition is enhanced. Unfortunately some women bodybuilders use male hormones to "bulk up." What long-term effects steroids will have on these athletes is unknown, since their use by females is a relatively new phenomenon.

Overall the results of strength-training prgrams for women have been positive. Not only have strength gains occurred, but the subjects have often lost girth in areas where girth loss is desirable. Weight-training programs for women usually lead to a significant loss of relative and total body fat with a gain in lean body mass. Women may actually show greater relative increases in strength due to lower initial strength levels. Despite early reports of the untrainability of females, current information supports equal trainability in males and females. There seems to be no reason to use special programs for developing strength in women, since they should respond positively to the same general guidelines used by athletes for many years.

OTHER DIFFERENCES

The total ATP and CP available for rapid energy usage is found in the same concentration in men and women. However, since women have relatively less muscle than men, they have a smaller total supply. Surprisingly, there is little difference in power measurements made using the Margaria-Kalamen power test.

Women are not able to develop blood lactic acid levels to the same extent as men, and are at their greatest disadvantage in events requiring high lactate development. This difference is also due to the greater muscle mass of the male. If expressed in relative values, the difference would be less.

A great deal of research has analyzed the differences in the muscle metabolism of male and female athletes. There appear to be greater differences between endurance and non-endurance athletes than between the sexes.

Men and women athletes in the same sport had almost exactly the same percentage of fast and slow twitch muscle fibers. However, the total fiber area is 68 to 85% smaller in women than men. There is little difference in the muscle concentrations of ATP-CP and scores on a stair-climbing test for power shows little difference between sexes.

THERMAL STRESS

One of the early arguments against women competing in long-distance running, was related to their response to thermal stress. Research in the 50s and 60s indicated that women could not tolerate heat as well as men. Researchers failed to account for the fact that these women were working at a higher % $\dot{V}O_2max$ and failed to acknowledge the relative low level of fitness of the women tested. Recent studies indicate that women working at the same relative percent $\dot{V}O_2max$ sweat less, have lower evaporative heat losses, and higher skin temperatures than men. All of these adjustments are advantageous since they reduce the total loss of body water. There is little evidence that heat is more of a problem for women than for men.

GYNECOLOGIC FACTORS

One area of potential concern to female athletes is the rather high incidence of *amenorrhea* (absence of menstruation) or *oligomenorrhea* (irregular menstruation). This phenomenon seems to be related to low levels of body fat, high levels of stress, high expenditures of energy, and is more prevalent in women who (1) experienced a late onset of menarche, (2) have not been pregnant, and (3) are currently taking contraceptive hormones. Certain athletes (long-distance runners, skiers, gymnasts, tennis players, and rowers) appear to be more prone to these disorders. One-third of all competitive long distance runners experience amenorrhea. These women often run 70 to 100 miles a week. When training is stopped either voluntarily or due to injury, the menses resumes a normal pattern. Supposedly these observations may apply to all sports. Whether the resumption of menses is through an increase in stored fat or a reduction in exercise-induced stress is still unknown.

Although the exact mechanism of exercise-induced amenorrhea is unknown, many researchers feel that heavy exercise training reduces the overall percent body fat and decreases serum levels of pituitary gonadotrophic hormones by stimulating the production of adrenal androgens. This results in reduced estrogen levels which directly affects menstruation. The low levels of body fat could also affect the peripheral production of estrogen.

Sports participation probably has little effect on the problem of *dysmenorrhea* (painful menstruation), although some studies have shown fewer complaints from athletes than non-athletes. Symptoms of dysmenorrhea include headaches, backaches, cramping, irritability, and nausea.

The question of whether to exercise or perform during the menstrual cycle often arises. The answer to this question depends on the effect of the cycle on the individual athlete. Some athletes are affected dramatically and others notice little difference. In one study, 69% of Olympic sportswomen always competed during menstruation. However, only 34% *trained* during menstruation. Similar findings occurred with a group of young female swimmers. In this group of 27 girls, only 7 trained during menstruation, whereas all competed during menstruation. From a physiologic standpoint, there is little reason to avoid participation during any of the stages of the menstrual cycle. A study with 8 trained and 9 untrained females looked at the physiologic responses during three phases of the menstrual cycle as follows: (1) 7 days after ovulation (premenstrual phase), (2) 3 days after the onset of bleeding (menstrual phase), and (3) 13 days after the onset of bleeding (postmenstrual phase). None of the physiologic responses was significantly affected at rest or during exercise during these phases.

Should athletes be encouraged to train during the cycle? As a general rule, those athletes who report no difference in performance should be encouraged to train and compete. However, no female athlete should be forced to train or compete during menstruation if she discovers some negative side effects from doing so.

PREGNANCY

Historically, a pregnant woman was treated as if she had an illness. She was advised to relax, to avoid higher levels of exertion, and to avoid stretching and bending for fear she would strangle or squash the baby. It is now clear that moderate exercise is good for both the mother and the baby. One question that is often asked is "should female athletes compete during pregnancy?" Some world-class athletes have competed successfully while pregnant. However, research shows a drop in $\dot{V}O_2$max during pregnancy (which could be related to decreased training mileage), and lifting activities could be dangerous. Decisions to compete or not compete should be made on an individual basis in consultation with the attending physician.

Does pregnancy and childbirth affect subsequent performance? There are many world-class athletes who have borne children without decreasing their performance following the birth. In fact, more than 30% of these women have better performance.

Should inactive women begin an exercise program after becoming pregnant? The answer is a resounding "yes." Moderate exercise seems to have a positive effect for both the mother and the baby. Moderate exercise during pregnancy can: (1) help maintain proper body weight, (2) decrease backaches, (3) decrease varicose veins, (4) relieve stress, (5) decrease constipation, and (6) help decrease the postpartum belly. Previously inactive women should probably choose activities such as walking or low impact aerobics where the energy expenditure is moderate and the stresses placed on the muscles and joints are minimal. They should also begin slowly and progress slowly just as other beginning exercisers. Women who are already active exercisers could probably continue their normal program through the second trimester but decrease intensity for the last 3 months.

Is exercise in any way unsafe during pregnancy? There is evidence that the baby's oxygen supply may be somewhat impaired by *unaccustomed* activity levels of the mother during the later stages of pregnancy because of the decreased blood flow to the uterus. Increased temperature from high levels of work or activity may also be a problem. If the mother-to-be is accustomed to moderate exercise, and other activities (racquetball, tennis, golf, etc.), there is probably no reason why she could not continue, realizing that there will be a progressive decrease in capacity as well as physical mobility as the pregnancy proceeds.

Generally, female athletes have few complications during childbirth. As a general rule, the length of labor is usually shorter mainly due to the fact that abdominal muscles are stronger and can exert more force. Athletes often experience fewer tissue ruptures during delivery, fewer cesarean sections, and fewer spontaneous abortions.

INJURIES

Problems common to all long-distance runners such as stress fractures, shinsplints, and knee pains occur in equal proportion in both men and women. Women are not excessively prone to injuries, but tolerate the physiologic stress induced by racing at least as well as men.

Injuries to the female reproductive organs seem to be rather rare. The breasts are the most vulnerable and should be protected during contact sports. It also may be wise for female water-skiers to wear rubber wet suits during competition or training to avoid forceful entry of water into the vagina, which could lead to several complications.

In summary, there is little difference in the way men and women respond to training and there is no reason why women cannot compete in almost any activity. The American College of Sports Medicine official statement on female participation in long distance running states: "It is the opinion of the American College of Sports Medicine that females should not be denied the opportunity to compete in long-distance running. There exists no conclusive scientific or medical evidence that long-distance running is contraindicated for the healthy, trained female athlete. The American College of Sports Medicine recommends that females be allowed to compete at the national and international level in the same distances in which male counterparts compete." Although there are differences, these differences should not restrict women from competing and enjoying the full range of activities available to them.

SELECTED READINGS

1. American College of Sports Medicine. Opinion statement on the participation of the female athlete in long distance running. Med. Sci. Sports *11*:ix–xi, 1979.
2. American College of Sports Medicine. Opinion statement on the participation of the female athlete in long-distance running. Sports Med. Bull. *15*(1):1, 4–5, 1980.
3. Astrand, I.: Aerobic work capacity in men and women with specific reference to age. Acta Physiol. Scand. *49*(Suppl):169, 1960.
4. Becklake, M.R., Frank, H., Dagenais, G.R., et al.: Influence of age and sex on exercise cardiac output. J. Appl. Physiol. *20*:938–947, 1965.
5. Brisson, G.R., Volle, M.A., Desharnais, M., et al.: Exercise-induced blood prolactin responses and sports habits in young women. Med. Sci. Sports *11*(1):91, 1979.
6. Brown, C., and Wilmore, J.: The effects of maximal resistance training on the strength and body composition of women athletes. Med. Sci. Sports *6*:174–177, 1974.
7. Cunningham, D.A., and Hill, S.: Effect of training on cardiovascular responses to exercise in women. J. Appl. Physiol. *39*(6):891–895, 1975.
8. Cureton, K.J., and Sparling, P.B.: Distance running performance and metabolic responses to running in men and women with excess weight experimentally equated. Med. Sci. Sports Exerc. *12*(4):288–294, 1980.
9. Dale, E., Gerlach, D.H., Martin, D.E., et al.: Physical fitness profiles and reproductive physiology of the female distance runner. Physician Sportsmed. *7*(1):83–95, 1979.
10. Dale, E., Gerlach, D.H., and Wilhite, A.L.: Menstrual dysfunction in distance runners. Obstet. Gynecol. *54*(1):47–53, 1979.
11. Drinkwater, B., Horvath, S., and Wells, C.: Aerobic power of females, ages 10 to 68. J. Gerontol. *30*(4):385–394, 1975.
12. Erdelyi, G.: Gynecological survey of female athletes. J. Sports Med. *2*:174–179, 1962.
13. Falls, H.B.: The physiological responses of females to endurance exercise, In Cundiff DE (ed): Implementation of Aerobic Programs. Washington DC, American Alliance for Health Physical Education and Recreation, 1980, pp. 36–51.
14. Feicht, C.B., Johnson, T.S., Martin, B.J., et al.: Secondary amenorrhea in athletes. Lancet *2*(8100):1145–1146; 1978.
15. Fox, E.L., Martin, F.L., and Bartels, R.L.: Metabolic and cardiorespiratory responses to exercise during the menstrual cycle in trained and untrained subjects. Med. Sci. Sports *9*(1):70, 1977.
16. Frisch, R.E., and McArthue, J.W.: Menstrual cycles: fatness as a determinant of minimum weight for height necessary for this maintenance or onset. Science *185*:949–951, 1974.
17. Hagerman, F., Fox, E., Conners, M., and Pompei, J.: Metabolic responses of women rowers during ergometric rowing. Med. Sci. Sports *6*(1):87, 1974.
18. Knuttgen, H., and Emerson, K.: Physiological response to pregnancy at rest and during exercise. J. Appl. Physiol. *36*:549–553, 1974.
19. Laubach, L.: Comparative muscular strength of men and women: a review of the literature. Aviat. Space Envir. Med. *47*(5):534–542, 1976.
20. Loucks, A.B., and S.M. Horvath: Athletic amenorrhea: a review. Med. Sci. Sports Exer. *17*(1):56–72, 1985.
21. Malina, R.M., Spirduso, W.W., Tate, C., et al.: Age at menarche and selected menstrual characteristics in athletes at different competitive levels and in different sports. Med. Sci. Sports *10*(3):218–222, 1978.
22. Noack, H.: Duet. Med. Wochenschr. Cited by Thomas, C. Special problems of the female athlete. In Ryan, A., and Allman, F. (eds.): *Sports Medicine*. New York, Academic Press, 1974, pp. 347–373.
23. Rowell, L.B.: Human cardiovascular adjustments to exercise and thermal stress. Physiol. Reviews *54*:75–159, 1978.
24. Schuster, K.: Equipment update: Jogging bras hit the street. Physician Sportsmed. *7*(4):125–128, 1979.
25. Sparling, P.B.: A meta analysis of studies comparing

maximal oxygen uptake in men and women. Res. Q. Exerc. Sport *51*:542–552, 1978.
26. Stager, J.M., Robershaw, D., and Miescher, E.: Delayed menarche in swimmers in relation to age at onset of training and athletic performance. Med. Sci. Sports. Exer. *16*(6):550–555, 1984.
27. Wells, C.L., Hecht, L.H., and Krahenbuhl, G.S.: Physical characteristics and oxygen utilization of male and female marathon runners. Res. Q. Exerc. Sport. *52*(3):281–285, 1981.
28. Wells, C.L., and Plowman, S.A.: Sexual differences in athletic performance: biological or behavioral. Physician Sports Med. *11*(8):52–63, Sept 1983.
29. Wells, C.L.: *Women, Sports, and Performance: A Physiological Perspective.* Champaign, Human Kinetics Publishers, 1985.

15

Measuring Athletic Characteristics

There are several reasons to include a section containing tests that measure certain athletic characteristics in a book of this type. First, coaches can sometimes stimulate excitement about training if they measure and record athletes' progress. They can also generate data allowing them to follow progress using the training programs they have chosen. Second, physical educators can use tests to help evaluate the progress of their students to help in program evaluation. In some cases, these tests can be used to help classify students into more homogeneous groups or to grade students on their progress as they are assigned to different training programs. These tests can also be used to teach principles relating to the physiology of activity. Students are often more interested in principles if they can see those principles applied. Third, these tests can be used as the basis of laboratory experiences for the undergraduate exercise physiology class. We considered organizing several laboratory experiences to be used in conjunction with the test, but felt that the individual instructor would be more able to choose the laboratory experiences to meet his and his students' specific needs if he had a group of tests relating to the various athletic characteristics. The following tests have been chosen because of their ease of administration and accuracy. Most can be used in almost any situation and by most people who have a basic background in exercise physiology. We will provide laboratory ideas for each section of tests to help instructors use these tests in exercise physiology classes.

It is recognized that practically all college students majoring in physical education or athletic coaching take a class in tests and measurements, and the experience of taking such a course should add significant meaning to the present content. Knowing that the reader has had or will have this kind of course, the material presented here is in condensed form, including only carefully selected information and short descriptions. See the reference list for more information.

TESTING STRENGTH

Although there are several different kinds of strength, there are only two basic ways to test strength—statically or dynamically. Static strength is easier to measure, but the measurements are less valuable to athletes and coaches because dynamic strength is the kind of strength that is most used in athletic performance. In fact, the relationship between isometric and dynamic strength measures are relatively low and one should not be predicted from the other. Results of most strength tests are also influenced by motivation. This factor should be controlled whenever possible.

Laboratory Ideas

1. Have students prepare a strength training outline for their favorite sport. Go to a strength training room and have them go through the program with each other. Teach

or have an athletic trainer teach the correct lifting techniques for various lifts.

2. Show students various types of strength training equipment and discuss the advantages and disadvantages of each.

3. Do static and/or dynamic strength tests. Set up several strength test stations, depending upon the available equipment, and have students rotate through these stations.

Static Strength Tests

Static strength of different body parts has been measured accurately using a cable tensiometer, a back and leg lift dynamometer, or a hand grip dynamometer (Fig. 15–1). More recent applications use a strain gauge and feed the information into a personal computer. With either application, it must be remembered that static strength varies at different points through the range of motion. Therefore, if comparisons are to be made, it is important that the strength be measured at exactly the same angle each time (see Fig. 7–10).

For any type of static strength measurement, the person being tested assumes the desired testing position. One end of the cable is attached to the body segment and the other end to a fixed object and the amount of force applied by the segment is measured. For accuracy, the body must be in stable position to allow for the application of maximal force by the body segment. Consistency of position and technique is critical for accurate results.

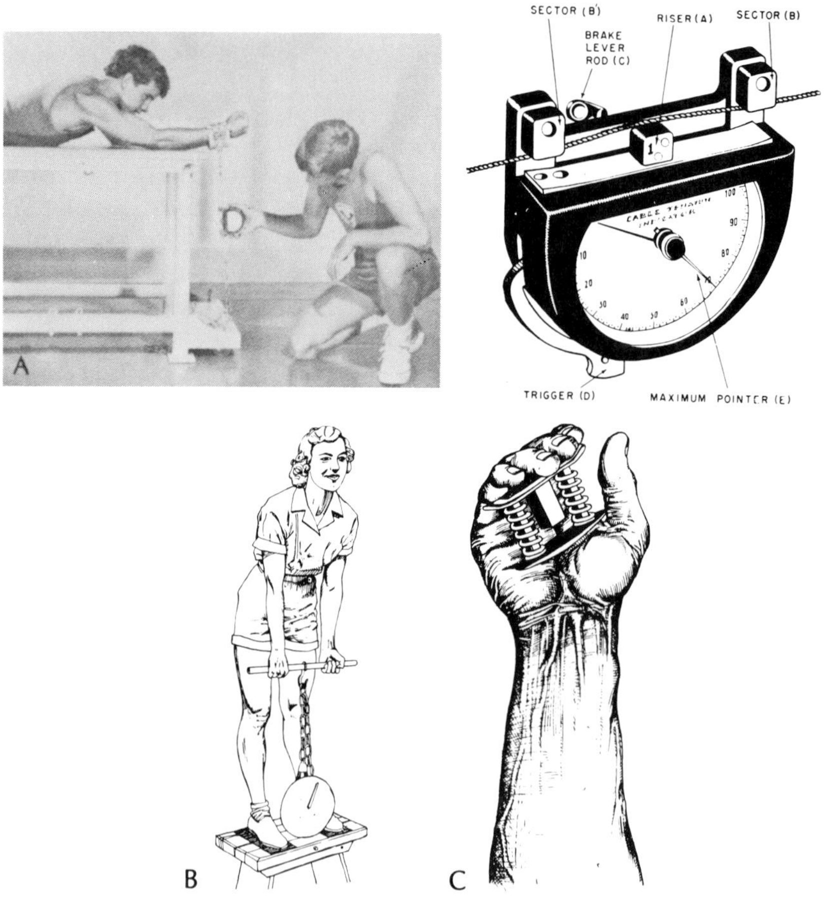

Fig. 15–1. Strength-testing instruments. *A.* Cable tensionmeter. *B.* Back and leg lift dynamometer. *C.* Handgrip dynamometer. (*A, left,* from Nielson, N.P. and Jensen, C.R. *Measurement and Statistics in Physical Education.* Courtesy of Wadsworth Publishing Co., Inc., 1972. *B,* from Mathews, D.K. and Fox, E.L. *Physiological Basis of Physical Education and Athletics,* 2nd Ed. Courtesy of W.B. Saunder Co., 1976. *A, right,* and *C,* from Mathews, D.K. *Measurement in Physical Education,* 4th Ed. Courtesy of W.B. Saunders Co., 1973.)

Back and Leg Lift Tests. For the *leg lift* test, the person stands on a platform and crouches to the desired leg bend position while he is strapped around the waist to the device. At a prescribed time he exerts a maximal force straight upward by *extending his legs.* He keeps his back straight, head erect, and chest high. Here again, a small amount of inconsistency can detract significantly from the reliability of the results.

For the *back lift* test the length of the resistance is properly adjusted and then the person bends forward and grasps the bar firmly with one palm upward and one palm downward, keeping his legs straight, feet flat on the platform, head up, and eyes straight forward. At the signal he lifts upward with maximal force by *straightening his trunk,* legs locked in the straight position.

Hand Grip Test. In performing the *hand grip* test, the grip dynamometer is placed in the palm of the hand with the dial toward the palm so that the convex edge is between the first and second joints of the fingers and the concave edge is against the base of the hand. The grip is started with the elbow slightly bent and the arm raised upward. The arm moves forward and downward while the hand grips with maximal force (Table 15–1).

Dynamic Strength Tests

Maximal lifts with different kinds of weight-training equipment provide some of the best measures of dynamic strength. A certain amount of experimentation is necessary to determine the maximal weight that can be lifted for one repetition, but when this is finally determined, it represents the dynamic strength for that particular movement. The two most commonly used tests of this kind among athletes are the bench press, and the squat or half-squat lift (Fig. 15–2). However, any of the exercise movements done with weights provides the opportunity for measuring dynamic strength for that particular movement. Strength can be measured by use of (1) free lifting equipment, (2) weight-lifting machines such as Nautilus or Universal gyms, and (3) isokinetic exercise devices such as the Cybex equipment.

Dynamic Strength–Endurance Tests. Often movements against one's body weight such as pull-ups or pushups have been used to measure dynamic strength. However, such tests actually measure a combination of strength and muscular endurance. A pure strength test involves only a single maximal muscle contraction; a second maximal contraction in succession would be weaker than the first, and a third contraction would be even weaker than the second. The degree to which either strength or endurance is the primary factor in a particular strength–endurance test depends on the number of times a person can repeat the movement. If an athlete is able to perform only one pull-up, then strength rather than endurance is measured. A failure to do even one pull-up results from insufficient strength, not lack of endurance. On the other hand, if an athlete performs 25 pull-ups, then the test is primarily one of endurance rather than of pure strength, although he would have to be unusually strong to do 25 pull-ups.

Many of the muscular strength–endurance tests are simple to administer, require limited space, and involve no unusual equipment. Among the more commonly used tests of this kind are *floor pushups, pull-ups* (or chin-ups), *dips* on the parallel bars, *sit-ups* (or body curls), and *squat jumps.*

Here again, precision and consistency in test administration are of the utmost importance, because if two people do slight variations of the same exercise, pull-ups for example, this can influence the results by 10% to 20%. Thus, the results cannot be compared meaningfully. (For women athletes, modified

Table 15–1. Grip Test Norms (kgs)

Fitness Category	*Men*	*Women*
I. Very Poor	Below 44	Below 25
II. Poor	44–48	25–28
III. Fair	49–52	29–31
IV. Good	53–58	32–34
V. Excellent	59+	35+

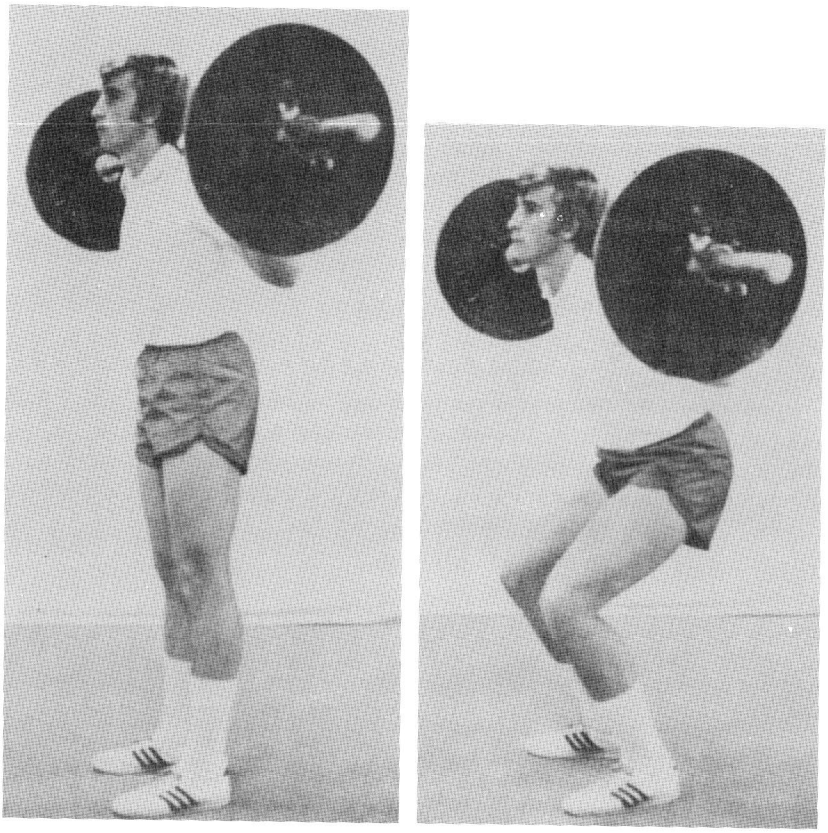

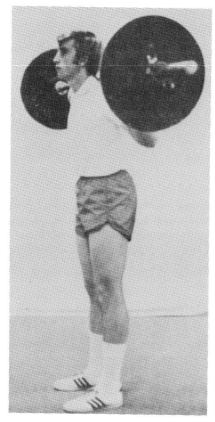

Fig. 15–2. Athlete doing a half squat with heavy weight, a form of dynamic strength testing. (From Robinson, C.F., Jensen, C.R., James, S.W., and Hirschi, W.M. *Modern Techniques of Track and Field*. Courtesy of Lea & Febiger, 1974.)

tests such as bench pushups or knee pushups, and modified low bar or diagonal pull-ups may be administered, if preferred.)

Another type of muscular strength–endurance test that can be easily used and is applicable to some situations is the "maximum repetitions of a standardized resistance test." A series of any of the basic lifts can be used and the weight to be lifted can be based on subject body weight. As shown in Table 15–2, the arm curl would use a weight as near one-third of total body weight as possible, and the bench press would use a body weight as near two-thirds body weight, etc. After calculating the weight, the subject would lift this weight as many times as possible. At the end of the treatment, the subject would again lift the same weight for each lift and the increase in the number of repetitions would be the gain in strength.

Isokinetic Tests. Several machines are available for measuring muscular strength accurately using the latest advances in computerized equipment and recording devices. Most of these machines can measure strength both isometrically and dynamically. Isometric

Table 15–2. Maximum Repetitions of a Standardized Resistance

Exercise	*Amount of Body Wt.*	*Weight*	*# of Reps*
Arm Curl	1/3	____	____
Bench Press	2/3	____	____
Lat Pulldown	2/3	____	____
Upright rowing	1/3	____	____
Quad lift	2/3	____	____

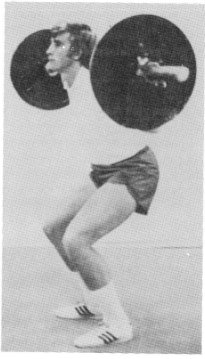

measurements are made by setting the speed dial to zero and recording maximum force on the readout/chart paper at any specified angle. Dynamic readings can be made at any given rotation speed. Graphs of these tests usually show a continuous relationship between the angle of the lever being tested and the force exerted at any angle. Since the force is exerted around an axis, the test measures applied torque and can be expressed several different ways (see Fig. 7–4). Most of these machines are computerized and can be used to prescribe carefully controlled resistance for rehabilitation.

MEASURING CARDIOVASCULAR ENDURANCE

The best test of cardiovascular endurance is the maximal oxygen uptake test described in Chapter 6 where expired air is measured and analyzed and the metabolic cost is calculated from these data. This test measures the actual oxidative capacity of the individual and should be used whenever a high level of accuracy is desired. However, there are many tests that can *estimate* cardiovascular endurance. These tests are valuable and can be used with large groups or to look at fitness levels in the school or spa setting. These tests can also be used by individuals to estimate their fitness levels and to evaluate changes in fitness associated with a training program.

Laboratory Ideas

1. Have students prepare a prescription for developing cardiovascular endurance for their parents or an older friend. Have them try using this prescription themselves for a period of time.
2. Have students write a prescription for developing cardiovascular endurance for a tri-athlete or marathon runner.
3. Have students measure their cardiovascular fitness using two or more of the tests in this section. The results from each test should be within a few ml/kg/min. from each other.

Cardiovascular Tests

Most fitness tests for cardiovascular endurance involve speed and distance relationships, or heart rate response to various work loads measured either during the work or in recovery. The following tests have been included because they give a fairly accurate estimate of fitness, and are easy to use.

Cooper's Test. One of the simplest ways to check cardiovascular endurance is to have a subject run a given distance for time or to run a given time to see how much distance he can cover. Table 15–3 shows the fitness categories for men and women who run various distances in 12 min. Table 15–4 presents fitness categories for the time it takes men to run 1.5 miles. These tables are based upon thousands of tests where time and distance information were compared to measure maximal oxygen consumption. The advantages of this kind of test are that (1) it is easy to administer to large groups, and (2) no specialized equipment is needed.

Astrand-Rhyming Test. This test requires the use of an accurate bicycle ergometer and metronome. A submaximal work load is performed at a level which will elicit a heart rate between 120 and 170 beats/minute. This range has been shown to be the most linear range of heart rate response.

To administer the test, adjust the bicycle seat height to fit the subject (leg should be nearly extended when pedal is in the down position) and set the metronome to 100 beats/minute (which is the same as 50 revolutions/minute with either leg). Calculate the maximum predicted heart rate by subtracting age from 220, and write down the 60 and 70% heart rate so that you can make decisions during the test concerning workload changes. Then, begin the test with a work load of 300 kgm/m (50 watts) for men, and 150 kgm/m (25 watts) for women. (Note: At 50 RPM the bike wheel travels 300 meters per minute. To set a workload of 300 kgm/min., the resistance wheel is set to 1 kg; for a workload of 150, the resistance is set to .5 kg. To increase the workload, use the same procedure—increase the resistance so that the resistance times 300 meters/min. equals the desired workload.)

Have the subject pedal for 2 minutes at the beginning workload and check the heart rate. If the heart rate is less than 60% of the maximum predicted heart rate that you have computed, increase the workload by 300 kgm/min. If the heart rate is between 60 and 70%

Table 15–3. 12-Minute Walking/Running Test
Distance (Miles) Covered in 12 Minutes

Fitness Category		Age (Years) 13–19	20–29	30–39	40–49	50–59	60+
I. Very poor	(men)	<1.30*	<1.22	<1.18	<1.14	<1.03	<.87
	(women)	<1.10	< .96	< .94	< .88	< .84	<.78
II. Poor	(men)	1.30–1.37	1.22–1.31	1.18–1.30	1.14–1.24	1.03–1.16	.87–1.02
	(women)	1.00–1.18	.96–1.11	.95–1.05	.88– .98	.84– .93	.78– .86
III. Fair	(men)	1.38–1.56	1.32–1.49	1.31–1.45	1.25–1.39	1.17–1.30	1.03–1.20
	(women)	1.19–1.29	1.12–1.22	1.06–1.18	.99–1.11	.94–1.05	.87– .98
IV. Good	(men)	1.57–1.72	1.50–1.64	1.46–1.56	1.40–1.53	1.31–1.44	1.21–1.32
	(women)	1.30–1.43	1.23–1.34	1.19–1.29	1.12–1.24	1.06–1.18	.99–1.09
V. Excellent	(men)	1.73–1.86	1.65–1.76	1.57–1.69	1.54–1.65	1.45–1.58	1.33–1.55
	(women)	1.44–1.51	1.35–1.45	1.30–1.39	1.25–1.34	1.19–1.30	1.10–1.18
VI. Superior	(men)	>1.87	>1.77	>1.70	>166	>1.59	>1.56
	(women)	>1.52	>1.46	>1.40	>1.35	>1.31	>1.19

*< Means "less than"; > means "more than."

From *The Aerobics Way* by Kenneth Cooper, M.D., M.P.H. Copyright © 1977 by Kenneth Cooper. Reprinted by permission of the publisher, M. Evans and Company, Inc., New York.

of the max predicted heart rate, increase the workload by 150 kgm/min. If the heart rate is greater than 70% of max predicted heart rate, leave the workload as it is and continue to check until the heart rate levels off. Follow the procedure above until the subject reaches a heart rate greater than 70% and then continue to check the rate until steady state occurs and two consecutive heart rates are within 5 beats of each other.

Enter Figure 15–3 with the last workload and the average steady-state heart rate to get predicted $\dot{V}O_2max$ in liters per minute. Be sure to use the *inside* edge of the workload box as the reference for the workload. Since heart rate decreases with age, use Table 15–5 to correct the predicted $\dot{V}O_2max$. To get $\dot{V}O_2max$ in ml/kg/min., multiply the liters/min. value from Figure 15–3 by 1,000 (to get ml), and divide by body weight in kg.

Fox's Test. A modification of the Astrand-Rhyming test was made by Fox who devised an equation using the heart rate during the fifth minute of a bicycle ergometer ride using 900 kg-m/minute work load. There might be a problem with untrained subjects who would reach maximal heart rate before 5 min. at this work load. The equation is:

$$\text{Pred. max } \dot{V}O_2 = 6.3 - (0.0193 \times \text{5th min. heart rate})$$

The Forest Service Step Test. The Forest Serv-

Table 15–4. 1.5-Mile Run Test
Time (Minutes)

Fitness Category		Age (Years) 13–19	20–29	30–39	40–49	50–59	60+
I. Very poor	(men)	>15:31*	>16:01	<16:31	>17:31	>19:01	>20:01
	(women)	>18:31	>19:01	>19:31	>20:01	>20:31	>21:01
II. Poor	(men)	12:11–15:30	14:01–16:00	14:44–16:30	15:36–17:30	17:01–19:00	19:01–20:00
	(women)	18:30–16:55	19:00–18:31	19:30–19:01	20:00–19:31	20:30–20:01	21:00–21:31
III. Fair	(men)	10:49–12:10	12:01–14:00	12:31–14:45	13:01–15:35	14:31–17:00	16:16–19:00
	(women)	16:54–14:31	18:30–15:55	19:00–16:31	19:30–17:31	20:00–19:01	20:30–19:31
IV. Good	(men)	9:31–10:48	10:46–12:00	11:01–12:30	11:31–13:00	12:31–14:30	14:00–16:15
	(women)	14:30–12:30	15:54–13:31	16:30–14:31	17:30–15:56	19:00–16:31	19:30–17:31
V. Excellent	(men)	8:37– 9:40	9:45–10:45	10:00–11:00	10:30–11:30	11:00–12:30	11:15–13:59
	(women)	12:29–11:50	13:30–12:30	14:30–13:00	15:55–13:45	16:30–14:30	17:30–16:30
VI. Superior	(men)	< 8:37	< 9:45	<10:00	<10:30	<11:00	<11:15
	(women)	<11:50	<12:30	<13:00	<13:45	<14:30	<16:30

*< Means "less than"; > means "more than."

From *The Aerobics Way* by Kenneth Cooper, M.D., M.P.H. Copyright © 1977 by Kenneth Cooper. Reprinted by permission of the publishers, M. Evans and Company, Inc., New York.

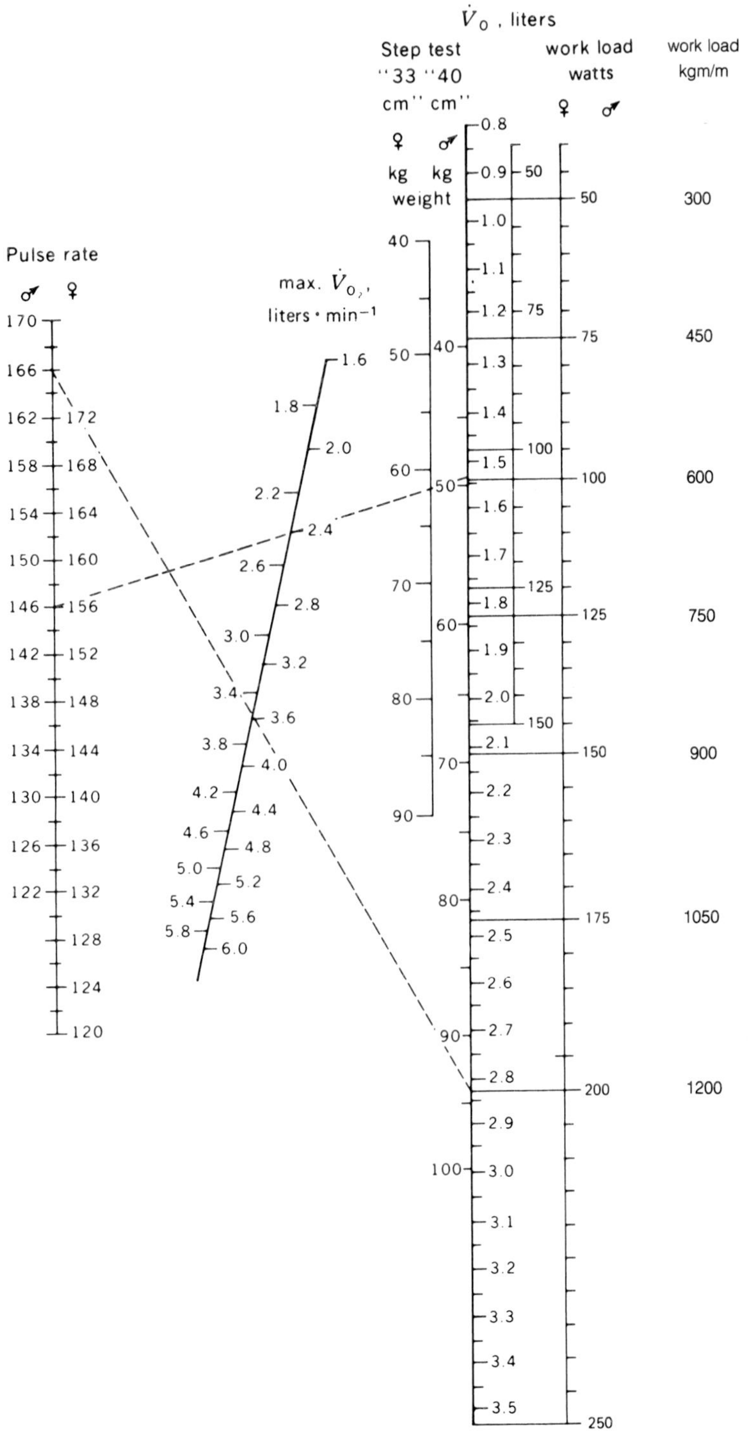

Fig. 15–3. Nomogram to determine the predictive maximal oxygen uptake. (From Astrand, P.O., and Rodahl, K. *Textbook of Work Physiology: Physiological Basis of Exercises*, 2nd Ed. Courtesy of McGraw Hill, 1986.)

Table 15–5. Factor to be Used for Correction of Predicted Maximal Oxygen Uptake

Age	*Factor*	*Max Heart Rate*	*Factor*
15	1.10	210	1.12
25	1.00	200	1.00
35	0.87	190	0.93
40	0.83	180	0.83
45	0.78	170	0.75
50	0.75	160	0.69
55	0.71	150	0.64
60	0.68		
65	0.65		

Astrand and Rodahl, *Textbook of Work Physiology,* 2nd ed. Courtesy of McGraw-Hill Book Company, 1972.

ice step test is an excellent test of cardiovascular fitness. A 15¾-inch bench is used for men and a 13-inch bench, for women. The subject steps up and down at 90 beats/minute (using a metronome) for exactly 5 min. The recovery pulse is counted for 15 sec starting exactly 15 sec from the end of the work bout. The 15-sec heart rate is multiplied by 4 and the result is entered into Table 15–6 or Table 15–7 using the nearest weight. The results are expressed as $\dot{V}O_2$ in milliliters/kilograms/minute. The fitness ratings for men or women, based upon the results of the test, are shown under the tables. An age adjustment should be made when necessary (see Table 15–5).

This test can be administered to large groups of subjects, such as physical education classes or adult fitness groups, if they are first taught to count pulse rate.

Fisher's Test. Using the prediction equations presented in Chapter 6, one can compute an estimated maximal oxygen uptake ($\dot{V}O_2$max) from the average speed a person can maintain for a run of 4 miles or more.

For instance, a person who can run 5 minutes in 40 min. averages 8 minute-miles or 7.5 mph (7.5 mph is equal to 201.15 m/minute). From the prediction equation for running, the cost of running at this rate is 43.73 ml/kg/min. (201.15 × 0.2 + 3.5). Since most moderately trained subjects can work for an extended period of time at about 75% of their maximum, the computed cost of the work is equal to 75% of their maximal $\dot{V}O_2$. A simple mathematical maneuver (43.75/75 = X/100) shows that the person described needs a maximal $\dot{V}O_2$ of about 58 ml/kg/min to accomplish the work he does.

MEASURING POWER

Power measurements can be extremely helpful in evaluating athletes who engage in sports that require them to jump, throw or strike. Interestingly, the power tests discussed in this section are the best tests available and only the Margaria-Kalamen test requires special equipment.

Laboratory Ideas

1. Have students write a prescription for developing power for their favorite power activity.
2. Test each student with as many of the power tests as you can set up and look at the correlation between the results.

Margaria-Kalamen Power Test. Margaria and his associates first published the Margaria leg power test; then Kalamen revised the test. The performer begins 6 meters from the bottom stair and runs up a flight of stairs as rapidly as possible, taking 3 steps at a time (Fig. 15–4). Switch mats are placed on the third and ninth steps. By stepping on the third stair, the performer activates a clock accurate to 1/100 sec; when he steps on the ninth stair, the clock is stopped. The time recorded by the clock represents the time required to move the body a height of 1.05 m (or the exact height of the stairs you use). Power is calculated by the formula:

$$\text{Power} = \frac{\text{Body weight (kg)} \times 1.05 \text{ m}}{\text{Elapsed time}}$$

Vertical Jump Test (Jump and Reach or Sargeant Jump). This test measures explosive power of the extensor muscles of the legs. However, other movements also contribute, such as the associated actions of the arms and shoulders. The athlete faces the wall with both feet flat on the floor and toes touching the wall, and then reaches as high as possible with either hand and makes a mark on the jump board (chalkboard). From the desired jump position with the preferred side to the wall, he jumps as high as possible, and at the peak of the jump makes another mark above the first one.

Table 15–6. Fitness Index for Men

	Body Weight 120	130	140	150	160	170	180	190	200	210	220	230	240	
180	33.0	32.8	32.8	32.6	32.6	32.3	32.3	32.3	32.3	32.1	32.1	31.9	31.9	180
175	34.8	33.9	33.9	33.7	33.4	33.4	33.4	33.0	33.0	33.0	32.8	32.8	32.8	175
170	35.4	34.8	34.8	34.8	34.3	34.3	34.3	34.3	34.1	34.1	34.1	34.1	34.1	170
165	36.7	36.7	35.9	35.6	35.6	35.6	35.2	35.2	35.2	35.2	35.0	34.8	34.8	165
160	37.2	37.2	37.2	37.2	37.0	36.7	36.7	36.7	36.5	36.5	36.5	35.9	35.9	160
155	38.7	38.5	38.3	38.1	37.8	37.8	37.8	37.8	37.8	37.8	37.6	37.4	37.4	155
150	40.3	39.8	39.8	39.6	38.9	38.9	38.9	38.9	38.7	38.7	38.7	38.7	38.5	150
145	41.6	40.9	40.7	40.3	40.3	40.3	40.0	40.0	40.0	40.0	40.0	40.0	40.0	145
140	42.9	42.7	42.0	41.8	41.8	41.8	41.6	41.6	41.6	41.6	41.6	41.6	41.6	140
135	44.4	44.0	43.3	43.1	43.1	43.1	43.1	43.1	43.1	42.9	42.9	42.7	42.5	135
130	46.2	45.8	45.5	45.3	45.1	44.9	44.9	44.9	44.7	44.7	44.7	44.2	44.2	130
125	48.0	47.3	47.1	46.9	46.6	46.6	46.6	46.6	46.4	46.4	46.4	46.4	46.4	125
120	49.7	49.3	49.1	48.8	48.6	48.6	48.4	48.4	48.4	48.4	48.4	48.4	48.4	120
115	51.7	51.7	51.5	51.0	51.0	51.0	51.0	51.0	50.6	50.6	50.6	50.4	49.5	115
110	53.7	53.7	53.5	53.2	53.2	53.0	52.8	52.8	52.8	52.6	52.6	51.7	51.3	110
105	56.1	56.1	56.1	55.7	55.4	55.2	55.2	55.0	55.0	55.0	53.9	53.5	53.0	105
100	59.0	58.7	58.3	58.1	58.1	58.1	57.4	57.4	57.6	56.5	56.1	55.3		100
95	64.2	61.8	61.2	61.2	61.2	60.9	60.7	60.7	59.4	58.7	57.2			95
90	67.3	65.1	64.7	64.7	64.5	64.2	64.0	62.5	61.6	60.1				90
85	69.3	69.3	68.2	67.8	67.8	67.8	65.8	64.9	63.7					85
80	72.8	72.6	71.9	71.9	71.9	69.5	68.4	67.2						80
	120	*130*	*140*	*150*	*160*	*170*	*180*	*190*	*200*	*210*	*220*	*230*	*240*	

Men's Fitness Rating as Calculated from the Above Table

NEAREST AGE	SUPERIOR	EXCELLENT	VERY GOOD	GOOD	FAIR	POOR	VERY POOR
25	55	50	45	40	35	30	25
35	53	48	43	38	33	28	23
45	51	46	41	36	31	26	21
55	49	44	39	34	29	24	19
65	47	42	37	32	27	22	17

Sharky, B.J.: *Physiological Fitness and Weight Control*. Missoula: Mountain Press Publishing Co., 1978, page 109.

The score is the difference in inches or centimeters between the two marks.

Standing Long Jump. This test measures essentially the same characteristics as the vertical jump; however, it depends on upper body movement a little more and leg extension a little less. Also, the standing long jump is slightly less reliable than the vertical jump because it is a more difficult and less common skill, and it improves more easily with practice.

The athlete stands with his feet a comfortable distance apart and his toes just behind the takeoff mark. He crouches, leans forward, swings his arms backward, and then jumps as far as possible horizontally, leaving from both feet and landing on both feet simultaneously. His score is the distance from the back of the

Table 15–7. Fitness Index for Women

	Body Weight 80	90	100	110	120	130	140	150	160	170	180	190	
175												31.2	175
170				31.9	31.9	32.1	32.1	32.1	32.1	32.1	32.1	32.3	170
165				32.3	32.6	33.0	33.0	33.2	33.2	33.2	33.2	33.2	165
160			33.4	33.7	33.9	34.1	34.3	34.3	34.3	34.3	34.3	34.3	160
155			34.5	34.8	35.2	35.4	35.4	35.4	35.4	35.4	35.4	35.4	155
150			35.6	36.1	36.3	36.3	36.7	36.7	36.7	36.7	36.7	36.7	150
145		37.2	37.4	38.1	38.1	38.1	38.1	38.1	38.3	38.3	38.9	38.9	145
140		38.7	39.4	39.4	39.4	39.6	39.6	39.6	39.6	39.6	39.6	39.6	140
135	39.6	39.8	40.0	40.3	40.3	40.9	40.9	41.1	41.1	41.4	41.6	41.6	135
130	40.5	41.1	41.8	42.0	42.2	42.9	42.9	43.1	43.3	43.3	43.6	43.6	130
125	41.4	43.6	43.8	44.0	44.0	44.4	44.7	44.9	44.9	45.3	45.3	45.3	125
120	42.5	45.3	45.8	46.0	46.0	46.4	46.9	47.1	47.1	47.3	47.5	47.5	120
115	44.4	47.7	48.0	48.0	48.0	48.0	49.3	49.3	49.3	49.3	49.3	49.3	115
110	48.0	50.2	51.5	51.7	51.7	51.7	51.9	52.4	52.4	52.8			110
105	51.7	53.7	53.7	53.9	54.1	54.6	55.4	55.7	55.7				105
100	55.2	56.8	57.0	57.6	58.3	58.3	59.4						100
95	58.1	60.7	61.2	61.6	62.3	62.3							95
90	62.7	64.7	65.6	67.5	67.5	68.6							90
	80	*90*	*100*	*110*	*120*	*130*	*140*	*150*	*160*	*170*	*180*	*190*	

Women's Fitness Rating as Calculated from the Above Table

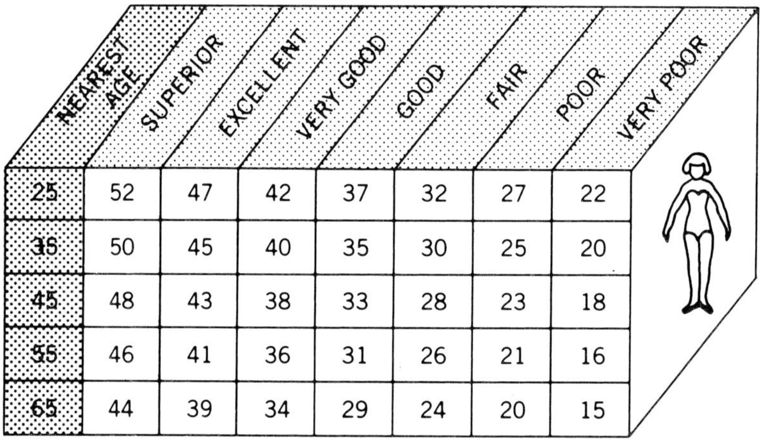

NEAREST AGE	SUPERIOR	EXCELLENT	VERY GOOD	GOOD	FAIR	POOR	VERY POOR
25	52	47	42	37	32	27	22
35	50	45	40	35	30	25	20
45	48	43	38	33	28	23	18
55	46	41	36	31	26	21	16
65	44	39	34	29	24	20	15

Sharky, B.J.: *Physiological Fitness and Weight Control*. Missoula: Mountain Press Publishing Co., 1978, page 108.

takeoff mark to the nearest point where any part of the body touches the floor at the completion of the jump. Obviously, the amount of friction between the feet and the jumping surface is important to success in this test.

Ball Throw for Distance. This test measures power of the total body with emphasis on the upper extremities. It can be done with one of several kinds of balls: softball, weighted softball, basketball, or medicine ball.

The athlete stands behind the restraining line, then using the desired approach, he projects the ball as far as possible using the overarm throwing technique and being careful not to cross the restraining line. The measurement is taken from behind the restraining line to the spot where the ball first strikes the surface.

Shot Put. As a test of power for noncompetitive shot-putters, the 12-pound (high school) shot is ordinarily used (8-pound shot for junior high school students). Starting from the back of a 7-foot shot-putting ring or between two lines 7 feet apart, the athlete pro-

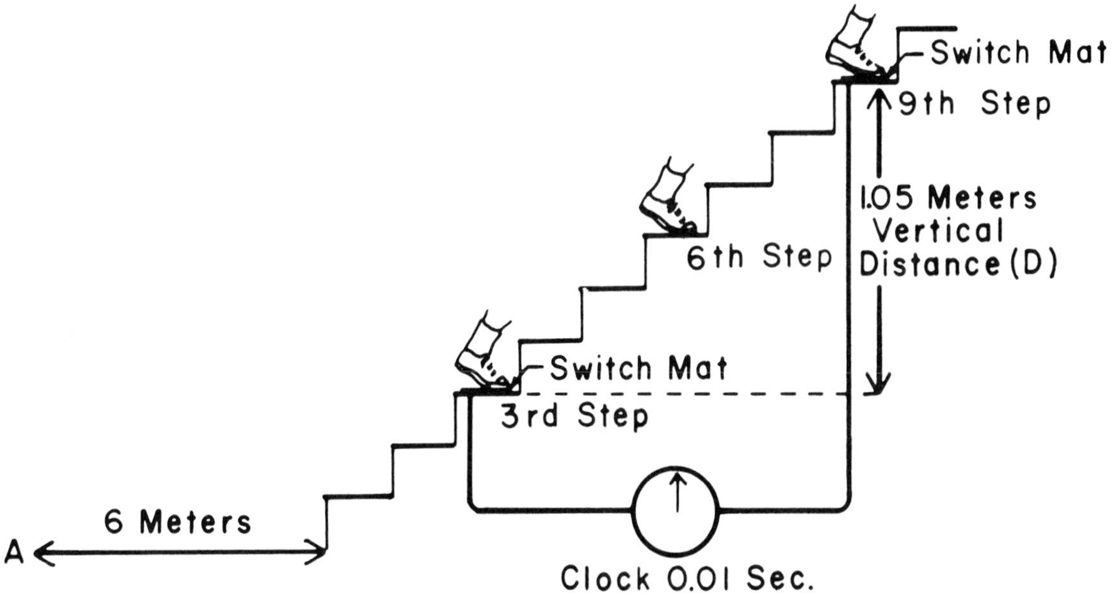

Fig. 15–4. Margaria-Kalamen power test. Subject commences at point A and runs as rapidly as possible up the stairs, taking them three at a time. The time it takes him to traverse the distance between stair 3 and stair 9 is recorded to the hundredth of a second. The power generated is a product of the subject's weight and the vertical distance (D) divided by the time. (From Mathews, D.K. and Fox, E.L. *Physiological Basis of Physical Education and Athletics,* 2nd Ed. Courtesy of W.B. Saunders Co., 1976.)

jects the shot by use of the usual shot-putting technique. The distance is measured from the back of the restraining line to the point where the shot first strikes the ground. This test involves a skill that is unfamiliar to many persons and in such cases, this detracts from its reliability.

MEASURING BODY FAT

There are many ways to determine the amount of fat on the body. Some medical people rely on the standard height-weight charts produced by insurance companies. Although helpful in some instances, height-weight tables are inaccurate because there is so much variability in body build among people. The gold standard for determining percent fat is hydrostatic weighing. This technique is based on the idea that different body components have different densities, and that fat is less dense than muscle or bone. Because of this, a person with more fat will weigh less in water because he or she has more low-density tissue.

Laboratory Ideas

1. Demonstrate hydrostatic weighing with a member of your class. Explain the principle behind this procedure.

2. Set up areas for estimating body fat and have students work in pairs to measure each other using the different techniques described below. Each technique should yield fairly consistent results with the other techniques.

Body Fat Tests

The following tests could be used for measuring body fat for an exercise physiology laboratory experience:

Skinfold Test. Measure the thickness of a skinfold on the right side of the body by pinching the skin (not including the muscle under the skin) between the thumb and index finger. Apply the caliper about 1 cm from the pinch site and hold the pinch while measuring. Release and try again.

For women, measure:

Triceps. Halfway between elbow and shoulder (vertical).

Thigh. Halfway between knee and hip (vertical).

Suprailium. On crest of ilium directly under axilla (measure at 45 degree angle).

Using the sum of the measures, enter nomogram (Fig. 15–5) with age and read percent body fat.

For men, measure:

Chest. Halfway between nipple and armpit

Abdomen. Just to the right of the umbilicus

Thigh. Same as for women

Using the sum of the measures, enter nomogram (Fig. 15–5) with age and read percent body fat.

NOTE: This is just one of hundreds of skinfold formulae that could be used for the skinfold percent fat.

Circumference Test. Measure circumference at the following points and enter Table 15–8 to get a *constant:*

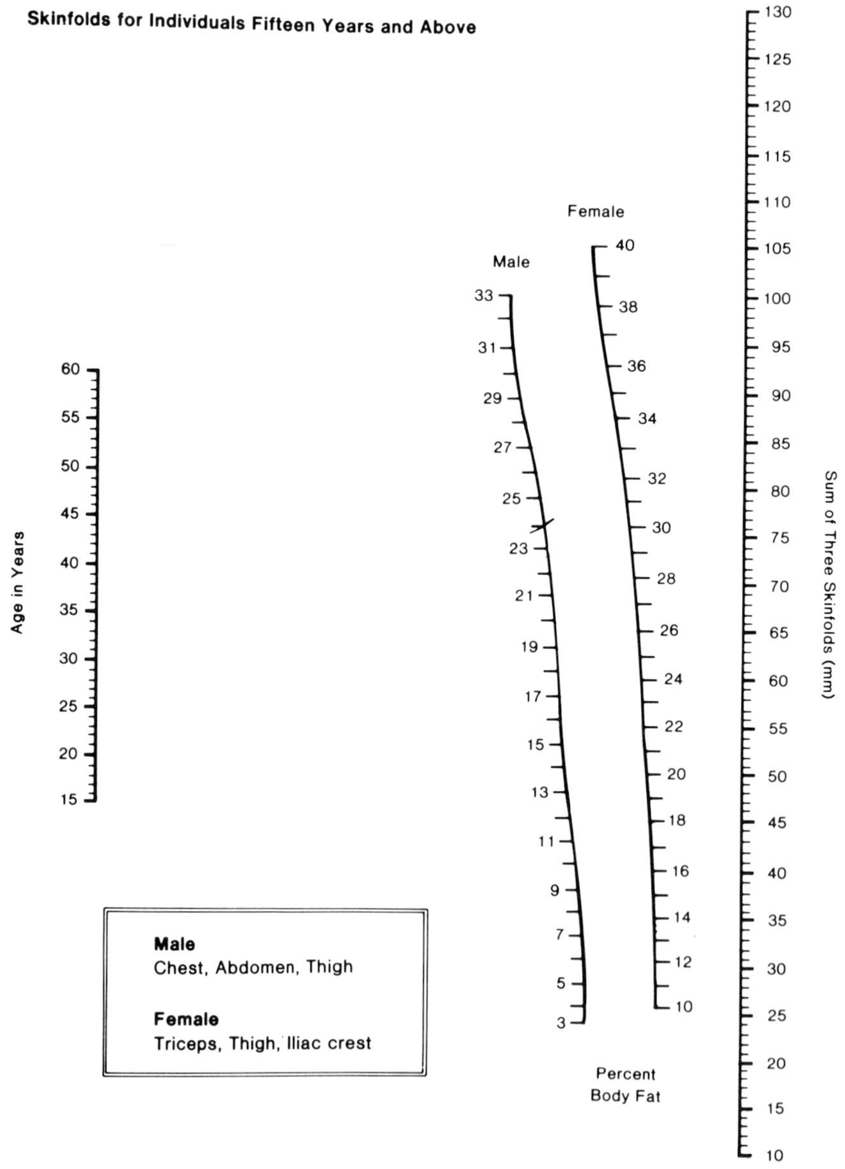

Fig. 15–5. A nomogram for the estimate of percent body fat from generalized equations. (From Baun, W.B., Baun, M.R., and Raven, P.B. *In* Res. Q. Exerc. Sport, *52*:380–384, 1981.)

Table 15–8. Conversion Constants to Predict Percent Body Fat (Women)

Hips *In.*	*Constant A*	*Abdomen* *In.*	*Constant B*	*Height* *In.*	*Constant C*
30	33.48	20	14.22	55	33.52
31	34.87	21	14.93	56	34.13
32	36.27	22	15.64	57	34.74
33	37.67	23	16.35	58	35.35
34	39.06	24	17.06	59	35.96
35	40.46	25	17.78	60	36.57
36	41.86	26	18.49	61	37.18
37	43.25	27	19.20	62	37.79
38	44.65	28	19.91	63	38.40
39	46.05	29	20.62	64	39.01
40	47.44	30	21.33	65	39.62
41	48.84	31	22.04	66	40.23
42	50.24	32	22.75	67	40.84
43	51.64	33	23.46	68	41.45
44	53.03	34	24.18	69	42.06
45	54.43	35	24.89	70	42.67
46	55.83	36	25.60	71	43.28
47	57.22	37	26.31	72	43.89
48	58.62	38	27.02	73	44.50
49	60.02	39	27.73	74	45.11
50	61.42	40	28.44	75	45.72
51	62.81	41	29.15	76	46.32
52	64.21	42	29.87	77	46.93
53	65.61	43	30.58	78	47.54
54	67.00	44	31.29	79	48.15
55	68.40	45	32.00	80	48.76
56	69.80	46	32.71	81	49.37
57	71.19	47	33.42	82	49.98
58	72.59	48	34.13	83	50.59
59	73.99	49	34.84	84	51.20
60	75.39	50	35.56	85	51.81

From: *How to Lower Your Fat Thermostat,* D.R. Remmington, A.G. Fisher and E.A. Parent, used by permission.

For women, measure:
Hips. (at the widest part).................. Constant A ___
Abdomen. (at level of umbilicus)............ Constant B ___
Add together ___
Now, get constant from Table 15–8 for height (in inches)............ Constant C ___
Subtract constant C from sum of A and B to get percent fat .... % fat ___
For men, measure:
Waist circumference (at umbilicus) ___
Subtract wrist circumference (just inside wrist next to hand) .... ___
Enter Table 15–9 with waist minus wrist measurement and body weight to get % fat.......:....... ___

Electrical Impedance. Some laboratories will have an electrical impedance device. Use the instructions with this device to cross-check with the percent fat calculated above.

OTHER TESTS

The following tests may be of interest to the exercise physiology student, but no laboratory suggestions are included. Use these tests however you like to support your teaching approach.

Running Acceleration Tests

The rate at which a person can accelerate is a measure of power with emphasis on the leg extensor muscles. Running is essentially a series of body projections from alternate legs. The rate at which a body is accelerated is directly proportional to the force causing it (muscular force in this case), according to Newton's second law of motion.

An electronic device is necessary to measure acceleration speed accurately over short distances up to 15 yards. Beyond 15 yards, measurements can be made fairly accurately with stopwatches. With proper equipment, acceleration tests of 5, 10, or 15 yards are meaningful measures of power, whereas tests of sprint speed for longer distances are less meaningful but still quite significant as measures of power.

It is true that most persons reach maximal sprint speed between 15 and 20 yards out of the blocks, and at this point, maximal running speed instead of acceleration speed becomes the dominant factor. Maximal running speed is dependent upon power but less so than acceleration speed.

In summary, measures of acceleration speed up to 15 yards timed with highly accurate equipment are good tests of power, and tests of sprint speed over longer distances (40 or 50 yards) are indicators of power. Many athletes in court and field games are measured by their coaches over the 40- or 50-yard distance. Football players especially are measured over the 40-yard distance. These measurements of acceleration speed combined with sprint speed are indicators of power but they are not pure power tests. However, such a test measures an important characteristic in this case, the ability to cover 40 yards in the shortest time possible from a stationary start.

Table 15–9. Body Fat Percentages From the Penrose-Nelson-Fisher Equations
Waist Minus Wrist (Inches)

Wt (lbs)	*22*	*22.5*	*23*	*23.5*	*24*	*24.5*	*25*	*25.5*	*26*	*26.5*	*27*	*27.5*	*28*	*28.5*
120	4	6	8	10	12	14	16	18	20	21	23	25	27	29
125	4	6	7	9	11	13	15	17	19	20	22	24	26	28
130	3	5	7	9	11	12	14	16	18	20	21	23	25	27
135	3	5	7	8	10	12	13	15	17	19	20	22	24	26
140	3	5	6	8	10	11	13	15	16	18	19	21	23	24
145	3	4	6	7	9	11	12	14	15	17	19	20	22	23
150	2	4	6	7	9	10	12	13	15	16	18	19	21	23
155	2	4	5	7	8	10	11	13	14	16	17	19	20	22
160	2	4	5	6	8	9	11	12	14	15	17	18	19	21
165	2	3	5	6	8	9	10	12	13	15	16	17	19	20
170	2	3	4	6	7	9	10	11	13	14	15	17	18	19
175	2	3	4	6	7	8	10	11	12	13	15	16	17	19
180	1	3	4	5	7	8	9	10	12	13	14	16	17	18
185	1	3	4	5	6	8	9	10	11	13	14	15	16	18
190	1	2	4	5	6	7	8	10	11	12	13	15	16	17
195	1	2	3	5	6	7	8	9	11	12	13	14	15	16
200	1	2	3	4	6	7	8	9	10	11	12	14	15	16
205	1	2	3	4	5	6	8	9	10	11	12	13	14	15
210	1	2	3	4	5	6	7	8	9	11	12	13	14	15
215	1	2	3	4	5	6	7	8	9	10	11	12	13	15
220	0	2	3	4	5	6	7	8	9	10	11	12	13	14
225	0	1	2	3	4	6	7	8	9	10	11	12	13	14
230	0	1	2	3	4	5	6	7	8	9	10	11	12	13
235	0	1	2	3	4	5	6	7	8	9	10	11	12	13
240	0	1	2	3	4	5	6	7	8	9	10	11	12	13
245	0	1	2	3	4	5	6	7	8	9	9	10	11	12
250	0	1	2	3	4	5	6	6	7	8	9	10	11	12
255	0	1	2	3	3	4	5	6	7	8	9	10	11	12
260	0	1	2	2	3	4	5	6	7	8	9	10	10	11
265	0	1	1	2	3	4	5	6	7	8	8	9	10	11
270	0	1	1	2	3	4	5	6	7	7	8	9	10	11
275	0	0	1	2	3	4	5	5	6	7	8	9	10	11
280	0	0	1	2	3	4	4	5	6	7	8	9	9	10
285	0	0	1	2	3	4	4	5	6	7	8	8	9	10
290	0	0	1	2	3	3	4	5	6	7	7	8	9	10
295	0	0	1	2	2	3	4	5	6	6	7	8	9	10
300	0	0	1	2	2	3	4	5	5	6	7	8	9	9

Penrose, Nelson and Fisher, Generalized Body Composition Prediction Equation for Men Using Simple Measurement Techniques. Med. Sci. Sports Exerc. *17*, No. 2, April, 1985.

Table 15–9. Continued

29	*29.5*	*30*	*30.5*	*31*	*31.5*	*32*	*32.5*	*33*	*33.5*	*34*	*34.5*	*35*	*35.5*	*36*
31	33	35	37	39	41	43	45	47	49	50	52	54	56	58
30	32	33	35	37	39	41	43	45	46	48	50	52	54	56
28	30	32	34	36	37	39	41	43	44	46	48	50	52	53
27	29	31	32	34	36	38	39	41	43	44	46	48	50	51
26	28	29	31	33	34	36	38	39	41	43	44	46	48	49
25	27	28	30	31	33	35	36	38	39	41	43	44	46	47
24	26	27	29	30	32	33	35	36	38	40	41	43	44	46
23	25	26	28	29	31	32	34	35	37	38	40	41	43	44
22	24	25	27	28	30	31	33	34	35	37	38	40	41	43
22	23	24	26	27	29	30	31	33	34	36	37	38	40	41
21	22	24	25	26	28	29	30	32	33	34	36	37	39	40
20	21	23	24	25	27	28	29	31	32	33	35	36	37	39
19	21	22	23	25	26	27	28	30	31	32	34	35	36	37
19	20	21	23	24	25	26	28	29	30	31	33	34	35	36
18	19	21	22	23	24	26	27	28	29	30	32	33	34	35
18	19	20	21	22	24	25	26	27	28	30	31	32	33	34
17	18	19	21	22	23	24	25	26	28	29	30	31	32	33
17	18	19	20	21	22	23	25	26	27	28	29	30	31	32
16	17	18	19	21	22	23	24	25	26	27	28	29	30	32
16	17	18	19	20	21	22	23	24	25	26	28	29	30	31
15	16	17	18	19	20	22	23	24	25	26	27	28	29	30
15	16	17	18	19	20	21	22	23	24	25	26	27	28	29
14	15	16	17	18	19	20	21	22	23	24	25	26	27	28
14	15	16	17	18	19	20	21	22	23	24	25	26	27	28
14	15	16	17	17	18	19	20	21	22	23	24	25	26	27
13	14	15	16	17	18	19	20	21	22	23	24	25	26	27
13	14	15	16	17	18	18	19	20	21	22	23	24	25	26
13	14	14	15	16	17	18	19	20	21	22	23	24	24	25
12	13	14	15	16	17	18	19	19	20	21	22	23	24	25
12	13	14	15	15	16	17	18	19	20	21	22	22	23	24
12	13	13	14	15	16	17	18	19	19	20	21	22	23	24
11	12	13	14	15	16	16	17	18	19	20	21	22	22	23
11	12	13	14	14	15	16	17	18	19	19	20	21	22	23
11	12	12	13	14	15	16	17	17	18	19	20	21	21	22
11	11	12	13	14	15	15	16	17	18	19	19	20	21	22
10	11	12	13	14	14	15	16	17	17	18	19	20	21	21
10	11	12	12	13	14	15	16	16	17	18	19	19	20	21

Table 15–9. Continued

Wt (lbs)	*36.5*	*37*	*37.5*	*38*	*38.5*	*39*	*39.5*	*40*	*40.5*	*41*	*41.5*	*42*	*42.5*	*43*
120	60	62	64	66	68	70	72	74	76	77	79	81	83	85
125	58	59	61	63	65	67	69	71	72	74	76	78	80	82
130	55	57	59	61	62	64	66	68	69	71	73	75	77	78
135	53	55	56	58	60	62	63	65	67	68	70	72	74	75
140	51	53	54	56	58	59	61	63	64	66	68	69	71	72
145	49	51	52	54	55	57	59	60	62	63	65	67	68	70
150	47	49	50	52	53	55	57	58	60	61	63	64	66	67
155	46	47	49	50	52	53	55	56	58	59	61	62	64	65
160	44	46	47	48	50	51	53	54	56	57	59	60	61	63
165	43	44	45	47	48	50	51	52	54	55	57	58	60	61
170	41	43	44	45	47	48	49	51	52	54	55	56	58	59
175	40	41	43	44	45	47	48	49	51	52	53	55	56	57
180	39	40	41	43	44	45	47	48	49	50	52	53	54	56
185	38	39	40	41	43	44	45	46	48	49	50	51	53	54
190	37	38	39	40	41	43	44	45	46	48	49	50	51	52
195	35	37	38	39	40	41	43	44	45	46	47	49	50	51
200	35	36	37	38	39	40	41	43	44	45	46	47	48	50
205	34	35	36	37	38	39	40	41	43	44	45	46	47	48
210	33	34	35	36	37	38	39	40	42	43	44	45	46	47
215	32	33	34	35	36	37	38	39	40	42	43	44	45	46
220	31	32	33	34	35	36	37	38	39	41	42	43	44	45
225	30	31	32	33	34	35	36	37	38	40	41	42	43	44
230	30	31	32	33	34	35	36	37	38	39	40	41	42	43
235	29	30	31	32	33	34	35	36	37	38	49	40	41	42
240	28	29	30	31	32	33	34	35	36	37	38	39	40	41
245	27	28	29	30	31	32	33	34	35	36	37	38	39	40
250	27	28	29	30	31	31	32	33	34	35	36	37	38	39
255	26	27	28	29	30	31	32	33	34	34	35	36	37	38
260	26	27	27	28	29	30	31	32	33	34	35	35	36	37
265	25	26	27	28	29	29	30	31	32	33	34	35	36	36
270	25	25	26	27	28	29	30	31	31	32	33	34	35	36
275	24	25	26	27	27	28	29	30	31	32	32	33	34	35
280	24	24	25	26	27	28	29	29	30	31	32	33	33	34
285	23	24	25	26	26	27	28	29	30	30	31	32	33	34
290	23	23	24	25	26	27	27	28	29	30	31	31	32	33
295	22	23	24	25	25	26	27	28	28	29	30	31	32	32
300	22	22	23	24	25	26	26	27	28	29	29	30	31	32

Table 15–9. Continued

43.5	*44*	*44.5*	*45*	*45.5*	*46*	*46.5*	*47*	*47.5*	*48*	*48.5*	*49*	*49.5*	*50*
87	89	91	93	95	97	99	99	99	99	99	99	99	99
84	85	87	89	91	93	95	96	98	99	99	99	99	99
80	82	84	86	87	89	91	93	94	96	98	99	99	99
77	79	80	82	84	86	87	89	91	92	94	96	98	99
74	76	77	79	81	82	84	86	87	89	91	92	94	96
71	73	75	76	78	79	81	83	84	86	87	89	91	92
69	70	72	74	75	77	78	80	81	83	84	86	87	89
67	68	70	71	73	74	76	77	79	80	82	83	85	86
64	66	67	69	70	72	73	75	76	77	79	80	82	83
62	64	65	67	68	69	71	72	74	75	76	78	79	81
60	62	63	64	66	67	69	70	71	73	74	75	77	78
59	60	61	63	64	65	66	68	69	70	72	73	74	76
57	58	59	61	62	63	65	66	67	68	70	71	72	74
55	56	58	59	60	61	63	64	65	66	68	69	70	71
54	55	56	57	58	60	61	62	63	65	66	67	68	69
52	53	55	56	57	58	59	60	62	63	64	65	66	68
51	52	53	54	55	57	58	59	60	61	62	63	65	66
49	51	52	53	54	55	56	57	58	60	61	62	63	64
48	49	50	51	53	54	55	56	57	58	59	60	61	62
47	48	49	50	51	52	53	54	56	57	58	59	60	61
46	47	48	49	50	51	52	53	54	55	56	57	58	59
45	46	47	48	49	50	51	52	53	54	55	56	57	58
44	45	46	47	48	49	50	51	52	53	54	55	56	57
43	44	45	46	47	48	49	50	51	51	52	53	54	55
42	43	44	45	46	46	47	48	49	50	51	52	53	54
41	42	43	44	44	45	46	47	48	49	50	51	52	53
40	41	42	43	44	44	45	46	47	48	49	50	51	52
39	40	41	42	43	44	44	45	46	47	48	49	50	51
38	39	40	41	42	43	43	44	45	46	47	48	49	50
37	38	39	40	41	42	43	43	44	45	46	47	48	49
37	37	38	39	40	41	42	43	43	44	45	46	47	48
36	37	38	38	39	40	41	42	43	43	44	45	46	47
35	36	37	38	38	39	40	41	42	43	43	44	45	46
34	35	36	37	38	39	39	40	41	42	43	43	44	45
34	35	35	36	37	38	39	39	40	41	42	43	43	44
33	34	35	36	36	37	38	39	39	40	41	42	43	43
33	33	34	35	36	36	37	38	39	39	40	41	42	43

Agility Tests

Agility is the characteristic of being able to change direction and position of the body and its parts rapidly. In athletics, we are mostly concerned about two kinds of agility: *running agility* and *total body maneuverability*. Running agility is tested by dodging and zigzag running, and total body maneuverability can be measured by the squat thrust test.

Squat Thrust Test–10 Seconds (Burpee Test). The performer stands erect at the start of the squat thrust test (Fig. 15–6). He then moves to the squat position with both hands on the floor, then thrusts his legs backward keeping his arms, back, and legs straight, then back to the squat position, and finally to the erect position. A complete cycle is counted as one squat thrust. If a person does not reach an acceptable position in any of the four phases, one fourth of a point is deducted. The objective is to do as many squat thrusts as possible in 10 seconds.

Even though the 10-sec test is the only agility test of this kind that has been standardized, many believe that for well-conditioned people, 10 sec is too short a time to get an accurate measurement, and that 20 sec gives a more correct indication of agility.

Incidentally, this same test held for 60 sec

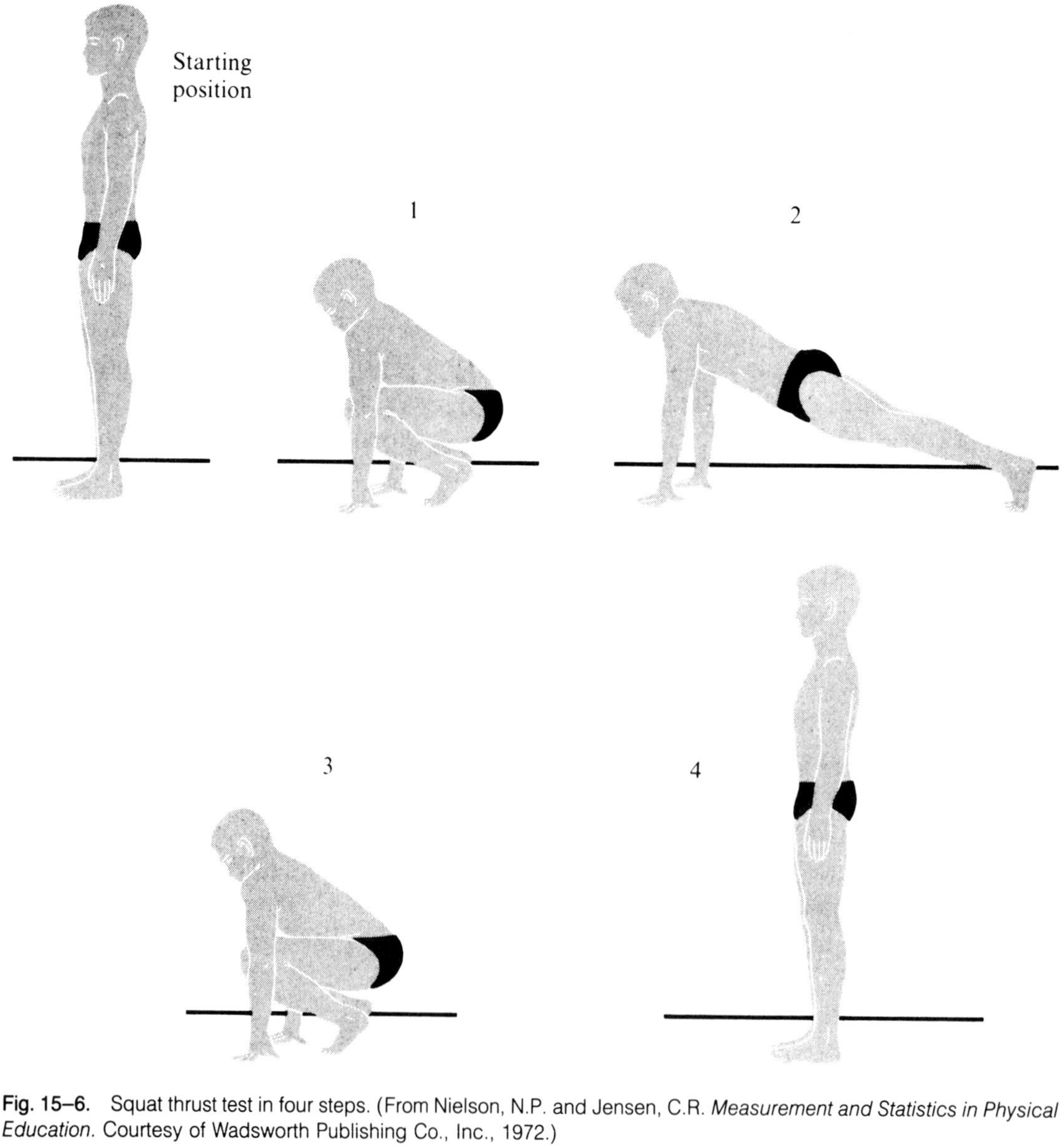

Fig. 15–6. Squat thrust test in four steps. (From Nielson, N.P. and Jensen, C.R. *Measurement and Statistics in Physical Education.* Courtesy of Wadsworth Publishing Co., Inc., 1972.)

is sometimes used as a measure of anaerobic endurance. Even though this crude measure of endurance does produce some meaningful results, it should be recognized that there are more useful and precise endurance tests available.

Shuttle Run. The standard shuttle run is done over a 30-foot course, however, it is possible to do it over a shorter course, and there is some argument that a shorter course provides a purer measure of agility with less emphasis on running speed. In order to do the standard agility test over a 30-foot course, two small blocks of wood are placed 30 feet from the starting line. At the signal the athlete starts from behind the starting line, retrieves one of the blocks and places it behind the starting line, then retrieves the second block and sprints back across the starting line. The run is measured to the nearest 1/10 sec. Lines on the surface can be used instead of blocks, if this is preferred.

Sidestep Test. This test measures agility in lateral movements. Three lines are placed parallel on the surface of the floor, 5 feet apart (Fig. 15–7). The athlete straddles the middle line. On signal, he sidesteps to the right until one foot crosses the right-hand line. Then he sidesteps to the left until one foot crosses the left-hand line. He repeats these lateral movements as rapidly as possible for 20 sec. His final score is the number of times that he crossed an outside line.

Right-Boomerang Test. This simple test has been popular for a long time and is still considered a good test of running agility. To establish the course, a jumping standard or similar object is placed at the center point with four smaller objects, such as Indian clubs, wastebaskets, and the like placed at the four outside points (Fig. 15–8). At the starting signal, the performer sprints toward the center point and then follows the course as indicated in the illustration. His time is recorded to the nearest 1/10 sec.

Measures of Flexibility

A large number of flexibility measures are possible because of the large number of specific movements that can occur in the body. Only three of the more commonly used tests are included here. They serve as examples of the kinds of flexibility measures that can be performed.

Hip and Trunk Flexion Test. The performer sits on a table or on the floor with his feet flat against the wall, hip width apart, and his legs straight and rigid. He bends his trunk forward and downward as far as possible extending his hands toward the heels of his feet. There are two important measurements that can be taken at this position: first, the distance the person's fingertips are from his heels, and second, the vertical distance from the top of his sternum to the surface of the table or floor. Lack of flexibility demonstrated in this test

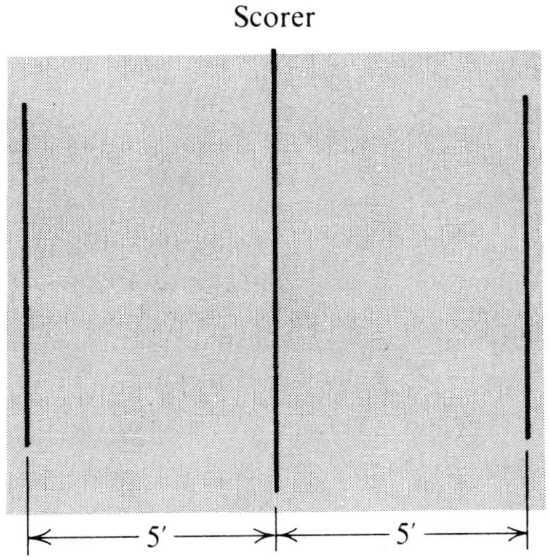

Fig. 15–7. Sidestep test floor plan. (From Nielson, N.P. and Jensen, C.R. *Measurement and Statistics in Physical Education.* Courtesy of Wadsworth Publishing Co., Inc., 1972.)

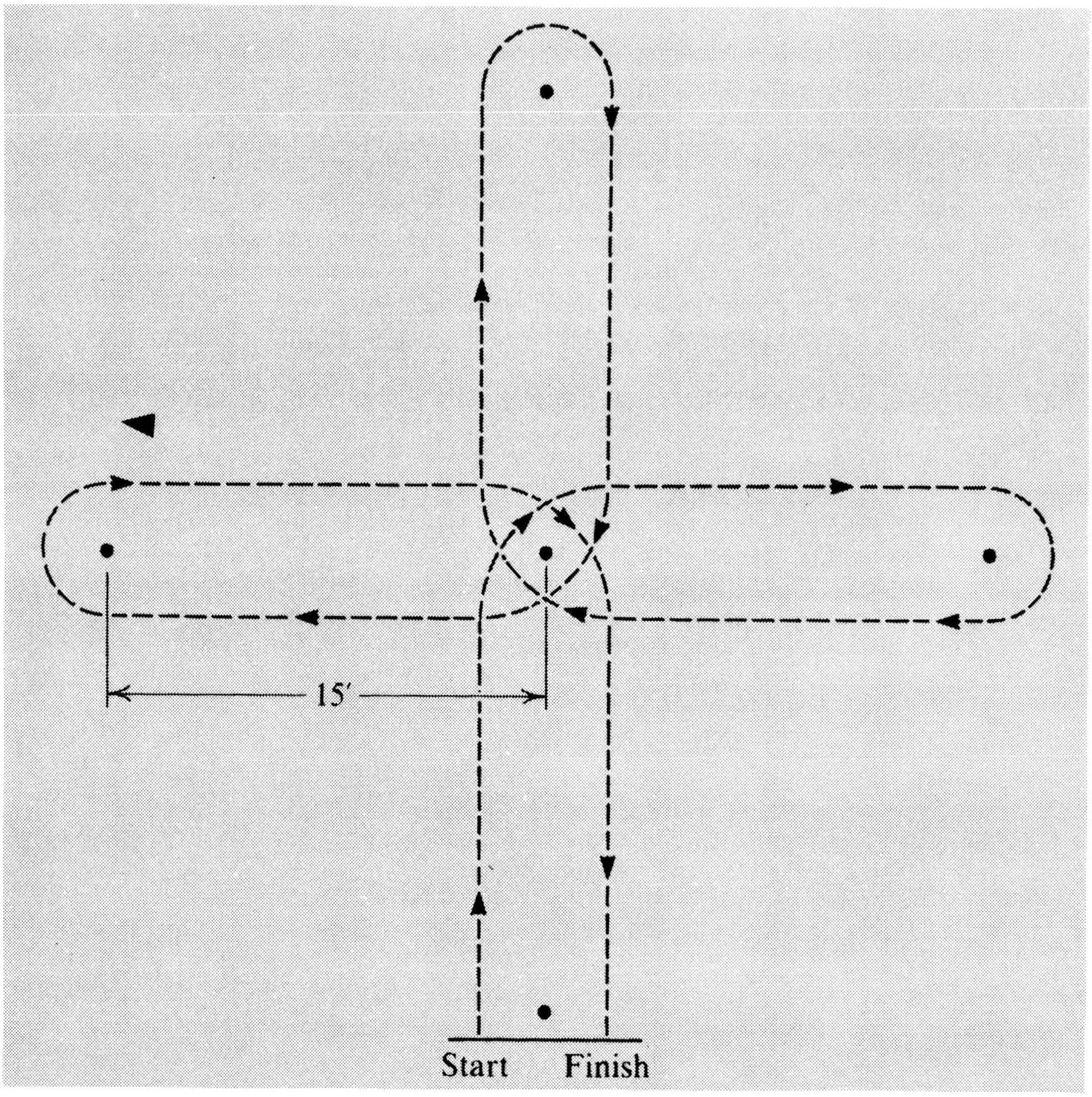

Fig. 15–8. Right-boomerang course. (From Nielson, N.P. and Jensen, C.R. *Measurement and Statistics in Physical Education.* Courtesy of Wadsworth Publishing Co., Inc., 1972.)

indicates tightness of the muscles and connective tissues that cross the back of the hip joints and the lower back.

Upward Arm Movement Test. The person lies prone on a table with his chin touching the table and his arms stretched forward directly in front of his shoulders. He holds a stick horizontally in both hands. Keeping his elbows and wrists straight and his chin on the table, he raises his arms upward as far as possible. The examiner measures the vertical distance from the bottom of the stick to the table. Insufficient flexibility in this movement indicates tightness of the muscles and connective tissues in the front of the shoulders and chest region.

Plantar-Dorsal Flexion Test. The subject sits on a table or on the floor with his leg straight. Keeping heel and back of knee on the table, he plantar flexes one foot as far as possible (Fig. 15–9). With a pad of paper placed in a vertical position as a backdrop to the foot, the examiner places a dot on the paper at the end of the toenail of the great toe. The subject dorsally flexes his foot as far as possible and the examiner again places a dot on the paper

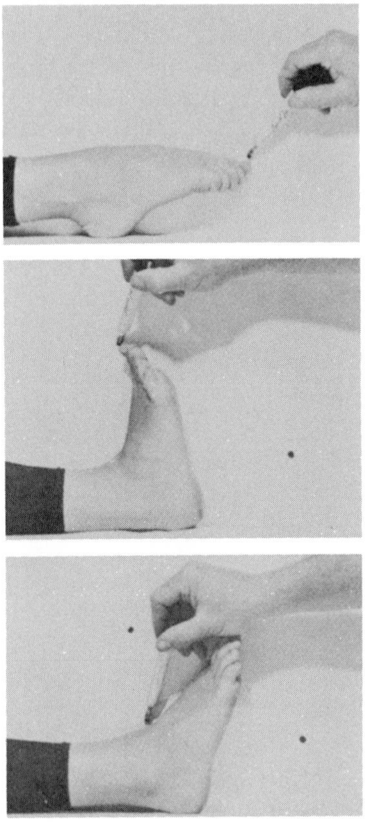

Fig. 15–9. Plantar-dorsal flexion test. (From Nielson, N.P. and Jensen, C.R. *Measurement and Statistics in Physical Education.* Courtesy of Wadsworh Publishing Co., Inc., 1972.)

at the end of the toenail of the great toe. Finally, the subject relaxes his ankle, and the examiner places a third dot on the paper where the ankle bends at the top of the instep. The pad is removed, and lines are drawn connecting the third dot to each of the other two. Using a protractor or a goniometer, the examiner determines the range of motion in degrees.

Measuring Speed

Running speed can be measured best by sprint tests. The most commonly used distances for such measures are 40 yards and 50 yards, but any distance to 100 yards would be satisfactory. If pure running speed is to be measured, the subject should have a running start, so that *acceleration* speed is not a factor. Whereas if running speed over a given distance including acceleration speed is to be determined, the subject should be stationary at the start. The importance of consistency in the conduct of such tests is apparent. When there is a high level of consistency, the test results can be compared meaningfully among individuals or among performances of the same individual.

SELECTED READINGS

1. Astrand, P., and Rhyming, I.: A nomogram for calculation of aerobic capacity (physical fitness) from pulse rate during submaximal work. J. Appl. Physiol., 7:218–221, 1954.
2. Cooper, K.H.: *Aerobics.* New York: Bantam Books, 1968.
3. Fox., E.: A simple, accurate technique for predicting maximal aerobic power. J. Appl. Physiol., *35*:914–916, 1973.
4. Margaria, R., Aghemo, I., and Rovelli, E.: Measurement of musclar power (anaerobic) in man. J. Appl. Physiol., *21*:1662–1664, 1966.
5. Neilson, N.P., and Jensen, C.R.: *Measurement and Statistics in Physical Education.* Belmont, Calif.: Wadsworth Publishing Co., Inc., 1972.
6. Remmington, D., et al.: *How to Lower Your Fat Thermostat.* Vitality House, 1982.
7. Sharkey, B.J.: *Physiological Fitness and Weight Control.* Missoula: Mountain Press Publishing Co., 1974.
8. Siconolfi, S., et al.: Assessing $\dot{V}O_2$max in Epidemiological Studies: Modification of the Astrand-Rhyming Test. Med. Sci. Sports Exerc., *14*:5, 1982.

Glossary

A Bands: The darkly striped areas seen in longitudinal slices of skeletal muscle tissue. A bands contain overlapping thick and thin filaments.

Acceleration: Rate of increase in velocity.

Acetyl Group: A two-carbon molecule produced by the removal of carbon dioxide from pyruvic acid; used to generate acetyl coenzyme A for use in the Krebs cycle.

Acetylcholine: A chemical mediator in the body, normally associated with depolarization of neurons.

Actin: A muscle protein which, with myosin, is responsible for muscle contraction and relaxation.

Action Potential: The electrical change that can be recorded during contraction.

Active Transport: The process of moving molecules against a concentration gradient.

Adaptation: A more or less persistent change in structure or function, especially as caused by repeated bouts of physical exercise.

Adenosine Diphosphate (ADP): One of the chemical products of the breakdown of adenosine triphosphate (ATP) for energy during muscle contraction.

Adenosine Triphosphate (ATP): A chemical that serves as the immediate source of chemical energy for most of the energy-consuming reactions of the body, especially for muscle contraction. ATP is split into adenosine diphosphate and phosphate to produce energy.

Adrenergic: Having to do with the release of epinephrine or norepinephrine.

Aerobic: Occurring in the presence of oxygen. Aerobic processes occur with oxygen present.

Aerobic Training: A training technique specifically designed to improve the aerobic processes of the body and thereby increase aerobic endurance.

Aerobic Endurance: The ability to persist in physical activities that rely heavily on oxygen for energy production.

Aerobic Power: The maximal volume of oxygen consumed per unit of time. Also known as maximal oxygen uptake or maximal oxygen consumption.

Afferent Fibers: Sensory nerve fibers, i.e., those that conduct impulses toward the central nervous system and especially the brain.

Afferent Nervous System: The bodily system that directs impulses from sensory receptors toward the spinal cord and brain; also called sensory nervous system.

Agility: The ability to change directions of the body or its parts rapidly, demonstrated in such movements as dodging, zigzagging, stopping, starting, and reversing direction of movement.

Agonistic Muscle: A muscle that contributes to the desired movement by its concentric contraction; a prime mover.

Alactacid: A process that provides energy without involving the glycolytic pathway.

Alactic Acid Oxygen Debt: That part of the oxygen debt which is not accompanied by an increase of lactic acid in the blood.

Alanine: An amino acid that is converted to blood glucose in the liver (See Glucose-alanine cycle).

Aldosterone: A hormone released from the adrenal cortex. Aldosterone causes sodium retention by the kidney.

All or None Law: A phenomenon whereby a motor unit either contracts maximally or not at all under similar environmental conditions.

Alpha Motor Neurons: Nerves that cause skeletal muscle fibers (extrafusal fibers) to contract.

Alveoli: The tiny air sacs in the lungs where gaseous exchange takes place.

Amino Acids: Compunds that are the building blocks of proteins.

Amphetamine: A synthetic drug related to epinephrine. Amphetamines cause stimulation of the central nervous system.

Amylases: Enzymes that digest carbohydrates.

Anabolic: Pertaining to the synthesis of complex substances from simpler substances, especially to the synthesis of body proteins from amino acids.

Anabolic Steroids: Chemical substances with a steroid structure that promote protein synthesis.

Anaerobic: Occurring in the absence of oxygen. Anaerobic processes occur with no oxygen present.

Anaerobic Capacity: The ability to persist at the maintenance or repetition of strenuous muscular contractions that rely substantially on anaerobic mechanisms of energy supply.

Anaerobic Power: The maximal rate at which energy can be produced for short periods of time.

Anaerobic Threshold: The point in exercise where significant lactate begins to accumulate in the blood.

Anaerobic Training: A training technique designed to increase the anaerobic processes of the body and thereby increase anaerobic endurance.

Anisotropic: Describing the movement of light through an opaque medium in which the velocity of the emerging light is not the same in all directions.

Annulospiral Endings: Specialized sensory neurons that surround the nuclear bag in stretch receptors and fire when the bag is stretched.

Antagonistic Muscle: A muscle that causes a movement opposite the desired movement. Resistance to the desired movement would occur if it were to contract.

Apneustic Center: A center in the brain that helps control breathing.

Arteriovenous Oxygen Difference (a-$\bar{v}$ O_2 Diff): The difference in oxygen content between the arterial blood and the mixed venous blood in the right atrium of the heart.

Artery: A vessel that carries blood away from the heart.

Atherosclerosis: A condition in which plaques occur inside blood vessels.

Atrium: An upper heart chamber.

Atrophy: Reduction in size of cells and tissues.

Attitude: Readiness to act in a particular way. Attitudes express different degrees of acceptance or rejection.

Autonomic Nervous System: That portion of the nervous system which controls the involuntary processes of the body, such as the functioning of the internal organs.

Autoregulation: The regulation of blood flow to an organ or tissue by direct effects of localized changes of chemicals or temperature in the organ or tissue.

a-$\bar{v}O_2$ Diff: See Arteriovenous oxygen difference.

Axon: Appendage of the neuron that conducts impulses away from the cell body.

Balance: Ability to keep the center of gravity over the base of support and to maintain equilibrium.

Basal Metabolic Rate: Energy expenditure at rest after a 12-hour fast and a good night's sleep.

Beta Oxidation: A metabolic pathway for the breakdown of long-chain fatty acids.

Biopsy: The extraction of small pieces of tissue for chemical analysis.

Blood Doping: The practice of injecting previously withdrawn and stored blood cells to increase the number of circulating red blood cells.

Boyle's Law: The law that states that the volume of gas is inversely proportional to the pressure exerted on it when the temperature is constant.

Buffers: Substances that decrease the chemical reaction otherwise produced by acids or alkalies.

Calcium Flux: The movement of calcium into the myocardium to cause contraction.

Calorie: A unit of heat used in metabolic studies.

Calorimeter: A machine to measure the number of calories used.

Capacity: The limits within which ability can be developed. Ability cannot extend beyond capacity.

Capillary: The smallest of the blood vessels.

Carbohydrate: A chemical compound consisting of carbon, hydrogen, and oxygen atoms in specified arrangements. Carbohydrates are major components of foods such as bread, potatoes, and rice.

Cardiac Output: Volume of blood pumped from the left ventricle in 1 minute.

Cardiorespiratory Endurance: See Aerobic endurance.

Cardiovascular Endurance: The endurance of the circulatory system; the ability of this system to carry on its functions efficiently under conditions of heavy work.

Catecholamines: A class of chemicals that includes epinephrine and norepinephrine.

Central Nervous System (CNS): That portion of the nervous system that includes the brain and spinal cord.

Cerebellum: A large bulbar structure at the rear of the brain that helps control voluntary movement and maintain balance.

Cerebral Cortex: The large outer portions of the cerebral hemispheres.

Chemoreceptors: Receptors sensitive to changes in certain chemicals in the body.

Cholinergic: Having to do with the release of acetylcholine.

Cholinesterase: An enzyme that is capable of destroying acetylcholine.

Chylomicrons: Lipoprotein molecules that carry fats to the bloodstream through the lymph.

Citric Acid Cycle: Krebs cycle.

Closed-Circuit Calorimetry: The method of estimating metabolic rate of the body using a spirometer to measure air taken into and expelled from the lungs.

Concentric Contraction: Shortening of a muscle due to nervous impulses.

Conditioned Reflex: A reflex pattern that is learned, as opposed to one that is inborn.

Conduction: The transfer of heat energy from a warm to a cooler object by direct physical contact.

Connective Tissue: Body tissue whose primary purpose is to connect one body part to another, such as ligaments connect bone to bone and tendons connect muscle to bone. There are several kinds of connective tissue.

Contractile Force: The amount of tension applied by a muscle or group of muscles during contraction.

Contractility: The ability to apply tension.

Convection: The transfer of heat by circulation or movement. Convective heat loss from the surface of the body to the surrounding air (or water, if one is swimming) is enhanced by increased air or water currents.

Coordination: The act of various muscles working together in a smooth, concerted way; correct and precise timing of muscle contractions.

Core Temperature: The temperature of the deep muscles and viscera of the body.

Cori Cycle: A sequence of metabolic reactions whereby lactic acid released by muscle is transported to the liver, transformed to glycogen, and then released from the liver as glucose to be transported back to the muscle.

Coronary System: The body system that includes the blood vessels that service the heart muscle.

Creatine Phosphate (Phosphocreatine): A high-energy chemical compound that transfers energy interchangeably with ATP.

Cristae: Shelf-like infoldings of the inner membrane of a mitochondrion.

Cross Bridges: The linkages between thick and thin filaments during muscle contraction.

Cross Training: The training effect that occurs in one side of the body as result of exercising the opposite side of the body.

Cyclic Adenosine Monophosphate (Cyclic AMP): A chemical implicated in the action of many hormones.

Dalton's Law: The law that states that the total pressure of a mixture of gases is equal to the sum of the partial pressures of the component gases.

Dehydration: The condition that results from excessive loss of water.

Dendrite: The appendage of a neuron that directs impulses toward the cell body.

Depolarization: The condition of the cell membrane when it has reached threshold and the sodium ion has rushed to the inside of the cell.

Diastole: The relaxation phase of each heartbeat.

Diastolic Pressure: The blood pressure during the relaxation of the ventricles.

Dicrotic Notch: A notch that occurs when recording the pressure after aortic valve closure in the cardiac cycle.

Diffusion: A movement of molecules through a membrane, from an area of high concentration to an area of low concentration.

Direct Calorimetry: A method used to estimate the metabolic rate of the body by measuring the heat released by the body.

Dynamic Contraction: See Isotonic contraction.

Dynamic Flexibility: Flexibility that can be exhibited as a result of contraction of the agonistic muscle and that does not result from the pull of gravity or from the body parts being moved by an outside force such as another person.

Dynamic Strength: Strength exhibited in motion.

Eccentric Contraction: Controlled lengthening of a muscle. The muscle becomes larger as it contracts because the resistance is greater than the contractile force.

Ectomorph: An individual who has a light or slender body build.

Efferent Nerve: A motor nerve.

Efferent System: The motor nervous system that directs impulses from the brain and spinal cord to muscles, glands, and organs.

Electrical Potential: An electrical difference between the outside and the inside of a cell, caused by a difference in the ionic composition on each side.

Electrocardiogram (EKG, ECG): A recording of the transmission of an action potential through the heart.

Electrolyte: Any substance that dissociates into positively and negatively charged ions when dissolved in water.

Electromyography (EMG): The recording of the electrical activity of muscles.

Electron Transport System: A series of biochemical reactions in the mitochondria whereby energy present in electrons is used to generate adenosine triphosphate.

Endocardium: A thin, smooth, shiny membrane covering the inside surfaces of the heart.

Endomorph: An individual who has a fat or heavy body build.

Endomysium: Connective tissue surrounding the muscle cell.

End Plate: That portion of a motor neuron that attaches to a muscle fiber.

Endurance: The ability to persist in performing some physical activity.

Energy: The capacity to perform work.

Enzyme: A protein molecule that serves as a catalyst for biochemical reactions.

Epicardium: A thin, shiny membrane covering the outer surface of the heart.

Epimysium: Connective tissue surrounding the whole muscle.

Epinephrine: A chemical liberated from the adrenal medulla and from sympathetic nerve endings. Important effects include cardiac stimulation and constriction of blood vessels with a consequent rise in blood pressure.

Ergometer: A device to measure work.

Estrogen: A class of hormones associated with feminine development.

Excitability: The ability to be excited by or respond to stimuli.

Expiratory Reserve Volume: A volume of air in the lungs that can be used to increase tidal volume.

Extracellular Fluid: Fluid not within the cells, e.g., interstitial fluid, blood plasma.

Extrafusal Muscle Fibers: Ordinary muscle fibers that lie outside muscle spindles.

Facilitation: The movement of the cell membrane toward the threshold.

Fascicle: A small group of muscle or nerve fibers.

Fasciculus (pl: Fasciculi): A bundle of muscle fibers bound together and connected to other fasciculi by connective tissue called the perimysium.

Fast Twitch Fibers: Skeletal muscle fibers most active in short-duration, intensive exercise, e.g., in sprints and jumps.

Fatigue: The inability to maintain a given level of physical performance.

Fatty Acids: Long-chain organic acids associated with glycerol in fat molecules. Fatty acids are used extensively for muscular fuel, especially in prolonged exercise.

Flavin Adenine Dinucleotide (FAD, FADH2): A coenzyme used to accept (FAD) or donate (FADH2) electrons in biochemical oxidation-reduction reactions.

Flexibility: Property of muscles and connective tissue that allows full range of motion.

Frank-Starling Effect: The increased contraction of the heart muscle caused by stretching of the muscle fibers upon increased filling of the chambers.

Free Fatty Acids: Fatty acids that circulate in the blood and are only loosely attached to proteins. Free fatty acids are used extensively for energy in long-duration exercise.

Functional Residual Capacity: The combination of residual volume and expiratory reserve volume.

Functional Syncytium: When one cell fires, the impulse spreads through all other cells.

Gamma Motor Nerve: A nerve that innervates the intrafusal fibers within muscle spindles.

Gamma Motor System: A motor system that causes movement through gamma efferent motor activity to the intrafusal fibers of the muscle spindle.

Gluconeogenesis: The synthesis of glycogen or glucose from amino acids and other substances.

Glucose: Blood sugar.

Glucose-Alanine Cycle: A series of metabolic reactions whereby pyruvic acid in the muscle is transformed into the amino acid, alanine. Alanine is delivered to the liver where it is changed to glucose. This glucose then can be delivered to the muscle for use in glycolysis.

Glycerol: A three-carbon compound associated with fatty acids in molecules of fat.

Glycogen: A polymer of glucose. Glycogen is the storage form of carbohydrate in animals.

Glycogen Loading: The filling of liver and muscle glycogen stores to greater than normal levels by consumption of a high-carbohydrate diet following the depletion of glycogen stores through exhaustive exercise and a low-carbohydrate diet.

Glycogenolysis: The breakdown of glycogen to glucose.

Glycogen Phosphorylase: An enzyme involved in the breakdown of glycogen.

Glycogen Supercompensation: See Glycogen loading.

Glycolysis: An anaerobic energy-producing pathway; the breaking down of sugars.

Golgi Tendon Organs: Receptors at the junctions of muscles and tendons that report force changes to the brain and spinal cord.

Grams Percent: A method of expressing concentration in grams per hundred milliliters of a substance.

Gray Matter: The tissue in the central nervous system made up of nerve cell bodies.

Growth Hormone: A hormone released from the anterior pituitary; causes growth of many body cells.

Heart Rate: The number of times the heart beats during 1 minute.

Heat Cramps: Muscle cramps associated with heat-induced changes in electrolyte balance in muscle tissue. May be relieved after administration of salt water.

Heat Exhaustion: Extreme fatigue, collapse, or fainting caused by heat-induced reduction in cardiac output.

Heat Stroke: Serious heat illness wherein the body loses its ability to regulate body temperature.

Hematocrit: The percentage of blood volume that is made up of red blood cells.

Hemoconcentration: An increase in the concentration of red blood cells in the total blood volume; usually caused by a loss of plasma water to the tissue spaces.

Hemodynamics: The basic physical principles of circulation.

Hemoglobin: A protein found in red blood cells. Hemoglobin combines with oxygen.

Hexokinase: The enzyme that changes blood glucose to glucose-6-phosphate in muscle.

High-Density Lipoproteins (HDL): Relatively heavy complexes of fat and protein in the blood; associated with a reduced incidence of coronary artery disease.

Homeostasis: The tendency of the body to maintain its internal environment within narrow ranges of temperature, acidity, osmolarity, etc.

Humoral: Found in body fluids.

Hydrogen-Electron Transport System: An energy scheme in which hydrogen atoms are passed through a series of oxidizing enzymes and are ionized with the release of energy.

Hydrolysis: The breakdown of a food particle by adding water at certain bonds.

Hydrophilic: Water loving.

Hydrophobic: Water hating.
Hydroxyl Ion: An OH molecule with an extra electron.
Hyperplasia: Increased cell number.
Hyperpnea: Significantly increased breathing.
Hypertension: A condition of persistently high arterial blood pressure.
Hypertrophy: Substantial increase in the overall size of a tissue; significant enlargement.
Hyperventilation: The state caused by hard breathing in which too much air pressure results in dizziness and/or unconsciousness.
Hypothalamus: A group of nerve cells at the base of the brain that has many complex functions, including regulation of temperature, appetite, emotional reactions, and hormonal responses.
Hypothermia: Lowering of the core temperature of the body.
Hypoxia: Below normal levels of oxygen in air.
H Zone: The central portion of an A band. The H zone contains only thick filaments at rest and usually disappears during contraction, when thin filaments overlap the central portions of thick filaments.
Indirect Calorimetry: A method of estimating metabolic rate by measuring the amount of oxygen used by the body.
Inhibitory Control: The control placed on muscle contractions as a result of inhibitory impulses that originate in the central nervous system.
Inhibitory Neurons: Neurons that inhibit other neurons, tending to keep the other neurons quiet.
Inotropic: An increase in the contractile condition of the myocardium.
Inspiratory Capacity: The combination of tidal volume and inspiratory reserve volume.
Inspiratory Reserve Volume: A volume of air in the lungs that can be used to increase tidal volume.
Insulin: A hormone secreted by the pancreas. Insulin lowers blood glucose by increasing the uptake of glucose by the tissues of the body.
Intercalated Discs: Cell membranes that separate individual cardiac muscle cells and allow the action potential to spread to all fibers.
Intermittent Exercise: Exercise sessions interrupted by rest sessions.
Internuncial Neuron: A neuron in the spinal cord that serves as a connection between motor and sensory neurons.
Interstitial Fluid: The fluid that lies between cells in the tissue spaces.
Interval Training: A training program that consists of short bouts of heavy work alternated with periods of rest or light work.
Intrafusal Muscle Fiber: Specialized muscle fibers within muscle spindles.
Ischemia: A lack of blood flow.
Isokinetic Contraction: A muscular contraction through a range of motion at a constant velocity.
Isometric (Static) Contraction: A muscular contraction in which there is no change in the angle of the involved joint(s) and little or no change in the length of the contracting muscle.
Isotonic Contraction: A contraction in which muscle fibers shorten as a result of stimulus.
Isotropic: Having like properties in all directions, as in movement of light through an opaque medium in which the velocity of the emerging light is the same in all directions.
Isovolumic: Occurring without an alteration in volume. This term is used to describe the isovolumic pressure line in the cardiac function curve.
Joint Receptors: Nerve receptor organs located in and around joints of the limbs. Joint receptors provide information about limb position to the brain and spinal cord.
Junctional Fibers: Specialized transmission fibers of the heart between the atrium and ventricle that delay the entrance of an electrical impulse into the AV node.
Kilocalorie: One thousand calories, sometimes called a large calorie.
Kilogram: A unit of mass equivalent to 2.2 pounds.
Kilopond-Meter (kpm): The work done when a mass of 1 kilogram is lifted 1 meter against the force of gravity.
Kinesthetic Sense: A sense of awareness, without the use of the other senses, of muscle and joint positions and actions.
Krebs Cycle: A sequence of chemical reac-

tions in the metabolic pathways in which the end products of glycolysis are degraded to carbon dioxide and hydrogen atoms; sometimes called the tricarboxylic acid cycle or citric acid cycle.

Lactic Acid (Lactate): The end product of anaerobic glycolysis.

Lactic Acid Oxygen Debt: Portion of the oxygen debt that is associated with a rise in blood lactic acid.

Laminar Flow: The flow of blood through vessels in which the velocity of flow in the center of the vessel is far greater than that toward the outer edges.

Ligament: Tough connective tissue that binds bones together, forming joints.

Lipases: Enzymes involved in the digestion of fats.

Lipid: Fat, especially triglycerides.

Lipoprotein Lipase: An enzyme that splits fatty acids from fat-protein complexes.

Lung Capacities: Lung measurements made up of at least two lung volumes.

Lung Volumes: Single measurements of primary lung subdivisions.

Maximal Oxygen Uptake: The maximal amount of oxygen that can be used by the body during heavy work.

Mesomorph: An individual who has a husky or muscular body build or a medium body build.

METS (Metabolic equivalents): An expression of energy cost relative to an individual's resting energy expenditure. One MET is equivalent to 3.5 milliliters of oxygen per kilogram of body weight.

Mitochondria: Cellular organelles that produce energy for cellular metabolism.

M-Lines: A protein structure muscle that anchors the myosin filaments.

Momentum: The property of a moving body that determines the force required to bring the body to rest. Momentum = mass × velocity.

Monosynaptic: Pertaining to or relayed through only one synapse.

Motor Cortex: Portion of the cerebral cortex that generates the nerve impulses leading to voluntary movement.

Motor End Plate: A connection between the nerve and muscle fiber.

Motor Neuron: A nerve cell that conducts an impulse from the central nervous system to muscles or glands.

Motor Unit: A group of muscle fibers dispersed throughout a muscle and supplied by a single motor nerve fiber.

Muscle Spindle: A group of specialized muscle tissues that are sensitive to changes of muscle length.

Muscular Endurance: Ability to continue muscular action.

Myocardium: Another name for the muscle tissue of the heart.

Myofibril: Element of muscle that contains the contractile actin and myosin proteins.

Myofilaments: Minute protein threads within a myofibril.

Myoglobin: Oxygen-binding protein in skeletal muscle.

Myoneural Junction: The intersection between the motor end plate of a nerve branch and the muscle fiber.

Myosin: A muscle protein that, with actin, is responsible for muscle contraction and relaxation.

Myosin ATPase: The name given to the activity of myosin in catalyzing the breakdown of adenosine triphosphate to adenosine diphosphate and phosphate during muscle contraction.

Nerve: A cable-like bundle of many nerve fibers.

Net Oxygen Cost of Exercise: The amount of oxygen consumed during both exercise and recovery less the oxygen that would have been consumed had the subject remained at rest during the period of exercise and recovery.

Neuromuscular Coordination: Coordination that results from nerve impulses reaching the proper muscles with sufficient intensity at the correct time.

Neuromuscular Fatigue: Inability to sustain or repeat the production of a given muscular force. Also, the inability to sustain the production of a given power.

Neuromuscular Junction (Motor End Plate): The junction between motor nerve ending and the sarcolemmal membrane of a muscle fiber.

Neuron: A complete nerve cell, including the cell body and all its appendages.

Neutralizer Muscle: A muscle that acts to equalize the action of another muscle.

Nicotinamide Adenine Dinucleotide (NAD, NADH): An electron acceptor (NAD) or donor (NADH) used in metabolic oxidation-reduction reactions.

Norepinephrine: A chemical secreted by sympathetic nerve endings and by the adrenal medulla. Norepinephrine increases cardiac output, vasoconstriction, and blood pressure.

Nuclear Bag: A specialized area of the muscle tissue inside the muscle spindle, surrounded by annulospiral endings.

Open-Circuit Calorimetry: The process of estimating metabolic rate by collecting and analyzing expired air.

Overload: The process of demanding more performance from a system than is ordinarily required.

Oxidation: The loss of electrons from an atom or molecule.

Oxidative Phosphorylation: The production of adenosine triphosphate dependent on oxidative processes in the electron transport system of the mitochondria.

Oxygen Debt: A condition that results when the demand for oxygen is greater than the supply.

Oxygen Deficit: The difference between the theoretical oxygen requirement of a physical activity and the oxygen actually used during the activity.

Oxygen Dissociation Curve: A curve that represents the percentage of saturation of the hemoglobin of the blood at various partial pressures of oxygen and blood CO_2 levels.

Oxygen Uptake: The oxygen used up by the mitochondria of all the body's cells.

Pacemaker: A small section of the heart located in the upper right portion, where the beat of the heart originates. The beat spreads from the pacemaker throughout the remainder of the heart.

Parasympathetic: Pertaining to a major subdivision of the autonomic nervous system.

Partial Pressure: In a mixture of gases, the pressure exerted by one of the gases in the mixture. The pressure is due to the heat energy of the gas molecules.

Perimysium: Connective tissue that surrounds fascicles of muscle fibers.

Peripheral Nervous System: The body system that includes all those parts of the nervous system not included in the brain and spinal cord.

pH: The relative acidity or basicity of body fluids. More exactly, pH is the negative logarithm of the hydrogen ion concentration.

Phosphorylase: An enzyme involved in the breakdown of glycogen to glucose-6-phosphate. Small changes in the activity of this enzyme help regulate the rate of glycogen breakdown.

Pneumotaxic Center: A center in the brain that helps control breathing.

Poiseuille's Law: The principle that attempts to explain the factors of blood flow, especially the velocity in relation to the size of the vessel.

Polyunsaturated Fat: A fat, many of whose fatty acid carbon atoms are not saturated with hydrogen atoms but are bonded together by double bonds. Polyunsaturated fats are usually liquid at room temperature and are derived from plant sources.

Power: The product of force and velocity; the ability to apply force at a rapid rate.

Precapillary Sphincters: Smooth muscle cells located at the entrances of many capillaries; they control blood flow into the capillaries.

Progressive Resistance: A muscle-training program in which the amount of resistance is systematically increased as the muscles gain in strength.

Ptyalin: An enzyme found in the mouth that hydrolizes starches.

Pyruvic Acid: A three-carbon molecule produced by the breakdown of glycogen or glucose.

Q: A standard symbol indicating blood flow, normally cardiac output.

Range of Motion: The amount of movement that can occur in a joint, expressed in degrees.

Reaction Time: Time between the reception of a signal to respond and the beginning of the response.

Reflex: An immediate response to a situation in which the thought process is bypassed.

Reflex Time: Time of nerve impulse travel in a reflex action.

Refractory Period: A period of time when muscle tissue is unable to be restimulated.

Repolarization: The condition of the membrane after depolarization when the ionic balance on each side of the cell has been restored.

Residual Volume: Amount of air in the lungs that cannot be expired.

Respiration: The movement of air into and out of the lungs.

Respiratory Exchange Ratio (R): The ratio between carbon dioxide produced and oxygen consumed as measured at the mouth. Often used as synonym for respiratory quotient (RQ) even though R may reflect processes other than foodstuff metabolism, e.g., hyperventilation due to acidosis.

Respiratory Quotient (RQ): The ratio of carbon dioxide produced to oxygen used at the tissue level.

Resting Potential: The electrical potential across a cell membrane during resting conditions.

Rest (Recovery) Intervals: In an interval training program, the periods of recovery between exercise intervals.

Reverse Potential: The electrical potential across a cell membrane at a given point following depolarization.

R.M. (Repetition Maximum): In weight training, the maximum number of repetitions that can be accomplished against a given amount of resistance.

Saltatory Conduction: The rapid high-speed conduction of myelinated fibers that occurs along the nodes of Ranvier.

Sarcolemma: Muscle-cell membrane.

Sarcomere: The functional unit of a muscle cell (from Z line to Z line).

Sarcoplasm: The cytoplasm of muscle fibers.

Sarcoplasmic Reticulum: A network of channels extending throughout muscle fibers; regulates the availability of calcium to the troponin molecules of the thin filaments.

Saturated Fat: A fat whose fatty acid carbon atoms are saturated with hydrogen atoms. Typically, saturated fats are solid at room temperature and are often derived from animal sources.

Sensory Fibers: Nerve fibers that conduct impulses from the periphery to the central nervous system.

Sinoatrial Node: Specialized cells in the right atrium of the heart that serve as the pacemaker of the heartbeat because of their rapid rates of depolarization and repolarization.

Skeletal Muscle: A muscle that attaches to and causes movement of the skeleton; also called striated, motor, and voluntary muscle.

Slow-Twitch Fibers: Skeletal muscle fibers characterized by relatively slow contraction times and great capacity for the aerobic production of adenosine triphosphate.

Smooth Muscle: A muscle located in the internal organs, with the exception of the heart; also called visceral and involuntary muscle.

Soma: Another name for a nerve cell body.

Spatial Summation: The movement of the membrane toward threshold as a result of two or more neurons firing in close proximity.

Sphincter: An opening that can be closed.

Sphygmomanometer: A device used to measure blood pressure.

Stabilizer Muscle: A muscle that contracts at a particular time to hold a body portion firmly in position.

Static Contraction: Same as tonic or isometric contraction.

Static Strength: Strength exhibited without overt motion.

Steady State: A condition in which the supply of oxygen to the tissues is equal to the demand for oxygen.

Steroids: Organic compounds including bile acids, sterols, and sex hormones.

Strength: The ability of the muscles to exert force against resistance.

Stretch Reflex: An automatic reflex to contract in skeletal muscles, brought on by sudden stretching of the muscles.

Stroke Volume: The volume of blood pumped out of the left ventricle with each contraction.

Submaximal Exercise: Usually exercise at less than maximal intensity, but may also refer to exercise of less than maximal duration.

Summation: A sustained muscular contraction caused by rapid firing of nerve impulses.

Sympathetic Nervous System: A major division of the autonomic nervous system.

Synapse: A web-like relay junction between neurons, which relays impulses in only one direction from axons to dendrites.

Synaptic Trough: A small area beneath the motor end plate.

Syncytium: A mass of cytoplasm with numerous nuclei. This term is used to describe the functional relationship of heart muscle cells.

Systole: The contracting phase of each heartbeat.

Systolic Pressure: The blood pressure during contraction (systole) of the heart.

Temporal Summation: The movement of the membrane toward threshold caused by increased frequency of firing by a single neuron.

Tendon: A tough, fibrous tissue that connects muscles to bones.

Terminal Cisternae: Structures adjacent to T-tubules that store CA^{++} for muscular contractions.

Testosterone: A hormone secreted by the testes; causes the secondary sex characteristics of the male and is involved in muscle growth.

Tetanic Contractions: Contractions of muscle fibers at such high frequencies that fibers do not have time to return to their resting lengths between contractions.

Tetanization: The increased contractile condition of muscle when stimulated by a high-frequency stimulation.

Tetanus: The state of apparently continuous contraction of a muscle fiber that is being stimulated at such high frequency that it does not have time to return to its resting length between contractions.

Threshold: The resistance level of a fiber to nerve impulses. If the fiber is to be activated, the impulses must be strong enough to exceed the fiber's threshold.

Tidal Volume: The amount of air inspired or expired during the normal breathing pattern of the lungs.

Transverse Tubules: See T-tubules.

Triglyceride: A form of fat containing one glycerol molecule and three fatty acids.

Tropomyosin: A protein molecule in the actin filament of muscle.

Troponin: A protein molecule in the actin filament of muscle.

T-Tubules: Channels that conduct action potentials from the surface of a muscle fiber to the interior of the fiber.

Twitch: A single, brief muscle contraction caused by a single stimulus.

Valsalva's Maneuver: The increase of pressures in the abdominal region associated with breath holding and extreme effort.

Vasoconstriction: Narrowing of the opening of blood vessels caused by contraction of the smooth muscle cells in the walls of the vessels.

Vasodilation: Widening of the opening of blood vessels caused by a relaxation of the smooth muscle cells in the walls of the vessels.

Vasomotor Tone: The tone of the muscles that line the walls of the blood vessels.

VE: Expiratory volume.

Vein: A vessel that returns blood to the heart.

Velocity: The rate at which an object travels in a given direction.

Ventilation: The exchange of air in and out of the lungs. The process of inhaling and exhaling.

Ventricle: A lower chamber of the heart.

V_I: Inspiratory volume.

Viscosity (Blood): The thickness of a fluid (e.g. blood); the resistance to flow.

Vital Capacity: The total amount of air that can be forced out of the lungs after a forced inhalation.

VO_2: Oxygen consumption in liters per minute (l/min).

Volume Percent: Method of expressing concentration in milliliters per hundred milliliters.

Voluntary Nervous System: That part of the nervous system which is consciously controlled.

White Matter: The tissue in the central nervous system made up of nerve fibers, not nerve cell bodies.

Wind-Kessel Vessel: A description of the aorta as it opens to receive blood and rebounds to push blood though the system.

Work: The result of muscle contractions. If the muscle contractions cause movement, the work is dynamic; if no movement occurs, the work is static.

Z Line or Disc: The structure that bisects the I bands of skeletal muscle and anchors the thin filaments.

Index

Page numbers in *italics* indicate illustrations; numbers followed by *t* indicate tables